AF818248

Pursuing the Origin of Pathogenic Bacterial Species

Pursuing the Origin of Pathogenic Bacterial Species

By

Shu-Lin Liu

Cambridge Scholars Publishing

Pursuing the Origin of Pathogenic Bacterial Species

By Shu-Lin Liu

This book first published 2022

Cambridge Scholars Publishing

Lady Stephenson Library, Newcastle upon Tyne, NE6 2PA, UK

British Library Cataloguing in Publication Data
A catalogue record for this book is available from the British Library

Copyright © 2022 by Shu-Lin Liu

All rights for this book reserved. No part of this book may be reproduced, stored in a retrieval system, or transmitted, in any form or by any means, electronic, mechanical, photocopying, recording or otherwise, without the prior permission of the copyright owner.

ISBN (10): 1-5275-8752-5
ISBN (13): 978-1-5275-8752-6

To my PhD supervisors Profs. Eiko Yabuuchi and Takayuki Ezaki and to all my students

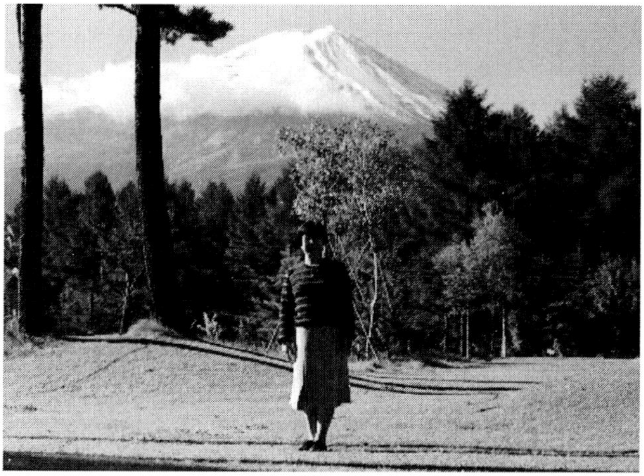

Professor Eiko Yabuuchi

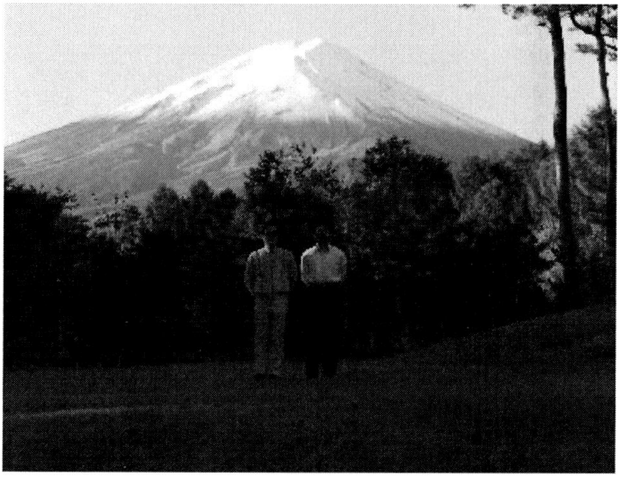

Professor Takayuki Ezaki (left) and me

学海无涯 逆水行舟乃是常态

书山有路 披荆斩棘方能成蹊

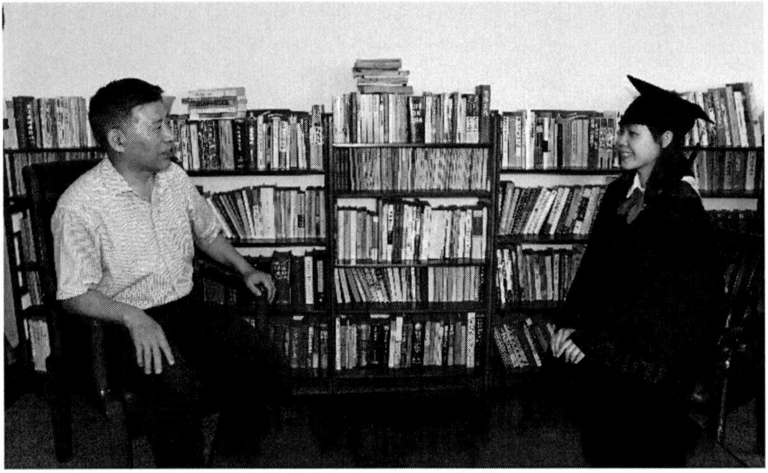

Flying higher after bachelor graduation

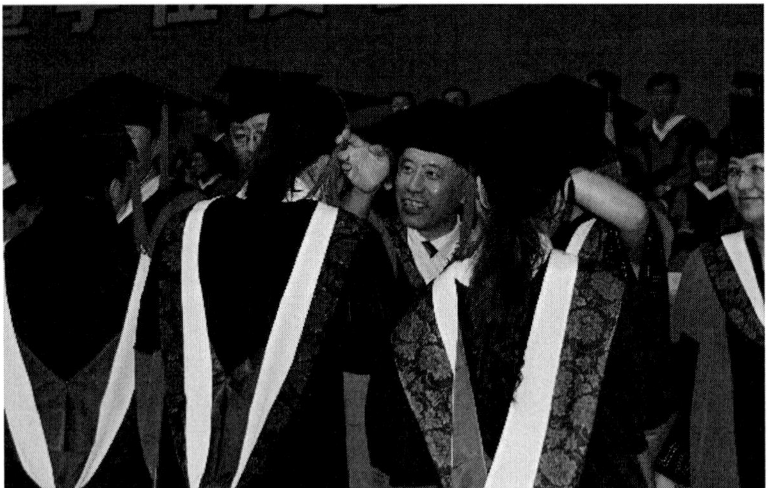

Marching to diverse professional fields after PhD graduation

TABLE OF CONTENTS

Part III: Genomic divergence of the *Salmonella* lineages: saltatory or gradual?

PREFACE BY THE AUTHOR

I have been haunted for over half century by mental illusions of a transformation fiction in which benign bacteria were turned into deadly pathogens. In reality, I have pursued the origins of pathogenic bacterial species for my entire career. I was curious about why some bacteria are pathogenic but many others are not. Or, more specifically, why closely related pathogenic bacteria may cause radically different diseases; how pathogenic bacteria branch out from commensal ancestors; and how we should control infections more appropriately.

Thousands of investigators in the fields of microbiology and infectious diseases have worked on these questions for hundreds of years and have, to date, built up solid foundations for continual and sustainable research toward answers to these questions. They have made great efforts to uncover the mysteries about pathogenic bacteria and have contributed enormously to human health. In ancient times, thousands of years ago, people had already felt the existence of live infectious agents that caused diseases and guessed that they might be too tiny to be seen by the naked eye. The first sight of live bacteria by Antony van Leeuwenhoek under the 200x lens of his microscope in the mid-1670s opened the window to the microbial world. Then Louis Pasteur started a new epoch in Microbiology, well-known as "the golden age of microbiology", from 1857. Beginning with Pasteur, scientists including Robert Koch and many others made a series of great discoveries, such as the association of microbes with diseases, immunity, vaccines, antibiotics, etc. The use of antibiotics has saved countless lives and vaccination has brought so many epidemics under control.

Therefore, human beings have fought with pathogenic microbes with great success across the centuries, especially over the past couple of centuries. However, deadly infections and disastrous pandemics are still threatening human health and taking numerous human lives. Penicillin was highly effective to kill cocci like *Neisseria* spp., but we do not have so many effective antibiotics against the large diversity of pathogenic bacteria. Additionally, initially effective antibiotics may soon become useless due to resistance arising in bacteria. In the mid-20th century, streptomycin and rimifon brought *Mycobacterium tuberculosis* under control. As a result, many people overoptimistically believed that tuberculosis would be eradicated. However, unfortunately, *M. tuberculosis* soon produced resistance to streptomycin and rimifon. Therefore, currently *M. tuberculosis* remains a huge problem worldwide.

Vaccines are extremely effective for prevention or treatment against many infectious diseases, such as measles and rabies, leading even to the eradication of some devastating diseases, such as smallpox and (almost) poliomyelitis. However, vaccination has not been sufficiently effective against certain diseases, such as tuberculosis or typhoid. Furthermore, tremendous efforts in developing vaccines against some microbial pathogens have ended in total failure, such as those against HIV. All the difficulties or failures in developing effective and sustainable antimicrobials and vaccines have resulted from insufficient knowledge about the pathogenic microbes.

Therefore, knowing how pathogenic bacteria have originated from their amiable ancestors is a prerequisite for the effective control of infectious diseases. This is truly urgent. An in-depth understanding of pathogenic microbes and novel insights into their evolution and biology will greatly facilitate the development of effective control strategies, in addition to antimicrobials and vaccines. New strategies would be based on non-killing measures, as killing will inevitably induce resistance in the microbes and stimulate cycles of an arms race between mankind and pathogens. The key idea is "change", as changes based on novel insights into the microbes or their hosts may lead to radical differences in host-pathogen relationships. Certainly, we cannot make changes on the pathogenic microbes themselves living in nature, but we may make changes to the way they approach their human host, such as by altering the environment by which the pathogenic microbes could contact human beings, or on the way they interact with the human host, such as by enhancing human resistance to microbial infections. Indeed, human society has greatly changed the environment that the pathogens use as the route to infecting human beings. For example, changes in environmental sanitation have remarkably reduced new annual cases of many epidemics, such as typhoid fever, and similar changes are continuing for better human health. Changes for enhancing the natural resistance of humans to microbial infections are the current topics of my research team. This is based on a concept of *elevating relative infectious doses* of pathogenic microbes by enhancing the human defensive functions. All pathogens have a natural infectious dose, below which a pathogen may hardly be able to establish infections in the host. In addition to normal functionalities of all anatomic and physiologic systems such as hemopoietic and immune systems, the intestinal microbiota plays key roles in defense against malignancies and infections. Our preliminary work has demonstrated that the population structure and biological functions of the intestinal microbiota can be dramatically improved for stronger defensive functions by several measures including the intake of dietary lignans. In animal experiments, the natural infectious dose of *Salmonella* could be increased by two orders of magnitude after ingestion of dietary lignans and we call the new and much higher infectious dose of *Salmonella* the "relative infectious dose" for mice.

The long journey of pursuing the origins of pathogenic bacterial species brings me a general picture of a bacterial cell budding from a benign ancestral tree to form a new and pathogenic branch by acquiring laterally transferred pathogenic traits and streamlining the genome through structural rebalancing and nucleotide amelioration. Once in a human host as a nascent pathogen, this new bacterial lineage may have the chance to co-evolve with the host through countless confronting interactions to become an "established" pathogen with a natural infectious dose. But scientific human beings may at a point of time repel them by enhancing resistance against infections, so that the pathogen may have to increase the infectious dose a hundredfold, or more, to possibly infect the host. At the community scale, such enhanced resistance may become a strong *herd resistance* against pandemics.

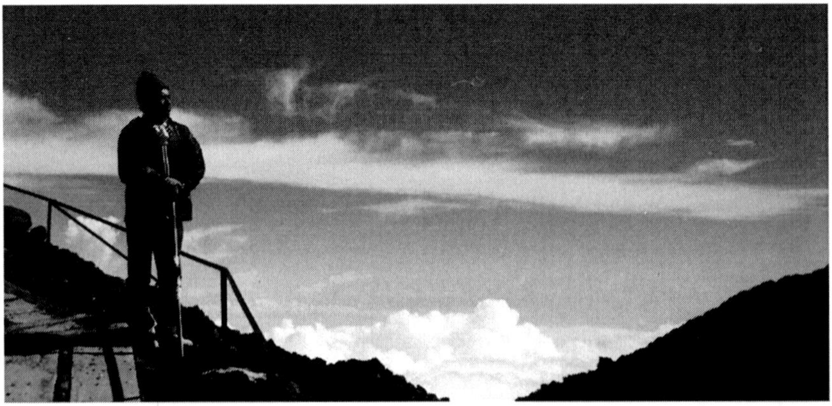

PREFACE BY DR. RANDAL N. JOHNSTON

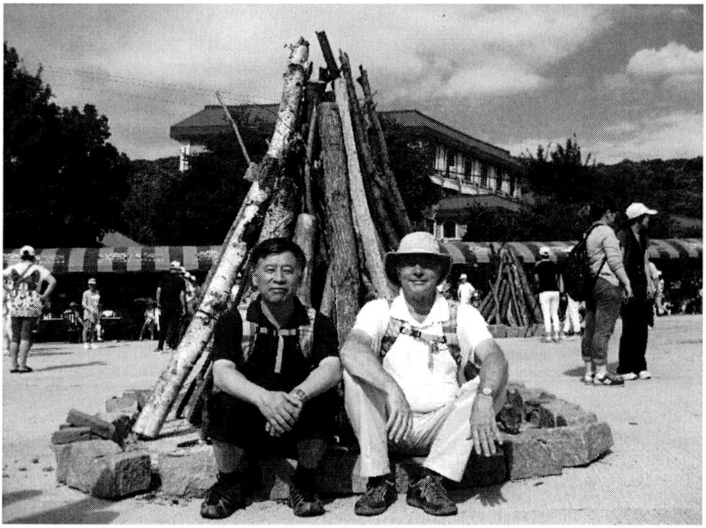

I am deeply honored that my dear friend and valued colleague Professor Liu has invited me to provide a second preface for this volume. When he told me that he was finally ready to begin working on "Pursuing The Origins of Pathogenic Bacterial Species", which he had been planning for many years, I anticipated that the result of this effort would be wonderfully satisfying – and in truth my high expectations have been greatly exceeded. Over the past several decades, I have held many long and enjoyable discussions with him about this book and the questions or theories behind it, so I had understood its general contents even before its completion. He first began working with me in the Southern Alberta Cancer Research Institute, University of Calgary, in the late 1990s, when I was the Director of the Institute. He was the first of the microbiology field to investigate bacterial evolution based on physical genomic parameters, employing the chromosome mapping strategy that he developed specifically for the comparative genomics of bacteria. These studies complemented very well my own interests in the genomics and rapid evolutionary changes observed in cancer cells as they become malignant and spread to multiple locations during metastasis. Even when I later assumed demanding positions as the Associate Vice President (Research) of the University of Calgary, and then as the President of Genome Prairie, and later as the Director of the Biomedical Technology Graduate Program, I frequently found opportunities to discuss bacterial evolution with him, because this research topic was so important and fascinating. His studies progressed swiftly during his time in Calgary and intensified even further after his move to Beijing and finally to Harbin, where he rejoined Harbin Medical University, the same institution where he had enjoyed some of his early formative education. It was my great pleasure to visit him and present research seminars (and continue our many discussions) once at Peking University and twice in Harbin, and to observe first-hand the rapid progress being made in China.

Professor Liu's discovery of genetic boundaries among discrete bacterial species will not only place bacterial taxonomy on a solid molecular foundation but may also greatly help research on the elucidation of structural genomic mechanisms involved in the emergence of pathogenic bacterial species from their benign ancestors. In fact, it has never in the past been clear precisely how bacteria diverge enough to become different species and how different they must be if they are to be defined as different. Thus, his discovery of genetic boundaries that circumscribe bacteria into discrete (rather than continual) phylogenetic clusters enables him to describe natural rather than arbitrary bacterial species.

In this book, Dr. Liu narrates his long educational and scientific march that begins with his initial surprise about the radical difference in pathogenic features among very closely related bacteria: he wondered whether they belonged to the same, or different, species and how one can rigorously establish that. Then he describes his stepwise decadal progress in searching for genomic parameters that can be used as common yardsticks to universally define natural species of bacteria. Finally, he describes the technical details of the genetic boundaries he proposes, interpreting these boundaries as the consequences of the independent accumulation of adaptive genomic rearrangements and variations plus the eventual formation of semi-closed gene pools once threshold differences have been reached. This book will be a key, and unique, contribution to the field of bacterial evolution and will be eagerly consulted by experts in the field worldwide. But in addition, it also provides a very touching and personal history of how one individual, through sheer hard work in difficult circumstances over many years, coupled with creative thought and critical analysis, has been able to achieve a conceptual breakthrough that will have ramifications and applications that are potentially far beyond bacterial evolution and include many other aspects of the evolution of life and the manifestation of disease. Finally, it should also be clear that Professor Liu has been able to set a shining example for his many students and colleagues, locally and internationally, and thus, to secure an enduring legacy for his life and his work.

ACKNOWLEDGMENTS

This long journey of pursuing the origins of pathogenic bacterial species would not have been possible without the support and encouragement of my family, mentors, friends, colleagues and students. More than sixty years ago, my parents sent me to elementary school and did their best to support my education at what was an extremely difficult time for them. My wife and son accompanied me all the way from my hometown Fujin, China, to Calgary, Canada, and provided all the assistance I needed for the forthcoming journey and for this book.

During my studies as a medical student, I had a burning enthusiasm for research in the field of microbiology and had the chance to join the research activities of Dr. Shao-Xian Li, who brought me from a virtually zero research background to several journal publications by the time of my graduation from medical school, showing me how to read literature, how to design research projects, how to conduct experiments, and how to analyze and summarize the results for publication. As a result, when I began my graduate study for the MSc degree, supervised by Drs. Zhen-Zhou Long and Wei-Feng Chen in Beijing, China, I quickly adapted to the pure research environment, compared to my medical school routines when I spent most of the time attending lectures or seeing patients.

My special thanks go to my PhD supervisors Profs. EikoYabuuchi and Takayuki Ezaki, who showed me new scientific horizons and brought me to the research of bacterial pathogenesis. After graduation with a PhD degree, I stayed for a few more months in Japan to focus on my research design for comparative genomic studies of *Salmonella* and sent the research plan to Dr. Kenneth Sanderson in Calgary, Canada, for him to make the necessary preparations for the research projects. Ken provided me with all the research conditions and materials needed, so the work went quite well.

I joined Dr. Randy Johnston in late 1996 to work on a cancer therapeutics project using genomics methods. Therefore, my research was then extended from bacterial genomics to human genomics. We had a common interest in molecular evolution, with a focus on the phylogenetic and pathogenic evolution of bacteria. We used to have long discussions together on the definition of bacterial species and the origins of pathogenic bacteria. His support and encouragement were key factors to bringing my research ideas to experimental tests and then to publication, including this book.

The latter parts of the research were conducted at Peking University and Harbin Medical University, where I received great support from Dr. Qi-De Han and Dr. Bao-Feng Yang and many colleagues of the two institutions, respectively. Finally, I thank all my students in Calgary, Beijing and Harbin – they did the experiments and collected the data. Many of them left my team decades ago but they have kept contact with me, mostly on Teachers' Day. My current students, including eight MSc and nine PhD students and eight postdoctoral fellows, are working mostly on genomics-related projects, with a focus on the phylogenetics of bacteria by genomic sequence analyses and microbial pathogenesis using both *in vitro* and *in vivo* experiments. One of the research groups in my lab is challenging lignan-treated animals with pathogenic bacteria to test the "*relative infectious dose*" concept and evaluate its role in enhancing the host resistance against infection. They all work hard and hope that such studies may lead to better control of microbial infections, including pandemics caused by viruses like SARS-CoV-2.

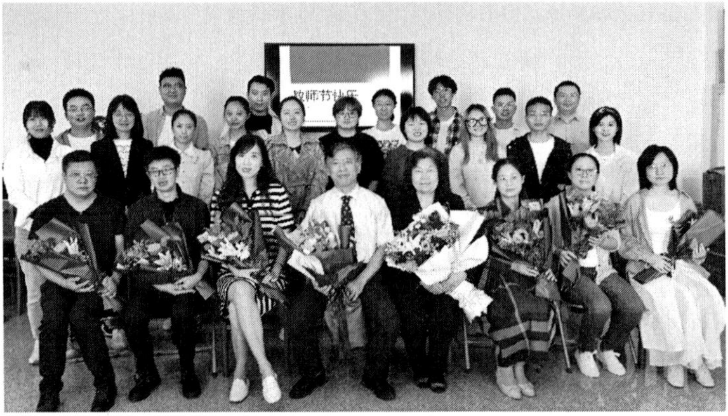

People of Liu lab, Teachers' Day of 2021 (Sept. 10, 2021)

My research has been supported by funding from the Natural Sciences and Engineering Research Council of Canada, the Medical Research Council of Canada, the Canadian Institutes of Health Research of Canada, the University of Calgary, Peking University, Harbin Medical University, and the National Natural Science Foundation of China (NSFC). This book was financed by NSFC 81871623 and 82020108022 and by a special funding from the College of Pharmacy, Harbin Medical University.

INTRODUCTION

Pathogenic bacteria originate from non-pathogenic ancestors, which has been very well documented by many generations of scientists, but whether the pathogens have become separate species from their ancestors or siblings was largely unclear. Elucidation of the phylogenetic status of a pathogen and the evolutionary scenarios leading to the transformation from benign to pathogenic bacteria helps in developing novel strategies for the control of infections. For this, the definition of bacterial species will have to be made unambiguous based on natural parameters without arbitrary judgements, which has been a serious challenge with many hardly resolvable questions. For example, man and chimpanzee belong to distinct species delineated by multiple decisive parameters, even though these two species share as much as 99% genetic similarity, whereas bacteria are classified by different standards with arbitrary cut-offs into species so that bacteria sharing as little as 70% genomic similarity may be categorized into the same species. As a result, bacterial species so defined often contain diverse bacteria with radically different biological or pathogenic traits. In this book, the author narrates the long journey towards finding natural parameters to define bacterial species, pursuing the origins of pathogenic bacterial species, and proposing a novel strategy, which is not antibiotics- or vaccine-based, for the control of pathogenic microbes.

PART I

BACTERIA AND HUMAN HEALTH: NON-PATHOGENIC, MILD PATHOGENIC OR DEADLY SPECIES

I tell my students to drop in any time to my office when they pass by to discuss research issues and they are encouraged to enter the office directly without having to knock at the door, even when they hear me meeting with any kind of VIPs – my students are more important than any other Very Important Persons.

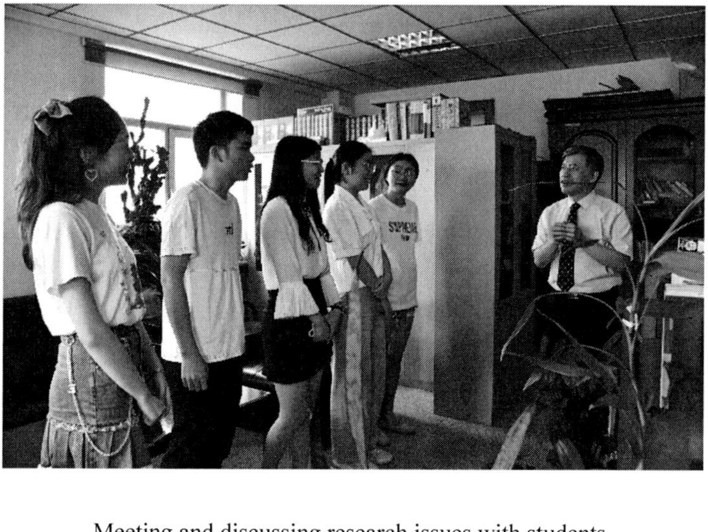

Meeting and discussing research issues with students.

CHAPTER 1

MANY BACTERIA ARE DEADLY PATHOGENS BUT MOST ARE FRIENDLY TO US

Parents pay great attention to the dirty hands of their babies – worrying about the bacteria carried by the dust and stains on the skin. They all hear so much about gastroenteritis, diarrhea, dysentery, enteric fever, cholera, plagues, and tuberculosis, so they wash their baby's hands before the child grabs the food to eat, or urge their three or four year olds to wash their hands by themselves before meals. It is the right thing to do, of course. I remember how stern I, like many parents and grandparents, was when urging children to wash their hands at eating times, and I am still stern. Many parents believe that it is the countless bacteria on unwashed hands that may cause infectious illnesses. It is true, in a way. However, most adults may not know the fact that only a tiny portion of the bacteria that scientists have so far documented may cause diseases and the rest (>99% of all known bacteria) are essentially harmless or, rather, even beneficial to human health, directly or indirectly. Bacteria are virtually everywhere around us – in nearly all kinds of environments and on the surface of us (skin and mucous membrane), except in the lava from erupting volcanoes. Despite some being notorious pathogens such as *Yersinia pestis* or *Mycobacterium tuberculosis*, most bacteria support our normal life, essentially by harnessing solar energy, converting inorganic substance to life compounds, recycling elements, producing oxygen, making nutrients, suppressing pathogens, stimulating our immune functions, and too many others to list. What readers are expected to know from this book are the general distinctions between pathogenic and non-pathogenic bacteria and how pathogens might have arisen from their non-pathogenic ancestors in evolution. As a result, readers may have a clearer understanding about how to protect endangered bacterial species in order to protect ourselves and how to live and co-evolve in the best possible harmony with our bacterial companions in and around us.

Bacteria in and around us

Quite often, in the Microbiology class, students yell or scream, all at once, when I show micrographs or plate cultures of the beautiful (but they call them awful or horrifying) bacteria on our skin or the mucous membrane of the tongue. “Don’t worry”, I then comfort them, “they usually do not hurt you but, rather, they protect you”. I show them a picture of *Staphylococcus aureus* colonies on a blood agar plate and say: “See the hemolysis zone around the *S. aureus* colonies?” I tell them that many hemolytic bacteria such as *S. aureus* have the excellent ability to cause infections. They are horrifying pathogens and may cause local skin or tissue infections, such as furuncles, but they may also elicit systemic illnesses, such as meningitis or sepsis. In the former cases, I continue, “you do not need any treatment, just let them go hot and mature, making you look beautiful in another way if they are on your face or neck, or torturing you by pain if they are on your waist or buttocks when you lie down to sleep”. Students usually laugh. “However”, I change to a serious face, “in the latter cases, you really need treatment as soon as possible, since most systemic infections are potentially fatal if not treated properly and timely enough”. People may think that such bacteria dwelling on your body surface may be extremely dangerous. They are, indeed, in a way. However, they are ordinary members of the normal human microbiota.

At this point, a small wave of low surprised noises often comes from the audience again. Students do not find it easy to relate *S. aureus* to “ordinary members” of their normal microbiota. *S. aureus* is a too familiar bacterial pathogen name for the students to accept as a close daily companion.

To this, I would continue: "they do not invade you unless you invite them by heavy smoking, staying up all night with your web games, or eating too many sweet or oily foods. Or you have compromised immune functions, such as in cases where you are under enormous stress before an exam for which you are not really prepared…"

Students laugh again. The course I teach is Systematic Bacteriology, not Medical Microbiology, which I also teach but for other classes. Whereas I also have a focus on pathogenic bacteria in the Systematic Bacteriology course as in Medical Microbiology, the difference is that I deliberate on how pathogenic bacteria cause infections in Medical Microbiology but on how new bacterial species, pathogenic or benign, arise in Systematic Bacteriology. Traditionally, medical students learn Medical Microbiology to deal with disease-related microbes in their medical career. However, I believe that they do also need to have at least a very brief introduction to other microorganisms in nature, such as Cyanobacteria producing oxygen and Rhizobia fixing nitrogen. Such non-medical bacteria do not cause infections but they nurture human health and even safety, by nourishing an optimal environmental setting suitable for life and thus, making the otherwise inorganic globe livable for humans and other creatures.

While encouraging the medical students to read General Bacteriology for more detailed information about such deemed "disease-irrelevant bacteria", I show a genealogical graph of known bacteria at the phylum level (Figure 1-1).

Among the documented phyla, three contain most of the known pathogenic bacteria, including Proteobacteria (e.g., *Salmonella typhi*), Firmicutes (e.g., *Clostridium tetani*), and Actinobacteria (e.g., *M. tuberculosis*).

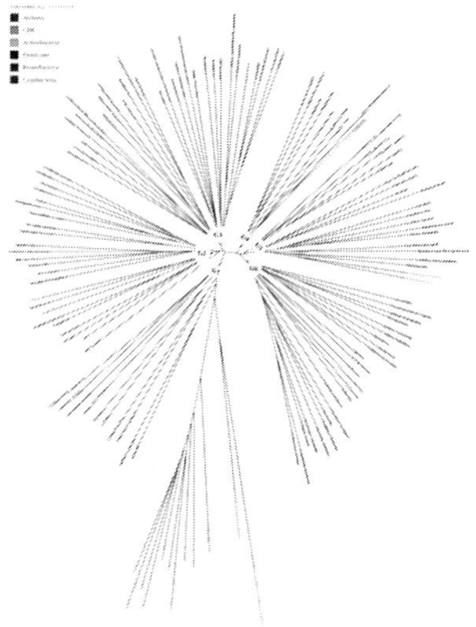

Figure 1-1. A phylogenetic tree showing the main phylogenetic lineages of bacteria at the phylum level. Branches represent phyla. Archaea lineages are included on the tree for a reference of genetic distances among the microbes. All phyla are clustered into six phylogenetic groups, G1-G6, which we call the six Kingdoms.

Pathogens: primary or opportunistic, causing mild or deadly diseases

Many textbooks divide pathogens into primary (or "true") and opportunistic pathogens. Primary or true pathogens are "professional" infectious agents, causing diseases in both vulnerable and healthy hosts by direct interaction using specialized "weapons" such as exotoxins or other virulence effectors. Illnesses caused by primary pathogens have specific disease names, specific symptoms and signs, and specific and mostly typical clinical patterns, such as typhoid fever caused by *S. typhi*, tetanus caused by *Clostridium tetani*, and tuberculosis caused by *M. tuberculosis*. Such diseases are generally called infectious diseases and have natural courses. In contrast, opportunistic pathogens infect individuals with compromised immune functions. Infections caused by opportunistic pathogens do not have specific disease names, specific symptoms or signs, nor typical courses, such as nosocomial infections by *Escherichia coli*, *Acinetobacter baumannii*, *Pseudomonas aeruginosa*, *etc*. In the lectures, I tell my students "please do not think that primary pathogens are deadlier than opportunistic pathogens in general". I usually use *Salmonella* gastroenteritis as an example, which is often caused by the primary pathogen *Salmonella typhimurium*. *Salmonella* gastroenteritis may, clinically, appear quite serious, with horrible vomiting and diarrhea, but usually does not require hospitalization or any medication. On the other hand, nosocomial infections caused by opportunistic pathogens could be fatal. I assign the students homework to make brief lists of primary and opportunistic pathogens causing mild or deadly diseases, telling them "I will compare a pair of closely related primary pathogens in the next lecture for you to have a better understanding about host-pathogen interactions and bacterial pathogenesis, one causing local infections without the need of medical treatment and the other eliciting systemic infections that are potentially fatal if not treated timely and properly". Then, in the next lecture, I usually make detailed comparisons between *S. typhimurium* and *S. typhi* for the students.

My first sight of real bacteria: some looking lovely but causing serious illnesses

My first glance at pathogenic bacteria was on October 22, 1971, when I began my career with bacteria in the clinical laboratory of Fujin Central Hospital in the small town of Fujin 富锦, in Heilongjiang Province, northeast China. I graduated from Fujin Second Middle School Class 1970 and was assigned to work in the Fujin Central Hospital. From the mid-1960s to late 1970s, most schools, including elementary and middle schools (which had junior high and senior high classes together), colleges and universities, stopped teaching. In the spring of 1970, when the schools had stopped producing graduates for a straight four-year period, the whole of society had an urgent workforce shortage. As a result, the hospital requested, and it was approved by the upper institution, the urgent recruitment from Senior High Class 1970 pre-graduates (dismissed from the school before the graduation time) and regular Class 1970 graduates (graduated according to the regular schedule; I was a graduate and so was in the latter group). Altogether, the hospital recruited about 60 youngsters from Fujin First, Second and Third Middle Schools and many of the young newcomers were assigned to the Departments of Internal Medicine, Pediatrics, Infectious Diseases, Surgery, Gynecology and Obstetrics, or Ophthalmology and Otorhinolaryngology, as assistants of nurses (many were promoted to nurses three years later). A few were assigned to Pharmacy as assistants of pharmacists, to Radiology as assistants of the technicians, or the Clinical Laboratory as junior staff. In general, the 60 of us were collectively referred to as "trainees" and we carried this label for about three years, as we had not received any medical education previously. We, as the Class 1970 Senior High graduates, received the diploma of senior high school education but the "pre-graduates" did not, as they did not have the chance to stay in the school according to the regular schedule and their school time was terminated prematurely. More striking is the fact that, being Senior High Class 1970 pre-graduates or even regular graduates, we all had only about five years of elementary school education. As a result, all 60 of us had to receive medical training on an educational background of Grade 5 or 6 elementary schooling. The training subjects included Anatomy, Histology, Physiology, Pathology, Pharmacology, Microbiology, Biochemistry, Internal Medicine, Pediatrics, Infectious Diseases, Surgery, Gynecology and Obstetrics, etc. The trainers were the best physicians in the hospital and the training was unbelievably successful. In another book, I provide moving details about this legendary history (Liu 2015).

I began my career at the hospital on March 1, 1971, and was assigned to work in the Clinical Laboratory on October 22, 1971. I met with the staff in the Laboratory on that day. I was very enthusiastically welcomed, because their workload had been so heavy that, unlike in a normal Clinical Laboratory where a person works either in Hematology, Biochemistry, Microbiology, or the Blood Bank, one had to work in all of these sections for daily routines and for night and weekend turns. They had night turns once in every two or three days and they did look pretty tired.

It was in the late afternoon when I was brought to the Clinical Laboratory to meet with the staff. They had just completed their daily work and Dr. Shu-You Wang (second from left, Fig. 1-2), Chair of the Clinical Laboratory, was the first to shake my hand. After asking my name and other general information, such as my father's profession (most mothers did not have a profession at that time) or my graduation middle school, he encouraged me to learn hard and work hard. A senior lab scientist, Dr. Song-Xue Wang (fifth from left, Fig 1-2), became my main mentor.

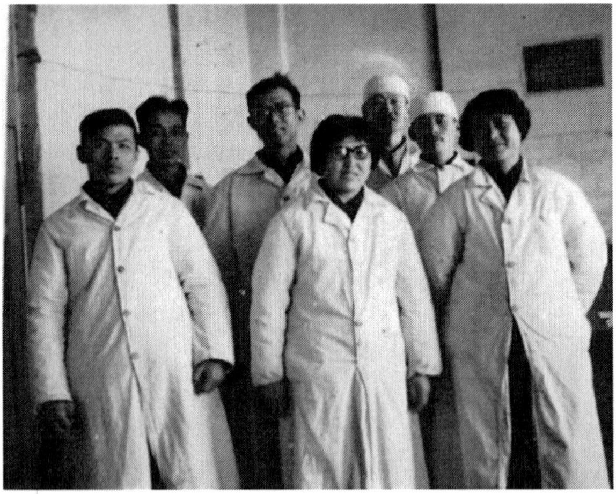

Figure 1-2. The staff of the Clinical Laboratory at Fujin Central Hospital. I am sixth from left. This photo was taken in the early winter of 1972.

Dr. Song-Xue Wang was extremely happy, as I was his first trainee in his career. He brought out a glass slide from a wooden case and put it under a microscope. He showed me tiny balls on the slide under the microscope, dark purple in color, telling me "these are *Staphylococcus* bacteria, or, grape-shaped bacteria". I was amazed and kept moving the stage to see more. "Look at this", he said and brought another glass slide to my eyes, "…these are *Salmonella* bacteria. Tell me whether you can see the difference between them."

It was my first time using a real microscope, which I had heard about before I attended the elementary school. As I did not know how to adjust the focus to find the field, Dr. Wang did all that and gestured to me to have another look through the eye piece of the microscope.

This time I saw short, pink rods, very tiny even under a microscope, and harder to see even than the *Staphylococcus* bacteria. "Yes, they are different", I reported to Dr. Wang, "*Staphylococcus* are dark purple and round but *Salmonella* are light pink and short-rod shaped." At this answer, Dr. Wang was very pleased. Then he put another glass slide under the microscope, encouraging me to adjust the focus and describe what I found. "*Salmonella*", I said to him. He smiled, asking "do you see any difference between the *Salmonella* in this and the previous slide?" I was at a loss and took another careful look. Then I put the previous *Salmonella* slide back under the lens. I watched and compared the images of the two slides. While I was making the comparisons, Dr. Wang told me that the bacteria on the first *Salmonella* slide cause gastroenteritis, which might make the patient appear quite sick, but special treatment would usually not be needed, as it is a self-limited local (gastrointestinal) infection; on the other hand, bacteria on the second *Salmonella* slide cause typhoid fever, which is potentially fatal and requires timely treatment with antibiotics. He asked me whether I could see any morphological differences between them. I said "No". "Surely they are both *Salmonella*, but they are very different *Salmonella* bacteria, causing totally different diseases in humans. You do not see any differences between them, eh?" I felt very ashamed, sheepishly grumbling "sorry, today it is my first time seeing real bacteria…" He laughed and tapped me on my right shoulder, saying "You are honest! Certainly it is not easy to distinguish between them and virtually impossible to tell one from the other by the morphology of their cells or the colonies they form on the agar plate." He brought two Petri dishes with tiny grains on the surface. "The grains are bacterial colonies. You cannot see single bacterial cells, as they are so tiny. They grow by fission, one growing into two and two becoming four. When they grow to millions together, as their motility and movement are limited on the surface of the solid culture medium, you can see the mass. Now can you see the differences between the colonies?" I said "No" and he nodded "Right, because they really form indistinguishable colonies."

He then showed me how to wipe and clean the oil lens after use.

I can never forget the excitement I experienced on that very first day of my career with microbes when I saw real bacteria by my own eye under a microscope (specifically, the left eye, because the right eye is to be used to draw the microscopic images by right hand) and by the naked eyes (both left and right) on the surface of an agar plate (in a Petri dish).

Dr. Song-Xue Wang advised me to look at the bacteria through a microscope using only the left eye with the right eye fully opened. Oddly enough, when I did so, i.e., opening both eyes, with the left one looking at the bacteria through the microscope and the right one looking at nothing, images arriving at my retina and visual cortex seemed to be coming only from the left eye. To be sure that there was nothing wrong with my right eye, I brought a pen and looked at it with my left eye closed, and I could see it very clearly.

Then a simple question came to me (I only knew, many years later, that it was not a simple but rather an extremely complex fundamental question): why are the two different kinds of *Salmonella* so similar in morphology – are they siblings or cousins? Further, if they are close relatives, why do they cause such different diseases? With such puzzles stuck in my brain since October 22, 1971, I worked with the senior lab scientists for many years (Fig. 1-3).

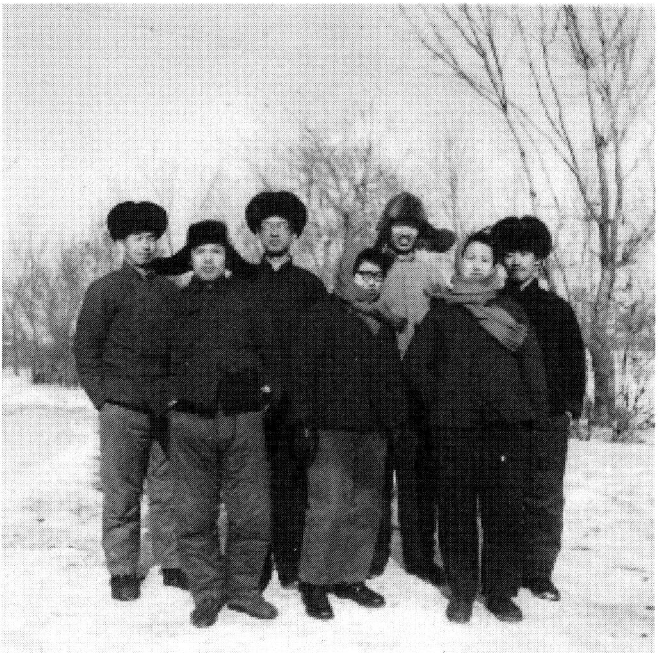

Figure 1-3. Members of the clinical lab in the early 1970s. I am first from the right.

CHAPTER 2

DETECTION OF THE TYPHOID AGENT: CULTURE AND SEROLOGICAL TESTS

Autumn is the season of many food-borne diseases, such as dysentery, gastroenteritis, or typhoid fever. Although a differential diagnosis among these illnesses was usually not difficult at that time, detection of pathogens was necessary and required. Indeed, patients with these illnesses may have similar clinical manifestations, such as fever, abdomen pain, diarrhea and vomiting, and obnubilation. In such cases, physicians would send fecal specimens to us for bacterial isolation and identification. We would then culture a small sample of the specimen and inspect the culture media to see whether the suspected bacteria might appear. Further examinations also included serological tests and biochemical assays. At that time, all culture media and fermentation tubes were made in the lab. We used to go to the slaughterhouse to buy beef or sheep blood for making the media.

Specimen collection and initial culture

I became an independent member of the laboratory staff in 1972 after the one-year training period - not only "independent" but also the only person when I worked in the clinical laboratory of the Outpatient Department in 1973. I came back to the main campus of the hospital in early 1974, when I became a mentor to train laboratory staff coming from some local clinics (Fig. 2-1).

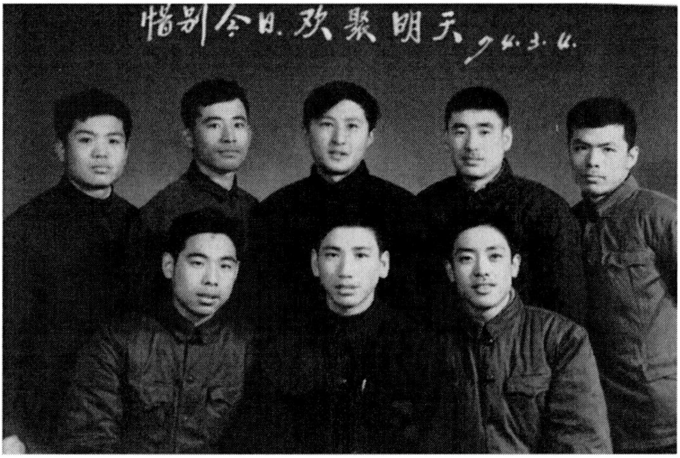

Figure 2-1. Young mentors and trainees in 1974. I am second from the left in the back row.

They were there mainly to learn blood cell counting, biochemical assays, microbiological examinations, serological tests, *etc*., but not bone marrow cell analysis for leukemia diagnosis – the latter requiring many years to learn and practice. They usually had only one year for the training. Therefore, they focused the one year of learning mostly on bacterial culture and identification procedures, and related knowledge. Occasionally, if they showed curiosity about bone marrow cells, I would then spend some time with them, showing them how to distinguish the immature blood cells and how to diagnose leukemia.

Upon admission to the hospital, patients were requested to have a fecal specimen collected. Usually, a nurse would bring the fecal specimen to the laboratory. We, in the daytime or night turn, would immediately streak the specimen out on an agar plate, which was often a selective plate called SS medium, with SS standing for *Shigella* and *Salmonella*, as it suppresses the growth of dominant gut bacteria such as *E. coli* so that the pathogenic bacteria *Shigella* or *Salmonella* would be more easily seen on the plate. The

SS agar plates, or sometimes other media for distinguishing *Shigella* and *Salmonella* from *E. coli* such as the MacConkey or eosin-methylene blue agar plates, contain lactose and a pH indicator, so that bacteria that can ferment lactose would turn the medium acidic and produce a purple or pink color on the bacterial colonies. *E. coli* ferment lactose, so their colonies are purple or pink in color, but *Shigella* and *Salmonella* colonies are colorless, as they do not ferment lactose. Of course, exceptions are known, as *Shigella* or *Salmonella* that carry lactose-fermenting enzymes on plasmids would produce purple or pink colonies. *Shigella* and *Salmonella* colonies are also smaller and flatter than those of *E. coli*, and more transparent.

Generally, all infectious agents have specific infectious doses, *i.e.*, the smallest number of the pathogenic microbes required to elicit infection in the host - the lower the infectious doses the higher the infectivity. The typhoid fever agent *S. typhi* has a pretty low infectious dose. Therefore, quite often, patients may manifest typical typhoid features, but detection of the *S. typhi* bacteria may not be easy. To maximize the chances of bacterial detection and isolation for identification and diagnosis, enrichment culture and blood culture are often needed. The enrichment culture procedure includes a pre-culture of the fecal specimen in a medium containing tetrasulfonate to suppress the growth of most intestinal bacteria, except *Salmonella*; after overnight incubation, a small aliquot of the tetrasulfonate culture is taken up and spread onto an SS plate. Blood, or occasionally bone marrow, culture may be conducted for higher detection chances. The colony morphology is inspected on the next day of plating. Suspected colonies will be picked up for identification by biochemical assays and serological tests.

Plate inspection and biochemical assays

Suspected colonies are usually easy to see on SS culture plates: greyish white, semitransparent, small to medium-sized flat colonies compared to the lactose-fermenting purple or pink medium to large flat-round colonies dominating the plate. Of course, many non-*Salmonella* bacteria have similar colony morphologies. Therefore, further tests will have to be performed to determine whether the suspected colonies are formed by *Salmonella*. This is simple: a well isolated suspected colony is picked up and inoculated into a Klinger iron agar slant, which contains glucose, lactose, ferrous sulfate, phenol red as the indicator, and rich nutrients. When the bottom part turns yellow (glucose is fermented), the slant part remains red (lactose is not fermented) and the part between the bottom and the slant turns shallow black (some ferrous sulfate is reduced to ferric salt by the hydrogen sulfite produced by the bacteria), it is possible that the growing bacteria are *S. typhi*; if the black part is very dark and wide (extending into both the bottom and the slant parts), it is possible that the growing bacteria are *S. typhimurium* (causing *Salmonella* gastroenteritis) or other salmonellae. However, a decisive identification of the bacteria is achieved by immunological reactions with techniques called serological tests.

Serological differentiation of *Salmonella* lineages and the Widal assay

Salmonella bacteria have O (somatic, polysaccharide) antigens on the surface of the cell wall, and most *Salmonella* bacteria have H (flagellar, protein) antigens on the flagellae; some *Salmonella* lineages, such as *S. typhi* and *S. paratyphi* C, also have another antigen, the Vi (standing for <u>vi</u>rulence, polysaccharide) antigen. Most *Salmonella* lineages have a unique combination of the O and H antigens. For example, the gastroenteritis agent *S. typhimurium* has the antigenic formula <u>1</u>,4,[5],12:i:1,2, meaning that *S. typhimurium* has four O antigens, including O<u>1</u> (the underline indicates that the O1 antigen is encoded by a phage whose DNA is incorporated into the bacterial chromosome), O4, O[5] (square brackets indicate that this antigen may, or may not, be detectable) and O12 antigens. Small characters between the two colons mean phase 1 H antigens, such as the single "i" in *S. typhimurium*; numerals after the second colon mean phase 2 H antigens, such as "1,2" in *S. typhimurium*. Another *Salmonella* lineage, *S. paratyphi* B, has an antigenic formula very similar to that of *S. typhimurium*, 1,4,[5],12:b:1,2, the only difference being the phase 1 flagellar antigen i in *S. typhimurium* but b in *S. paratyphi* B. As they share O4, they are categorized into the same O4 group.

The first step of serological tests on a bacterial isolate preliminarily determined as *Salmonella* by biochemical assays is the use of O grouping antisera to identify the isolate into an O group. Most often, the *Salmonella* isolate is first tested by slide agglutination with antisera against O groups O2 to O1, 3, 19 (previously called O groups A to E, respectively), as most clinical *Salmonella* isolates belong to one of these O groups. If the agglutination test is negative, the *Salmonella* isolate will be tested by pools of antisera against O groups 11 to 67. The second step is to use appropriate O single-factor antisera on the isolate to identify the bacteria down to a specific serotype.

Although most antigenic formulae are unique to individual *Salmonella* lineages, a few of them are shared by several *Salmonella* lineages, such as 1,4,[5],12:b:1,2 shared by *S. paratyphi* B and *S. java,* or 6,7:c:1,5 shared by *S. paratyphi* C, *S. choleraesuis* and *S. typhisuis*. Therefore, if a *Salmonella* isolate is identified to a serotype such as 1,4,[5],12:b:1,2 or 6,7:c:1,5, further differentiation is necessary.

False negative results of *Salmonella* detection were possible, because the infectious dose or the load of the bacteria, such as *S. typhi*, may be low. Therefore, for the timely diagnosis and treatment of the potentially fatal typhoid disease, the detection of antibodies in the serum of the patient against *S. typhi* (or the paratyphoid agents *S. paratyphi* A, B or C) by Widal assay is often performed. In cases in which the patients had typical typhoid manifestations, but the culture of *S. typhi* was negative, typhoid could still be diagnosed if the Widal assay was positive.

Starting from 1972, the Clinical Laboratory where I worked kept accepting trainees. Gradually, the trainees undertook most of the routine laboratory work, so that I as a mentor had more free time. The Chair of the Clinical Laboratory, Dr. Shu-You Wang, was doing some research and asked me to join him as his only assistant (Fig. 2-2). His main research was on the antibacterial effects of local herbs. I used to accompany him to the mountains by bicycle to collect known and unknown herbs and extract the components for analysis. In the process, I really learnt a great deal about the herbs and, more importantly, about research. Now, nearly a half century has passed and my current research is still on herbs and bacteria.

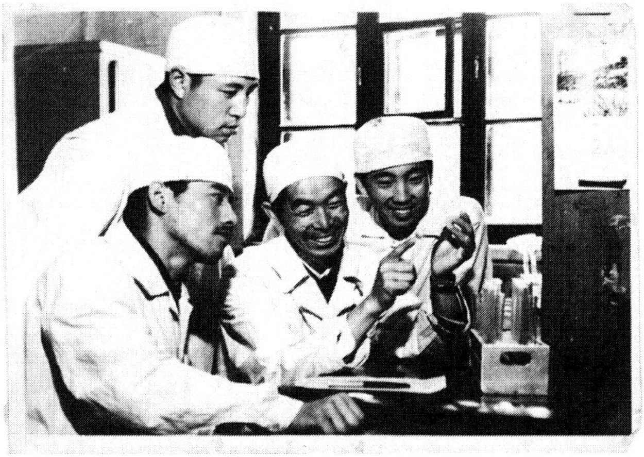

Figure 2-2. Dr. Shu-You Wang analyzing the research results. Front row from left: me, Dr. Shu-You Wang, and Peng Bai (a trainee from Huama Clinic, whom I was mentoring). The one in the back: Dr. Tie-Jun Jiang, a physician and one of my best friends.

CHAPTER 3

SALMONELLA SEROTYPES: VASTLY DIFFERENT PATHOGENIC FEATURES AND HOST RANGES

When I came to work in the mornings of the late summer to early autumn days of the 1970s, the first thing I used to do was to go directly to the Bacteriology Lab, open the incubator and inspect the SS plates that I had streaked the day before to see whether there might be *Salmonella*-like colonies between the hundreds of *E. coli*-like purple or pink colonies. On the left front corner of the bench where I and others in the lab streaked bacteria on the plates and inspected the colonies, there was a very thick book titled "Manual of Clinical Microbiology", in which there was a long table listing the more than 800 *Salmonella* serotypes (Note: the number of recognized *Salmonella* serotypes is about 2700 in March, 2022); each *Salmonella* serotype has an antigenic formula in the table. I was very curious about why, among the 800 *Salmonella* serotypes, only *S. typhi* causes typhoid fever. At that time, so many patients died of typhoid fever every year and I wanted to know more about the bacteria and about the disease. I was certain that *S. typhi* must have very special genetic traits that encode the unusual pathogenic properties not seen in the other 800 *Salmonella* lineages. But what might they be?

Salmonella typhi in the lab: how to distinguish this pathogen from the other 800 *Salmonella* serotypes?

Salmonella bacteria have indistinguishable cell or colony morphology among the serotypes, many of which cause human diseases, with *S. typhi* being the deadliest. Therefore, I would most often presume the *Salmonella*-

like bacteria to be *S. typhi* and go directly to the identification of *S. typhi*. Routinely, I would pick up a suspected colony and inoculate a Klinger iron agar slant; at the same time, I would conduct slide agglutination with antisera against *S. typhi*. *S. typhi* bacteria have two O antigens, O9 and O12, and a phase 1 H antigen d, or z66 in some strains; there is no phase 2 H antigen on *S. typhi*. Sometimes, the agglutination test results may be ambiguous, as the Vi antigen may mask the O antigens. In such cases, a brief heating of the bacterial suspension may help and make the O antigen agglutination results easier to judge, as the Vi antigen is heat-labile but O antigens are heat-stable. If the O antigen agglutination result is still not unambiguous, H antigen agglutination tests combined with Klinger iron agar slant fermentation assay results would provide key information for the bacterial identification.

Salmonella typhi isolated as the typhoid agent: many names

The typhoid agent was first isolated in 1880 from a typhoid patient. Soon after, this infectious agent was frequently isolated worldwide from typhoid patients. Authors reporting on the bacteria proposed different names, most of which have the meaning ''the typhoid-causing bacteria''. Among the names are Typhusbacillen, Eberth; Typhus abdominalis, Gaffky; Bacterium typhosum, Zopf; Bacillus typhosus, Zopf; Bacillus typhi, Schroeter; Bacillus typhi abdominalis, Flugge; Bacillus typhicus, Da Camara Mello; Bacterium typhi, Chester; Acystia typhi, Enderlein; Bacterium (Eberthella) typhi, Buchanan; Eberthus typhosus, Castellani and Chalmers; Eberthella typhi, Bergey et al.; Eberthella typhosa, Weldin; *Salmonella typhi*, Warren and Scott; Salmonella typhosus, White; Typus Typhus, Kauffmann; and Salmonella typhosa, Haupt. When the name *Salmonella typhi* was used in 1929, it was gradually accepted as the most widely used name until the 1980s. Initially, I was amazed to know that a bacterial lineage, species or serotype, whichever it might be, may have so many interesting names, but I later had it clear that eventually a bacterial species should have only one unique scientific name, according to the rules in the book "International Code of Nomenclature of Bacteria". (Fig. 3-1).

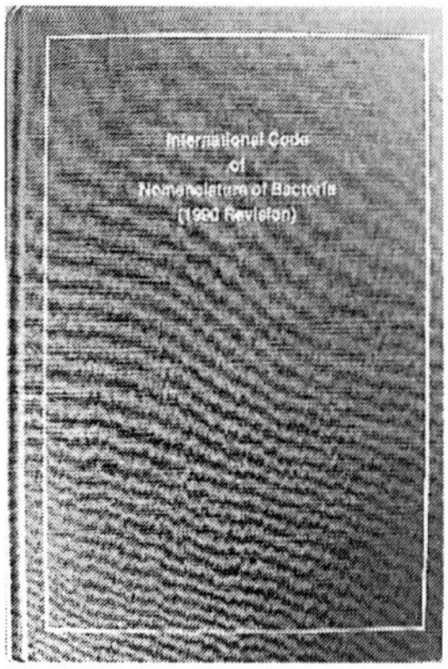

Figure 3-1. International Code of Nomenclature of Bacteria. (1990 Revision).

Salmonella serotypes: morphologically and biochemically similar but pathogenically distinct bacteria

Following the isolation of *S. typhi* in 1880, many morphologically and biochemically similar bacteria were increasingly isolated, subsequently categorized as *Salmonella enteritidis*, *Salmonella typhimurium*, *Salmonella choleraesuis*, *etc*. By 1914, a total of twelve species were documented. In 1928, the number was 24; in 1934, the number was 44. Fortunately, most of the newer species do not cause typhoid; they either cause gastroenteritis or hardly infect humans. Many of them can infect a broad range of hosts or cause different diseases in different hosts. For example, *S. typhimurium* can infect humans, primates, rodents, cattle, birds, *etc*., causing gastroenteritis in humans but typhoid-like disease in mice. On the other hand, *S. typhi* cause typhoid in humans but do not naturally infect any other hosts. For example, you may use *S. typhi* to experimentally infect chimpanzees, but not rodents. Similarly, *S. paratyphi* A, a *Salmonella* lineage that causes paratyphoid fever, cannot infect any host species except humans. *S. gallinarum* and *S. pullorum* share the same antigenic formula, 1,9,12:-:-, and have been treated as different biovars or pathovars of the same serotype; they are both adapted to fowl but cause totally different diseases, with the former causing typhoid-like disease and the latter causing dysentery.

I worked with *Salmonella* and other bacteria in the Clinical Laboratory of Fujin Central Hospital until March of 1978, when all schools were re-opened and I was admitted to Harbin Medical University (Fig. 3-2). The University admission rate was low: 5.7 million people took the admission exams and 0.27 million people passed the exams – a rate of less than 5%. As a medical student, I kept my interest in *Salmonella* throughout the medical school years. In fact, my interest in *Salmonella* has continued for the following four decades and, even now in the 2020s, I am still working on *Salmonella*.

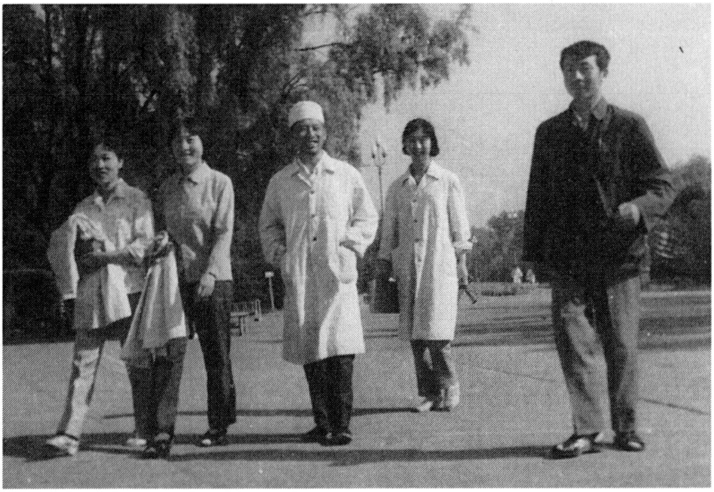

Figure 3-2. My classmates and I (middle) at Harbin Medical University. Photo taken in the summer of 1980.

CHAPTER 4

DYNAMIC *SALMONELLA* CLASSIFICATION AND A DILEMMA IN TAXONOMY

As described above, many *Salmonella* lineages had typical binominal scientific names, with the first word indicating the genus and the second word indicating the species, both being italicized, with the first letter of the genus name capitalized. Therefore, each of the *Salmonella* lineages was treated as a species. Since these bacteria are so similar in their morphology and biochemistry, a rapid and unambiguous identification method would be needed, especially to distinguish systemic infection agents from the gastroenteritis pathogens and those that do not normally infect warm-blooded hosts. The serological tests based on the Kauffmann-White scheme almost perfectly solved this issue.

The Kauffmann-White scheme: serological and phylogenetic classification

The Kauffmann-White scheme began to be used in 1934 for classifying these bacteria into serotypes based on their antigenic formulae (Fig. 4-1).

Beginning with Supplement I in 1957, the Kauffmann-White scheme has been updated annually (Kauffmann and Edwards 1957; Popoff, *et al.* 2004). There are two outstanding merits in the Kauffmann-White scheme, including 1, rapid and unambiguous identification of the *Salmonella* bacteria; and 2, phylogenetic classification of the *Salmonella* bacteria. Therefore, *Salmonella* serotypes were reasonably treated as species at that time (and even now by many researchers). According to different levels of relatedness, the *Salmonella* serotypes were divided into eight subgroups, including Subgroups I, II, IIIa, IIIb, IV, V, VI and VII. Among these, Subgroup I is quite special, as it is the only subgroup of *Salmonella* serotypes that infect warm-blooded hosts, and there are more than 1600 serotypes in *Salmonella* Subgroup I. The bacteria of the remaining seven subgroups mostly dwell in cold-blooded hosts but, occasionally, may also infect humans or other warm-blooded hosts.

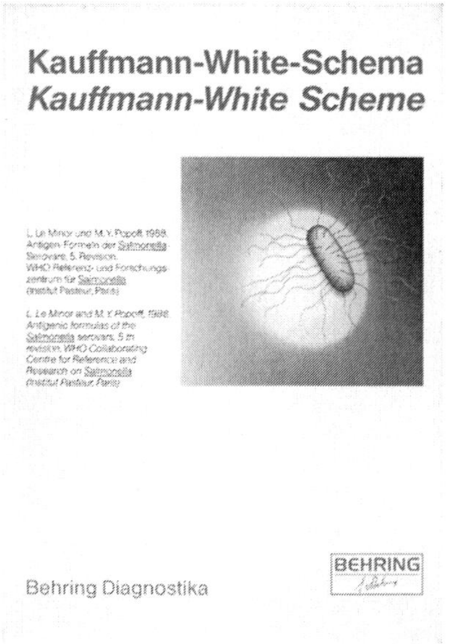

Figure 4-1. The Kauffmann-White scheme; edition of 1988.

Salmonella taxonomic changes in the 1980s

All *Salmonella* species across the eight subgroups are closely related, which was initially validated at the genomic level by DNA-DNA re-association assays (Crosa, *et al.* 1973). As a result of such high levels of close relatedness among them, all *Salmonella* species were categorized into a single species in the mid-1980s and given the taxonomic name *Salmonella enterica* (Le Minor and Popoff 1987); later, *Salmonella bongori* was recommended to regain the species status (Reeves, et al. 1989). So the *Salmonella* genus was *made* to contain two species, *Salmonella enterica* and *Salmonella bongori*, and all previous *Salmonella* species, except *S. bongori*, at once became serovars of *S. enterica*. In the changed nomenclature, the previous specific epithet was used as the serovar name, with the first letter capitalized and the whole word not italicized. The previous Subgroups I, II, IIIa, IIIb, IV and VI became subspecies of *Salmonella enterica*, and Subgroup V regained the species status as *Salmonella bongori*; Subgroup VII was not given a subspecies status (Table 4-1).

Table 4-1. Species and subspecies of *Salmonella* after the taxonomic changes in the 1980s.

Species	Subgroup	Subspecies
Salmonella enterica	I	*enterica*
	II	*salamae*
	IIIa	*arizonae*
	IIIb	*diarizonae*
	IV	*houtenae*
	VI	*indica*
Salmonella bongori	V	-

Consequently, the two representative and distinct pathogenic species *S. typhi* and *S. typhimurium* became members of the same species (*S. enterica*) and even of the same subspecies (*S. enterica* subsp. *enterica*), although they have as much as >10% genetic differences (note that the genetic difference between man and chimpanzee is only about 1% and that man and chimpanzee belong to different species, genera and families), dwell in different niches (mucosa vs deep tissues), and cause drastically different (local vs systemic) diseases in humans. Accordingly, their taxonomic names became *Salmonella enterica* subsp. *enterica* Typhi and *Salmonella enterica* subsp. *enterica* Typhimurium, respectively. In fact, the two nomenclature systems have both been in use, *e.g.*, the typhoid agent has been referred to as *Salmonella typhi* by some authors and as *Salmonella enterica* subsp. *enterica* Typhi by others, in publications.

Enthusiasm for pathogenesis research

There was a sharp drop in typhoid morbidity in the late 1970s. Then afterwards, only sporadic cases could be seen and outbreaks have been very rare, due mostly to the significant improvement of environmental sanitation. In the hospital, I very seldom saw patients with *Salmonella* infections (Fig. 4-2).

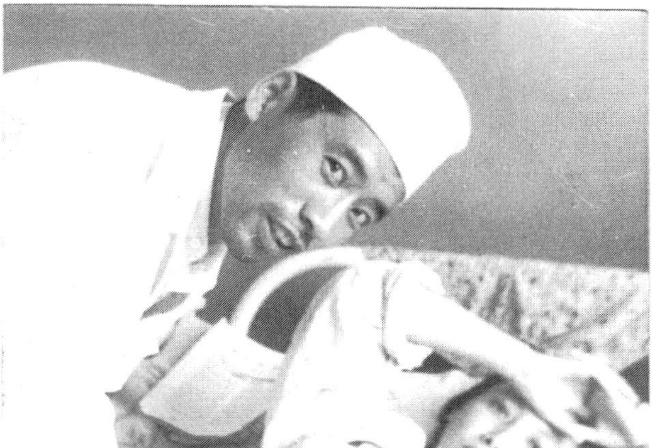

Figure 4-2. Examining a recovering patient in a morning round in the Department of Infectious Diseases. Photo from 1981.

The changes in *Salmonella* taxonomy and nomenclature often cause considerable confusion in basic research as well as in clinical practice. I sometimes tried to interpret the changes in *Salmonella* taxonomy to my classmates or colleagues, but in most cases would make things worse. However, investigators and clinical practitioners seemed more interested in *Salmonella* pathogenesis. Investigators wanted to know how pathogenic bacteria may cause diseases rather than what the bacteria should be called, or what name would be more correct than others. They sometimes joked: "a rose by any other name would smell as sweet, and *Salmonella* bacteria by any other names would sound as pathogenic". Enthusiasm for studies about the virulence factors of *Salmonella* was widespread, globally, at about the same time as the taxonomic and nomenclature changes of *Salmonella*.

To establish an infection in the host, pathogenic bacteria first need to break through the protective layers of the body, including not only the skin and the gastrointestinal and pulmonary mucous membranes, but also the normal microbiota covering the surfaces, as well as the immune network underlining the body surface. From the outside inward, there are three basic layers of protection: normal microbiota, mostly biological; skin and mucous membrane (often covered by a thin film of glycosylated proteins and glycolipids), mostly mechanical or physical; and phagocytes (e.g., macrophages) and cytokines right beneath the skin and mucous membrane, mostly cellular and chemical. These three layers of protection can ward off most microbial invasions and are extremely effective, unless the invading microbes are equipped with special virulence traits.

The usual entrance of many pathogenic bacteria, such as *Salmonella*, is the epithelium of the gastrointestinal tract. The epithelial cells, along with the glycosylated protein and glycolipid covering, provide the platform for active interactions between the host inner environment and the intestinal microbes. As the surface of the gastrointestinal epithelium is heavily occupied by bacteria of the normal microbiota, pathogenic bacteria like *Salmonella* usually do not have much chance to invade the epithelium and elicit infections, unless the number of invading *Salmonella* cells is significantly greater than the infectious dose, or, otherwise, the intestinal micro-ecological environment is impaired, such as in cases of intestinal micro-dysbiosis due to stress, ingestion of improper food, or abusive use of antimicrobials.

Salmonella may enter the host tissue through any of three cell types: M cells, enterocytes or dendritic cells, with M cells as the main portal. Once in the intestine, *Salmonella* interact with the mucins secreted by Goblet cells, immune molecules, and other defensive substances. In the *Salmonella*-mucin interactions, the *Salmonella* adhesin protein, called giant SiiE, plays a crucial role. SiiE is expressed in most documented *Salmonella* species but, interestingly, is decayed in *S. typhi*, along with many other ancestral *Salmonella* genes such as *gtgE*, the loss of which has made *S. typhi* incapable of invading any host species except humans (Spanò and Galán 2012).

My PhD supervisor Professor Eiko Yabuuchi had been curious about the striking pathogenic distinction of *S. typhi* from other *Salmonella* pathogens for many years when I joined the lab in October, 1985 (Fig. 4-3). She had hoped to elucidate why *S. typhi* would behave so differently in pathogenesis, wondering what had made *S. typhi* the only *Salmonella* lineage among thousands of others that infects only humans and causes typhoid fever. This question led me to ponder what would the genetic differences be between *S. typhi* and other *Salmonella* pathogens. I then set out to tackle the *S. typhi* pathogenesis issues as my PhD research project, supervised by Professor Yabuuchi and mentored by Dr. Ezaki, who helped me throughout my PhD thesis studies.

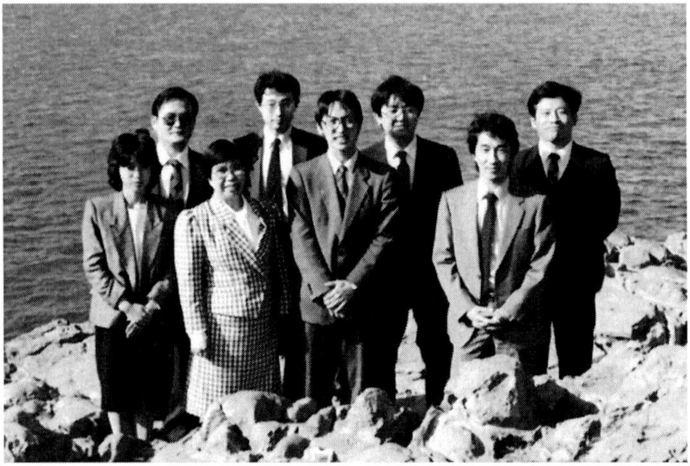

Figure 4-3. Professor Eiko Yabuuchi's team. Prof. Ezaki, 2nd from left; Prof. Yabuuchi, 3rd from left. I am 1st from right.

We used the Tn*5* mutagenesis method to randomly disrupt the genes of *S. typhi* and screen the mutants by HeLa cell invasion experiments for those that could no longer invade the HeLa cell. So the research design was simple. We inspected thousands of HeLa cell culture chambers under a microscope and obtained several *S. typhi* mutants that could not be internalized into the HeLa cells. These mutants stirred up enormous excitement in the lab and we designed the next step of the investigation: the characterization of these mutants and identification of the mutated genes. Fermentation and nutrient assimilation assays did not bring any clues about the particular pathogenic properties of *S. typhi*, so we focused our attention on the invasion-associated traits of the bacteria.

Salmonella, like many other bacterial pathogens, had been presumed to use three key systems for host invasion: flagellae, fimbriae and non-fimbrial adhesins, although not much had been documented on these systems by the 1980s. We characterized the mutants and were very surprised to find that most of the invasion mutants had impaired flagellar structures or functions, including total loss of flagellae, morphologically intact but entirely non-motile flagella, and motile but chemotaxis-defective flagella (Fig. 4-4). Through genetic analysis, we pinpointed the Tn*5*-inactivated genes and found that these genes were all associated with flagellae or chemotaxis (Liu, et al. 1988).

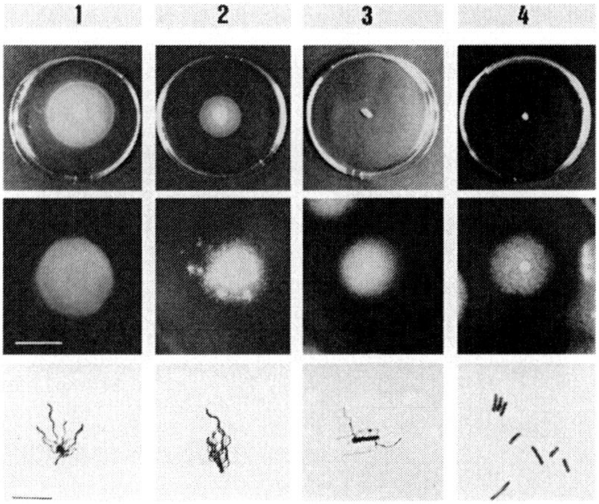

Figure 4-4. Morphology and motility of representative *S. typhi* invasion mutants. From top to bottom: semi-solid agar plate; semi-solid gelatin plate; bacterial cells showing the morphology of flagellae. From left to right: 1, wild-type strain with intact flagellar morphology and function, spreading on the semi-solid agar plate and semi-solid gelatin plate normally; 2, chemotaxis-defect mutant, flagellated but with limited spreading on the semi-solid agar plate and "crippled" swarming on the semi-solid gelatin plate (some bacteria cease moving forward and make tiny colonies where they stop); 3, flagellar gene mutant with paralyzed flagella, non-motile; 4, flagellar gene mutant with no flagellae produced, non-motile.

This finding indicates that *Salmonella* invasion of host tissues requires not only the physical structure of the flagellae but also intact motility, as bacteria with paralyzed or chemotaxis-defective flagellae would not be able to invade the cultured cells unless complemented with wild-type flagellar genes (Liu, et al. 1988). This fact further emphasizes the role of flagellae, not only as a swimming apparatus toward the target intestinal cells, but also as a bacterial organ for invasion.

Among the structural flagellar proteins, FliC is the most abundant (Chevance and Hughes 2008; Evans, et al. 2014). The binding of FliC, even by a single antibody fragment against it, would completely abolish the invasiveness of the bacteria (Huen, et al. 2019). Additionally, FimZ, as a regulator of the fimbrial *fim* operon, is also involved in the regulation of motility – its overexpression is associated with the decreased motility and weaker invasiveness of the bacteria (Clegg and Hughes 2002).

So organs for "civil" use of bacteria, like flagellae for the motility of *Salmonella*, could also be involved in pathogenesis such as flagella in invasiveness, but, obviously, pathogenic bacteria must also have professional pathogenicity traits to elicit diseases in the host. Additionally, the professional pathogenicity traits should be pathogen-specific, providing the bacterial pathogen specific pathogenic properties, such as different hosts that the bacteria may infect or the nature of the infectious diseases that the bacteria may cause. Therefore, such studies would have to be performed right from the "root", *i.e.*, the genetic differences among the bacteria that code for their pathogenic distinctness. For this, I needed to fly to Calgary, Canada, where there was a *Salmonella* Genetic Stock Center that I hoped could provide me with all the materials needed for the research. I wrote to Dr. Kenneth E. Sanderson, Director of the *Salmonella* Genetic Stock Center, telling him that I wanted to compare the genetic differences between *S. typhi* and many other *Salmonella* lineages to know why *S. typhi* may elicit the deadly typhoid fever but others could not. Specifically, I told him that I would construct physical genome maps on *S. typhi* and other *Salmonella* lineages and make direct comparisons to identify their genetic differences that may account for their pathogenic differences. The term “genome”, coined by the German scientist Hans Winkes, of the University of Hamburg, by combining the two words “gene” and “chromosome” to indicate the whole set of genes of an organism, was not familiar to Dr. Sanderson at that time; in addition, he asked me how to construct “physical maps”. I gave him all the necessary details and he was very happy to accept me in his laboratory as a postdoctoral fellow (Fig. 4-5).

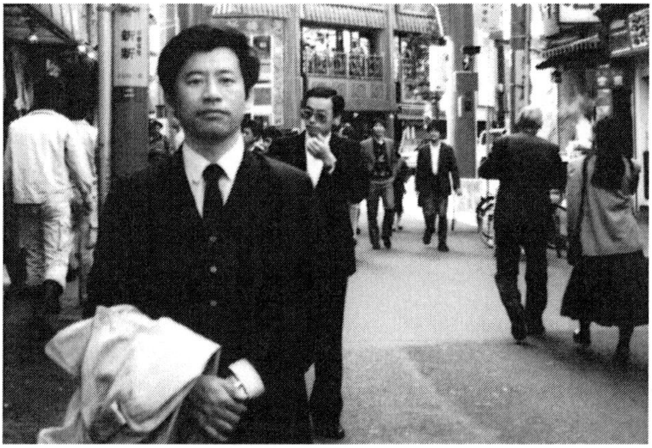

Figure 4-5. Leaving Japan for Canada to start genomic comparative studies on *Salmonella*.

PART II

GENOMIC DIFFERENCES AMONG THE *SALMONELLA* PATHOGENS

The blue sky and broad horizon in Canada gave me a feeling that this was the right place for me to pursue the origins of pathogenic bacterial species.

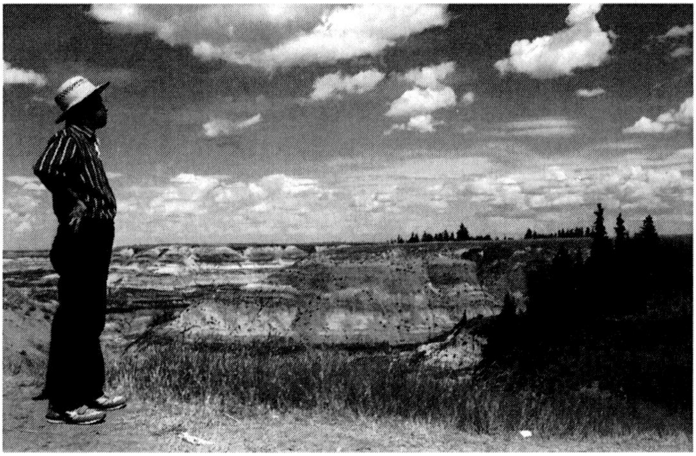

Summer, early 1990s, Canada

CHAPTER 5

GENETIC DIVERGENCE OF *SALMONELLA* FROM *E. COLI* AND THE BEGINNING OF COMPARATIVE GENOMICS

Most of the human knowledge on molecular biology began with studies of *E. coli*; specifically, the strain most frequently used was K12. Later on, other model bacterial strains have also been extensively studied, including *Salmonella*, which is very closely related to *E. coli*, and *Bacillus subtilis*, which is a Gram positive bacterial lineage, very remotely related to *E. coli*. As a lactose fermenter, *E. coli* emerged at about the time when mammals first appeared and since then has co-evolved with mammals as commensals. *Salmonella* lineages, as "professional" pathogens, have diverged from a common ancestor with *E. coli*. So, genetic comparisons between pathogenic and commensal descendants of a common ancestor are supposed to give clues to the origins and evolution of the pathogenic bacterial species.

Genetic comparison of *S. typhimurium* LT2 with *E. coli* K12 by linkage mapping

When numerous genes were identified in *E. coli*, investigators wondered how these genes might be arranged on the bacterial chromosome. A genetic map of *E. coli* K12 was then constructed, based on the techniques of F-Prime plasmid mediated conjugation and P1 phage mediated transduction. The first version of the map was published in 1964 by Taylor and Thoman (Taylor and Thoman 1964), followed by the map of *S. typhimurium* LT2 in the following year by Sanderson and Demerec (Sanderson and Demerec 1965). In *S. typhimurium* LT2, phage P22, instead of P1, was used for the generalized transduction experiments. Since then, the maps have been updated every few years, with more genes mapped, until 1996, when the ninth version of the *E. coli* K12 linkage map and the eighth version of the *S. typhimurium* LT2 linkage map were published as symbols of the end of the genetic linkage map era (Berlyn, et al. 1996; Sanderson, et al. 1996).

The availability of genetic maps made it possible to compare pairs of bacterial strains, one being commensal and the other being pathogenic, to elucidate their genetic similarities and differences for studies, say, of the origins and evolution of the pathogenic bacterial species. However, the genetic linkage methods could determine the chromosomal locations of only a very small number of genes, which would have to have readily detectable phenotypes. Additionally, gene locations on the chromosome could not be determined by physical parameters. Actually, only relative orders of adjacent genes could be estimated, but their physical distances on the DNA molecule could not be measured. Therefore, physical mapping methods were desired.

Physical mapping of *E. coli* K12: Kohara and Smith maps

Dr. Yuji Kohara and colleagues used a highly complex method to physically map *E. coli* K12 and for the first time in history laid out the bacterial genes on a physical framework. They employed 3400 λ phage clones containing the *E. coli* chromosomal DNA segments, made cleavages with eight six-base-recognizing enzymes by a rapid mass-analysis method, and finally, constructed a 4700 kb long integrated restriction map. This map had several merits: 1, both the genome size and the distances between genes were provided in physical dimensions; 2, the map had a relatively high resolution at that time; and 3, the λ clones used for the mapping could be exploited for the isolation of genes for those with known map positions. I was amazed by their work and planned to develop a similar method to map *Salmonella*.

After I finished my dissertation defense and received the PhD Degree at Gifu University, I was to leave for Canada. Before the trip, I contacted Dr. Kohara to ask for a set of his λ clones, thinking that they might be useful for my *Salmonella* mapping project. Dr. Kohara arranged this for me and I picked up the set from Dr. Mitsio Futota of Nagoya University. Dr. Futota knew me, because we had attended Microbiology conferences several times. I remember, at the 1987 Annual Meeting of the Japanese Society for Microbiology, I gave a presentation on the association of the *Salmonella* flagella with the invasiveness of the bacteria into the HeLa cells. As a foreigner in Japan, I was allowed to use English in the oral presentation, but I chose to speak Japanese in order that a broader audience range would understand my work and communicate with me more conveniently at question time. Dr. Futota was extremely interested in my work and asked a question: "Do *Salmonella* bacteria penetrate into the HeLa cells the way a loach in hot water penetrates into cold tofu?" A wave of loud laughter came from the audience. "In a way, you are right, because the loach would feel more comfortable in the cold tofu than in the hot water. Similarly, the *Salmonella* bacteria would prefer the home-like epithelial cells than the hostile extracellular fecal environment." I paused for a moment, waiting for louder laughter, which instantly came from the audience. "However, as you may know, the loach uses its tail to move forward, because it is not flagellated." This sentence invited a burst of applause.

I stayed in the laboratory of Dr. Futota for a whole afternoon, dispensing the set of λ clones; I brought the set of λ clones to Calgary on March 18, 1990.

At around the same time, Dr. Cassandra Smith constructed another kind of physical map on *E. coli* K12, using rare-cutting endonucleases and the pulsed field gel electrophoresis (PFGE) technique (Smith, et al. 1987). This kind of map has two obvious merits: 1, greater time- and labor-saving in mapping and data analysis; and 2, more intuitive in the comparisons among different bacteria. These advantages of rare-cutter mapping attracted my high attention, as I needed to construct a large number of genome maps for comparative studies. Obviously, therefore, the Kohara map strategy would not fit my project, as it would require quite a few years to construct just a single map.

I thus decided to use the rare-cutter enzyme and PFGE technique for the *Salmonella* genomic comparative studies.

Physical and genetic mapping: the pulsed field gel electrophoresis technique and gene locator

Dr. Sanderson met with me at Calgary airport the afternoon of March 18, 1990, with a few books under his left arm. He extended his right hand to me: "Dr. Liu?" I was standing beside the conveyor belt, waiting for my luggage. I was quite surprised to see him, since, usually, individuals who come to the airport to meet with arriving passengers would not be allowed to enter this part of the airport. Maybe he somehow sneaked in, like Kevin McCallister in the TV drama "Home Alone II", who sneaked onto a passenger airplane and flew to New York City, I thought. But I was very happy: "Yes. Dr. Sanderson?" Holding the three or four books with both hands now, he said: "Yes. Please wait here and I will go and get my car."

In his car, running from the airport to the campus of the University of Calgary, we talked a lot and the conversation was really information intensive. I provided details about the PFGE principle and techniques, rare cutters, physical mapping, and comparisons of the *Salmonella* genomes. He kept nodding and occasionally asked some questions, such as different brands of PFGE machines and how they work, high GC and low GC rare cutters for the *Salmonella* genome, and what would be the rough budget to complete such a project. My answers seemed to be pleasing, as he looked delighted when I said the rough budget. I could fully understand, as I had heard that research grants were very difficult to obtain in Canada at that time.

The next day, March 19, 1990, I walked out of the house in the early morning and saw heavy snow turning the world brilliantly white under the street light. It was about 3 o'clock, probably 6 o'clock in China or 7 o'clock in Japan in the evening, I thought. I lay awake the whole night recalling the memorable five years in Japan and imagining the coming days in Canada, hoping to have the genomes of *S. typhi* and *S. typhimurium* compared as soon as possible. I did not get any sleep the very first night in Canada, partly because of jet lag and partly because of the excitement. I then went back to the room and picked up a pen to make a list of the required materials, including a PFGE machine; rare cutters, including XbaI, BlnI, and a few eight base cutters; agarose and other chemicals; a long roll of paper, a long ruler, and pens and pencils.

The PFGE machine was initially a problem. First, this kind of machinery had been invented only a couple of years earlier, so not many institutions had such equipment yet; second, what the PFGE could do was not in the consideration of most investigators of the biomedical research fields; and third, the PFGE set was relatively expensive. By chance, Dr. Manju Kapoor of the neighboring laboratory had one, and fortunately she did not have a plan to use it yet. So Dr. Sanderson borrowed it from Dr. Kapoor. The core issue seemed to have been solved.

Then we discussed the rare cutter issue. "Conventional" restriction endonucleases cleave the genomic DNA very frequently. For example, Dr. Kohara used a set of eight restriction endonucleases to cleave or "cut" the genomic DNA of *E. coli* K12 into thousands of fragments, because all the eight restriction endonucleases are six-nucleotide sequence cutters. They all have numerous cut sites on the *E. coli* K12 genome so are also called "frequent" cutters. In contrast, some restriction endonucleases recognize a sequence of more than six nucleotides and so cut the genomic DNA much more rarely; they are called "rare cutters". For example, Dr. Smith used the restriction endonuclease NotI, which cuts the genome of *E. coli* K12 into only 22 DNA fragments, which could be well separated by PFGE and ordered by using available genetic information and partial digestion data. As *Salmonella* lineages are closely related to *E. coli*, I assumed that NotI may also be suitable for *Salmonella*.

Then, finally, we discussed the issue of a long roll of paper, a long ruler, and pens and pencils. As Dr. Sanderson had just purchased a laser printer, so the old fashioned printer became obsolete and the old printer paper, continual with holes on both edges, could be used as the "long roll of paper" for drawing the physical map. A long ruler, and pens and pencils were no problem, as he had many to spare. "Here, the rubber eraser", he said, smiling and handing me one, which I did need but had forgotten to request. All set. I began installing the brand new PFGE apparatus right away.

The PFGE apparatus was a great invention. Unlike the conventional electrophoresis apparatus, which can separate DNA segments no larger than about 25 kb (kilo bases), or a maximal 40 kb (if the voltage, temperature and agarose gel concentration are all set very low), the PFGE can separate much larger DNA segments, routinely 2000 kb or smaller, or the range of 2000–4000 kb if the voltage, temperature and agarose gel concentration are set properly low. The electric current goes forward and then backward, with the forward running time longer than the backward running time. Or the current goes in one direction for a while and then reorients to another direction, with the directions having various angles. If the angles are set narrowly, say 90°, the electrophoresis goes faster but the resolution of separation will be lower; conversely, if the angles are set widely, say 160°, the resolution of separation will be higher but the electrophoresis will go slower. When the electric current reorients, either going between forward and backward or between two directions, the DNA segments in the agarose gel will also have to reorient, and the larger the DNA segments the longer time they require for the reorientation and the slower they move forward in the gel. I was so looking forward to getting my hands on the PFGE apparatus to run the bacterial genomic DNA fragments.

I then had to think about another issue, the gene locator, as I needed not only to arrange the restriction cleavage fragments but, perhaps more importantly, also to locate the genes on the genome. Nevertheless, setting up the PFGE apparatus was the first thing to do.

The first PFGE gel for the XbaI cleaved genome of *S. typhimurium* was quite beautiful and exciting. I was then pulled deep into the genomic world of *Salmonella*.

CHAPTER 6

THE BEGINNING OF THE PHYSICAL MAPPING ERA OF *SALMONELLA*

The physical mapping of *Salmonella* lineages revealed many previously unknown facts about bacterial evolution. For example, the overall physical structure of the bacterial genomes could be highly conserved for hundreds of millions of years. Of more personal interest, the main genomic differences among the *Salmonella* lineages were the species-specific insertions, deletions and endonuclease cleavage patterns. Very strikingly, the extent of the genomic nucleotide sequence degeneracy after the divergence of the *Salmonella* lineages was beyond imagination, which brought unprecedented insights into the adaptive processes of nascent bacterial species into novel niches.

Ordering the DNA fragments and genes: probe hybridization and Tn*10* insertion mutation

I was familiar, in a way, with the PFGE technique, because I played around with the equipment after my dissertation defense, but before my departure from Japan for Canada. It was at that time that I decided to use the rare cutters and the PFGE technique, rather than the frequent cutter strategy as used by Dr. Kohara, to map the *Salmonella* genomes for their comparisons. I tried running the PFGE apparatus borrowed from the Kapoor lab and found that it could hardly work – it could manage to separate the rare cutter fragments but the separation resolution was very low. I found that the PFGE machine was smaller than the one that I had used in Japan and it needed an external computer to run it. As I recalled, the machine that I used in Japan was the Bio-Rad brand and I requested Dr. Sanderson to purchase one. He told me that he could not afford it, due to the lack of research money; he had some funds from the National Science and Engineering Research Council of Canada (NSERC), but that was for maintaining the SGSC and not for conducting research. "We do need a Bio-Rad PFGE machine very badly, Ken. Could you go and get a loan from a bank? When we have the machine, we will publish good papers, then you can obtain research money from NSERC or the MRC (Medical Research Council of Canada) to pay back the loan", I suggested, clearly knowing that no man with a normal mind would do that. He laughed hysterically and repeated what I had said to many of his colleagues, and they also laughed hysterically. I judged that they all had normal and healthy brains.

I managed to use the smaller PFGE machine to separate the rare-cutter fragments. I tested it on NotI and found that this restriction enzyme cut the *Salmonella* genomic DNA into too many fragments, rather than 22 fragments as in *E. coli*, even though the two kinds of bacteria were so closely related in phylogeny. I then had to try other rare cutters. Usually, rare cutters recognize a sequence of eight or more nucleotides, but there are exceptions. For example, XbaI and BlnI are both six-base cutters but they cut the *Salmonella* genomic DNA infrequently, with only about 15-35 cut sites per genome, which is because both of their cut sites contain CTAG, a four nucleotide sequence that is very rare in the *Salmonella* genome.

After playing around with several rare cutters, I finalized XbaI as the tool enzyme in the genomic analysis; BlnI was good too, but it was much more expensive. Next, I needed to put the XbaI cleavage fragments back into the genome and arrange them in their natural order. The first method I used was probe hybridization by cloned DNA, containing known genes labeled with the radioisotope P^{32}. This method was very effective, producing highly reproducible and unambiguous results, but was, on the other hand, quite tedious. More seriously, such useful probes were not readily available. Dr. Cassandra Smith described the partial digestion method, but it was very hard to find the concentration range of XbaI in order to produce partial DNA digests. Quite often, when the right concentration range of XbaI was obtained for partial digestion, after many titration tests, the tube of enzyme was nearly used up and a new batch of XbaI, similarly diluted, would usually not produce any partial digests.

Fortunately, there was a large number of the transposon Tn*10* insertion mutants in the SGSC with Tn*10* inserted in known genes and, even more fortunately, the Tn*10* sequence contained a cleavage site for XbaI. So, if a gene is inactivated by Tn*10* insertion, the XbaI fragment that carries that gene would be cleaved into two fragments (Fig. 6-1).

Since many of the genes with Tn*10* insertion had previously been located on the genetic linkage map of *S. typhimurium* LT2, XbaI analysis could order the fragments and, in the meantime, locate a gene; so the previously characterized Tn*10* insertion mutants played the role of gene locators, thanks to so many previous *Salmonella* investigators, who produced and characterized the Tn*10* insertion mutants and stocked them to SGSC.

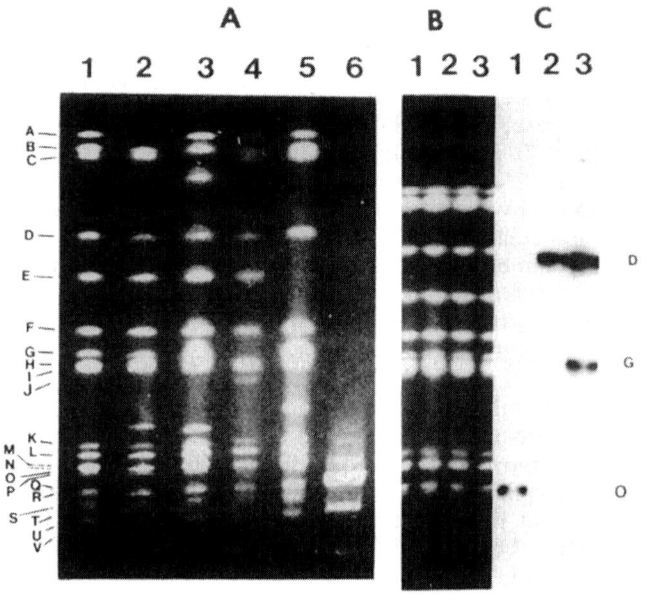

Figure 6-1. PFGE patterns of XbaI cleaved *S. typhimurium* LT2 genome and illustration of fragment identification strategies by Tn*10* insertion and probe hybridization. A, XbaI cleavage pattern. Lanes: 1, wild-type LT2; 2, fragment A cleaved into two smaller fragments (see the appearing DNA bands not present in lane 1); 3, fragment C cleaved into two smaller fragments; 4, fragment G cleaved into two smaller fragments; 5, fragment E cleaved into two smaller fragments; 6, λ DNA as the molecular size marker. In lanes 2-5, the addition of the two newly appearing fragments comes to the size of the missing fragment, plus 9 kb (wild-type Tn*10*) or 4 kb (modified Tn*10*). B, a gel of XbaI cleaved wild-type *S. typhimurium* LT2 genome after PFGE to be used for Southern hybridization. C, probe hybridization with DNA containing known genes, exemplified by lane 1, plasmid DNA containing the gene *pyrE* hybridizing with fragment O; lane 2, phage P22-carried DNA containing the gene *pyrF* hybridizing with fragment D; and 3, phage P22-carried DNA containing the gene *pyrF*, and many other genes, as a linking probe showing that fragments D and G are contiguous on the genome.

The first physical *Salmonella* map with gene locations

Finally, in late 1991, with resource support from Dr. Sanderson and technical assistance from Mrs. Donna Douey, I finished the mapping and sent the draft to Dr. Sanderson, who was on sabbatical at the University of Leicester, UK. He suggested the Journal of Bacteriology for the publication. The reviewers gave it a pretty high evaluation, saying that, as the first physical map of *Salmonella*, every investigator in the field of *Salmonella* research should have it on their desk. Dr. Sanderson was very pleased with the reviewers' comments, enthusiastically telling me "I bet one of the reviewers is John Roth!" Dr. John Roth was a member of the National Academy of Science, USA, and one of the most well-known *Salmonella* research experts. This LT2 map showed the physical size of the genome as 4807 kb, which was later confirmed to be surprisingly accurate considering the "macro" physical mapping technology used at that time, and for the first time brought the genetic linkage between genes to a physical foundation (Liu and Sanderson 1992). The XbaI map also corrected some errors in spatial relationships between some genes and confirmed the overall correctness of the linkage map in terms of gene order (Fig. 6-2). This map was used at the turn of this century as a template of the *S. typhimurium* LT2 genome sequencing project for pinning sequence contigs and determining gaps between the contigs. Most importantly, the accuracy of a finished genome had to be confirmed by a high resolution physical map at that time.

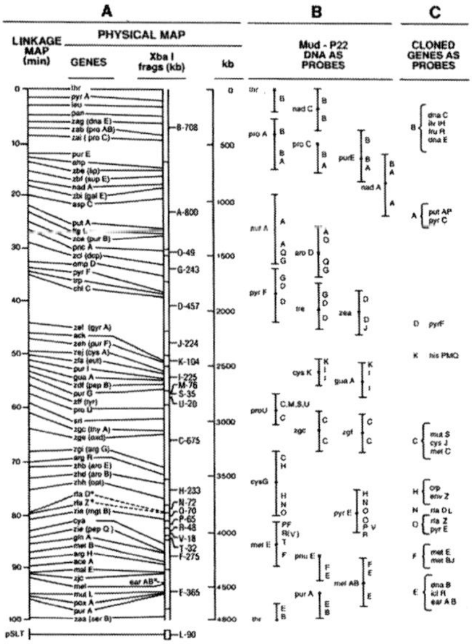

Figure 6-2. The first edition of the *S. typhimurium* LT2 physical map and its comparison with the seventh edition of the LT2 genetic linkage map.

This map took me 15 months to construct. I anticipated that other *Salmonella* maps would be constructed in a similar way, but would require much less time due to my experience with the first map. However, I actually worked on the map of *S. typhi* for two whole years without seeing a sign of completion. For those painful two years, I just earned salaries and wasted so many expensive reagents, including PFGE quality agarose, endonucleases, and various salts. Dr. Sanderson could not hide his anxiety any longer – spending a straight two years without a publication was nearly suicidal and may lead to the failure of grant applications for many years to come or for good. Naturally, I was under enormous pressure too – the *S. typhimurium* genome as a “reference” was mapped and waiting there, but the *S. typhi* genome map as the “goal” just would not come. I therefore tried other rare cutters, hoping to somehow get over the difficulties, although I had no idea on earth what the difficulties might be – for unknown reasons I just could not put the XbaI digest fragments back to close a perfectly ordered circular DNA molecule. Among the many rare cutters I tried, I found the endonuclease I-CeuI very interesting, as it cleaves the *S. typhimurium* LT2 genome into only seven fragments and the fragments are well separated on a PFGE gel (Fig. 6-3).

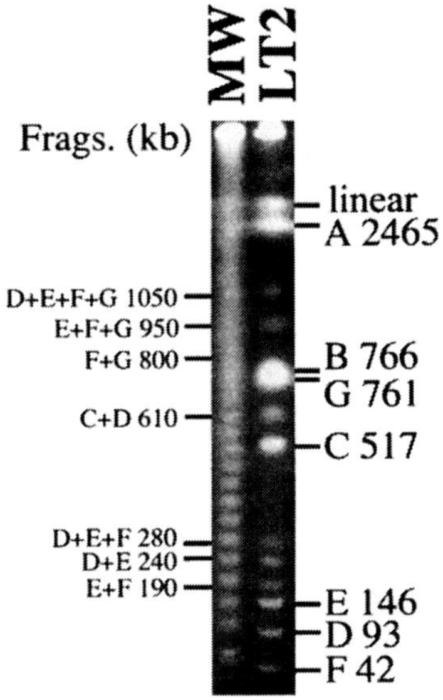

Figure 6-3. I-CeuI cleavage of the *S. typhimurium* LT2 genome. The molecular weight maker (MW) is a concatemer of λ genomic DNA with a monomer size of 48.5 kb. I-CeuI cleaves the *S. typhimurim* LT2 genome into seven fragments with sizes as shown. In addition, there are faint bands, the sizes of which are indicated on the left side of the gel photo. They are the products of partial I-CeuI cleavages, with adjacent segments of the genomic DNA remaining jointed by incomplete I-CeuI cleavages, which are very useful for determining the natural order of the seven fragments on the genome.

Very interestingly, *Salmonella* strains of all eight subgroups show extremely similar I-CeuI cleavage patterns (Fig. 6-4).

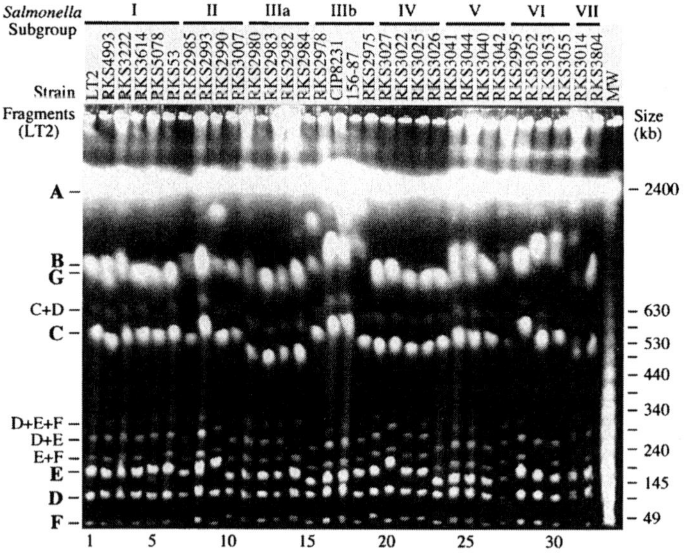

Figure 6-4. I-CeuI cleavage of *Salmonella* strains representing all eight subgroups, showing extremely similar patterns.

I almost lost my mind with extreme excitement and brought the picture to Dr. Sanderson, saying that the I-CeuI enzyme must have recognized evolutionarily highly conserved genomic loci; if so, this enzyme would greatly accelerate the comparative genomic studies among the *Salmonella* species. Specifically, I told him, with I-CeuI revealing the overall similarity amongst the bacteria, we could use the other endonucleases to dig out their specific differences. "I cannot judge whether it might be so useful…" he looked at the picture and continued: "Evolutionarily conserved genomic loci, eh? Recognized by a restriction enzyme? Ha, ha, ha, Shu-Lin!" He tapped my left shoulder with a cheeky grin after the laughter and said: "You have been so tired recently, Shu-Lin", he showed some sympathy on his face behind the grin, "Go home and take a hot bath. Do not analyze any data tonight and just have a very good sleep. Tomorrow, you will feel very refreshed and will not mention a restriction enzyme cutting evolutionarily conserved genomic loci again". I felt a little offended but did not feel so frustrated, as I believed deeply that I would soon convince him.

I-CeuI: a homing enzyme rather than a restriction endonuclease

I-CeuI is special in several ways. First, it is not a restriction endonuclease: it is not for bacterial defense but rather for homing of an intron to the right genomic location. It is encoded by a group I intron in the large subunit rRNA gene of the alga *Chlamydomonas eugametos*; as a homing enzyme, it brings the intron back to the large subunit rRNA gene of the alga (Gauthier, et al. 1991; Marshall and Lemieux 1991). Second, I-CeuI has a peculiar behavior: it creates partial cleavage at a very broad range of concentrations (see Fig 6-3), which allowed me to make an I-CeuI map instantly. Interestingly, and more importantly, the seven I-CeuI cleavage sites were co-located with the rRNA gene loci (Fig. 6-5).

Ribosomal RNA genes are the most highly conserved genomic DNA sequences among not only bacteria but also all cellular life forms; the American scientist Dr. Carl Woese reclassified life on Earth from five Kingdoms to three Domains based on the comparisons of ribosomal RNA molecules (Fox, *et al.* 1980; Woese 1987; Woese, *et al.* 1990).

In fact, the I-CeuI cleavage site is right in the *rrl* gene (Fig. 6-6).

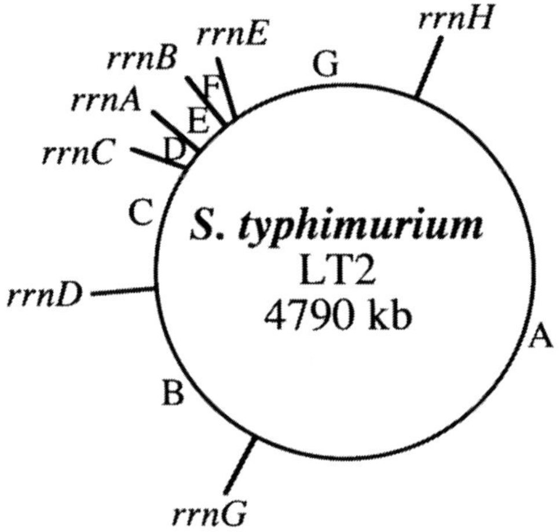

Figure 6-5. The I-CeuI map of *S. typhimurium* LT2, with the seven cleavage sites being co-localized with the seven *rrn* operons.

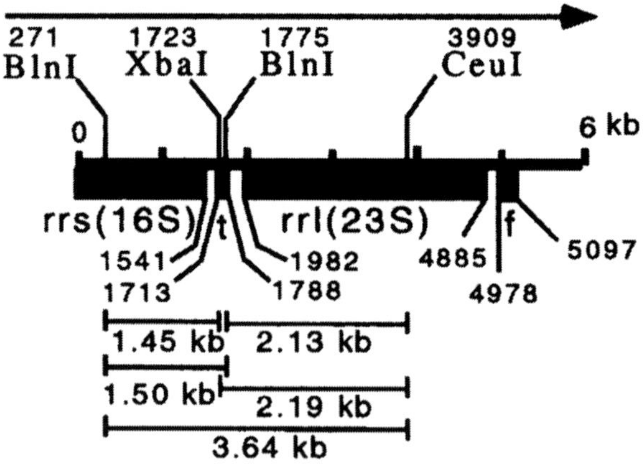

Figure 6-6. The structure of a representative *rrn* operon, containing genes *rrs, rrl* and *rrf*, encoding 16S, 23S and 5S ribosomal RNA, respectively.

The revelation of genomic locations of *rrn* operons is of great interest and of enormous importance for the comparative genomics of bacteria. We therefore updated the physical map of *S. typhimurium* LT2 for a higher resolution and more detailed genomic information, including the locations of the *rrn* operons and also a larger number of genes. In the updated version of the LT2 map, we also used another rare cutter, BlnI, which has cleavage sites both in the *rrn* genes and in Tn*10*, so that data from XbaI and those from BlnI can make mutual corrections and refinements, significantly improving the resolution and accuracy of the updated LT2 map (Fig. 6-7).

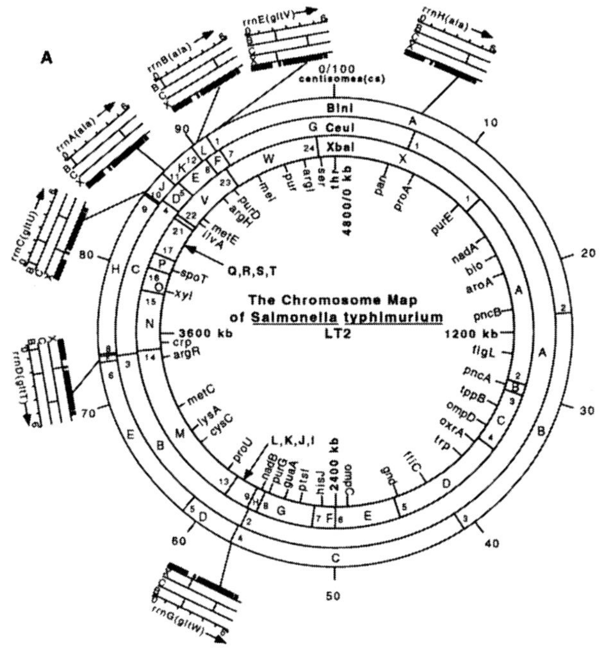

Figure 6-7. The 1993 version of the *S. typhimurium* LT2 physical map. Starting from the gene *thr* clockwise, the *rrn* operons are *rrnH, rrnG, rrnD, rrnC, rrnA, rrnB* and *rrnE.*

We had known about BlnI for a couple of years, but it was so expensive that we could not afford to use it for mapping until Dr. Sanderson obtained another grant from NSERC.

CHAPTER 7

THE EVOLVING BACTERIAL GENOMES: HIGHLY STABLE PHYSICAL STRUCTURE AND SALTATORY DIVERGENCE

Before the physical mapping era, it was not easy to determine, or even imagine, the geometrical parameters of the bacterial genomes. At international conferences, speakers often reported their "discoveries" about bacterial genomes, such as "very different genome sizes" among bacterial strains of the same species, such as those among *S. typhi* or *Helicobacter pylori*, *etc*. Genomic similarity, or differences, among bacteria of different species, genera or families was of course even farther beyond the ability of determination before the physical mapping time. Therefore, in fact, PFGE and I-CeuI, along with other endonucleases, opened the era of the comparative genomics of bacteria for studies in the fields of bacterial evolution, speciation, pathogenesis, epidemiology, ecology, and many other applied areas.

Co-linearity of the *Enterobacteriaceae* bacterial genomes: a common framework for 200 million years

Such high levels of evolutionary conservation of *rrn* genomic locations among all eight *Salmonella* subgroups prompted me to look into the situation at the higher ranks of taxa, such as different genera of the family *Enterobacteriaceae*. Surprisingly, *E. coli* had a highly co-lineal physical structure with *Salmonella* (Liu, *et al*. 1993a). *E. coli* emerged about 200 million years ago, together with mammals, as lactose fermenters; *Salmonella* had a common ancestor with *E. coli* (Doolittle, *et al*. 1996;

Doolittle 1999; Feng, *et al*. 1997; Ochman and Bergthorsson 1995; Ochman and Wilson 1987). Even the *Klebsiella* species, phylogenetically more distant to *E. coli* or *Salmonella* than *E. coli* to *Salmonella*, also had highly conserved physical structures similar to those of *E. coli* and *Salmonella* (Liu, *et al*. 2002b), as exemplified by *K. pneumoniae* and *K. oxtoca* (Fig. 7-1).

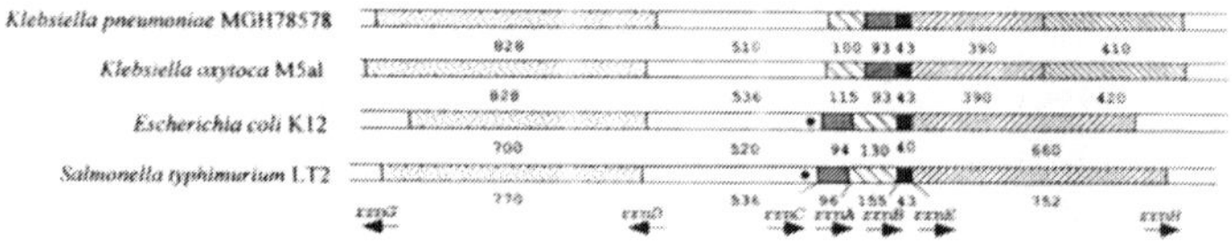

Figure 7-1. Highly conserved physical structure of bacteria among different genera in the family *Enterobacteriaceae.*

Structure of other *Salmonella* genomes: species-specific constructions

The unprecedented findings about bacterial genomes, such as the highly conserved physical genomic framework for hundreds of millions of years among bacteria of different genera, were very encouraging. Having proven to be a successful strategy in revealing the genomic features arising during the evolution of the bacteria, physical mapping was anticipated to bring insights into the genomic divergent events that might have transformed closely related bacteria into different pathogens: infecting different hosts or causing different diseases in the same host. Taking advantage of the much improved mapping techniques and the additional rare cutters, in addition to my experience accumulated over the previous years in PFGE data analysis and physical map construction, I thought this time I should be able to make the map of *S. typhi*, on which I had spent more than two years, but ended up once again with a total failure.

The *S. typhi* map could still not be made. The core problem remained the repeatedly unsuccessful tries in joining the "fragment contigs" into a single chromosomal DNA circle. Readers may be able to imagine my frustration, which, as I can recall, had reached my limit of tolerance.

I struggled on for another while in vain and so had no choice but to put aside the map of *S. typhi* once again.

I had to force myself to forget about *S. typhi* for another moment and decided to embark on other *Salmonella* lineages, such as *S. enteritidis*, *S. paratyphi* A, B and C, *S. gallinarum*, *S. pullorum*, *etc*. I found that all three rare cutters cleaved *Salmonella* genomes into relatively small numbers of fragments – both XbaI and BlnI producing around 30 fragments and I-CeuI producing seven in all these bacteria, making the analysis and ordering of the fragments quite straightforward.

The kind of physical map we made should be called a "physical genetic map", not a simple physical map, as we also determined the locations of many genes on the *Salmonella* genome. We could do this simply on *S. typhimurium* because we had a very large pool of Tn*10* insertion mutants with the transposon inserted in known genes – when we located the Tn*10* insertion, we had, in the meantime, located that gene. But for the other *Salmonella* species, we did not have such Tn*10* insertion mutants.

This issue, however, was something that could not be easier – it just needed some blocks of time to move the Tn*10* insertions from *S. typhimurium* to the other *Salmonella* genome to be mapped by phage P22-mediated generalized transduction. I thus selected a set of insertion mutants from the *S. typhimurium* Tn*10* pool, grew them in an LB broth with tetracycline pressure (Tn*10* contains the tetracycline resistance gene), infected them with phage P22, and made lysates from them. Next, I spread an overnight culture of the *Salmonella* strain to be mapped onto an LB plate containing tetracycline along with a lysate of a particular *S. typhimurium* Tn*10* mutant.

Colonies appearing on the plate contain the Tn*10* insertion in the gene of interest.

I began with *S. enteritidis*, using the three endonucleases XbaI, BlnI and I-CeuI, and the set of selected Tn*10* insertion mutants.

After cleavages by I-CeuI, XbaI and BlnI, the DNA fragments were separated by PFGE, and I began the mapping with the I-CeuI cleavage products. As in *S. typhimurium* LT2, where I-CeuI cleaved the genome into seven fragments, which were ordered on the genome as A, 2465 kb; B, 766 kb; C, 517 kb; D, 93 kb; E, 146 kb; F, 42 kb; and G, 761 kb (see Fig. 6-3), I ordered the seven I-CeuI fragments of *S. enteritidis* (Fig. 7-2), similarly, according to the sizes of the fragments, assuming that I-CeuI fragments of

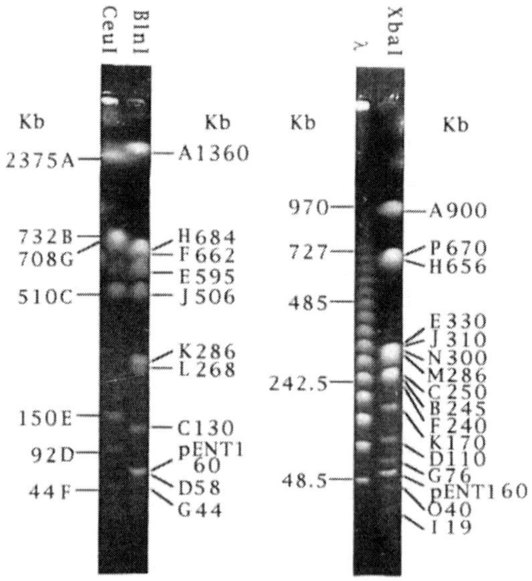

Figure 7-2. Cleavage patterns of the *S. enteritidis* genome by I-CeuI, BlnI and XbaI.

similar sizes were homologous among different *Salmonella* bacteria (see Fig. 6-4). I was right, because the mapping of fragments of all three endonucleases was completed very quickly and smoothly, without having to take as long as 15 months, as in *S. typhimurium* LT2. In fact, the *S. enteritidis* mapping took me only three months, thanks to I-CeuI. In contrast to *S. typhimurium* LT2, where everything, including suitable endonucleases, techniques, a protocol, and analysis methods, was new to me, except for a pre-existing linkage map as a reference, *S. enteritidis* had all of the above available for me to embark on the mapping, especially the experience in data analysis. For example, as soon as the I-CeuI data became available, I constructed the *S. enteritidis* I-CeuI map, literally, within one minute of the analysis, by analogy to the I-CeuI map of *S. typhimurium* LT2 (see Fig. 6-5).

Next, I just needed to arrange the XbaI and BlnI fragments onto the already existing I-CeuI map. I took two steps for this: 1, assigning the XbaI and BlnI fragments roughly to the genomic regions using the Tn*10* data by reference to the *S. typhimurium* LT2 map; and 2, mutual double cleavages to make adjustments for the spatial relationships of cleavage sites between pairs of endonucleases, e.g., between I-CeuI and XbaI, between I-CeuI and BlnI, between XbaI and BlnI, etc. For example, I-CeuI fragment A excised from the gel and re-cleaved by XbaI would produce XbaI fragments A through E and truncated XbaI fragments at the two ends of I-CeuI A; similarly, BlnI fragment K excised from the gel and re-cleaved by I-CeuI would produce I-CeuI fragments D, E and F. In such mutual dual cleavage processes, XbaI or BlnI fragments that did not have Tn*10* insertions can be roughly located on a genomic region and later their locations can be refined by additional data. The second cleavage on the excised DNA fragment usually produces very faint bandings on the ethidium stained agarose gel, so I would end-label the fragments with radioisotope P^{32} and expose the gel on an X-ray film after drying the gel. I did all of the wet manipulations, including labeling the DNA cleavage fragments with radioisotopes, developing and fixing the X-ray films, *etc.*, manually, all by myself for many years, until I had graduate or undergraduate students, postdoctoral fellows and research assistants. That was an unforgettable and "tearing" period of time, which I often recall and greatly treasure, although the word "tearing" is not literal. In our traditional culture, there is a saying "men do not easily shed tears", so as a man I do treasure such good, old, and touching memories, but I do not cry. Having obtained all the necessary ethidium bromide or X-ray images, I would conduct the recording, calculating, drawing, erasing, re-drawing and mapping processes by pencil on the long and continual piece of printer paper, and finalize the map on a computer (Fig. 7-3).

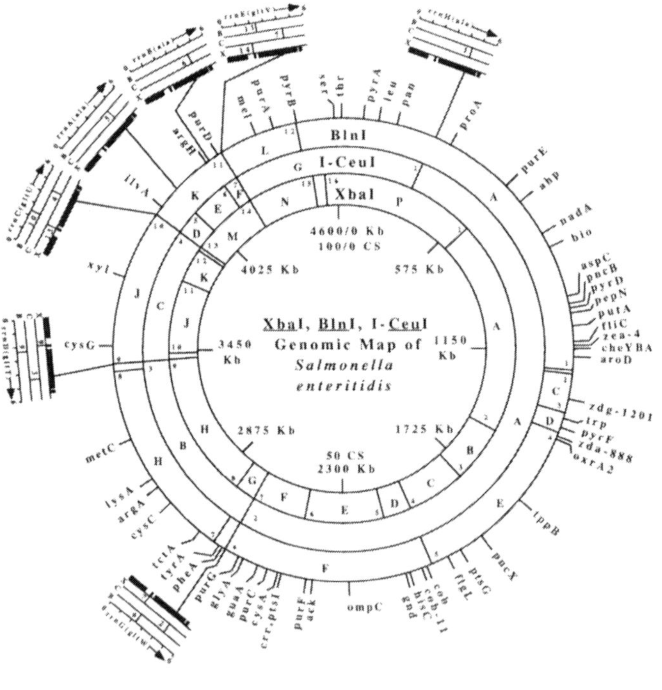

Figure 7-3. Genome map of *S. enteritidis*. This map closely resembles the map of LT2, except an inversion of 815 kb around *terC* (Liu, *et al.* 1993b).

The next genome mapped was on *S. paratyphi* B (Liu, *et al.* 1994), which contains a large insertion (Fig. 7-4). This map took me one month to construct.

At this point, thinking that I had become so experienced in mapping a *Salmonella* genome, spending from as much as 15 months on *S. typhimurium* to merely one month on *S. paratyphi* B, I felt I would be able to map any *Salmonella* genome, including, maybe, *S. typhi*. So, I tried mapping *S. typhi* for the third time.

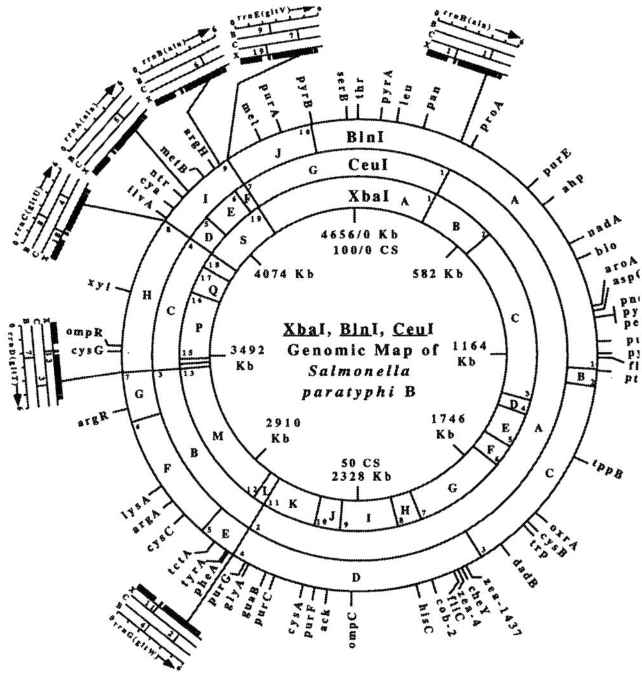

Figure 7-4. Genome map of *S. paratyphi* B.

The peculiar physical structure of the *S. typhi* genome: multiple rearrangements

I brought together all the previous *S. typhi* genome data, obtained in the first and second tries for the mapping, pondering how to re-proceed. Like in mapping *S. enteritidis* and *S. paratyphi* B, I first joined the seven I-CeuI fragments to make an I-CeuI map. This process took me no more than one minute in *S. enteritidis* or *S. paratyphi* B, because I knew how to make an I-CeuI map based on my previous experience with *S. typhimurium*. Similarly, I made the *S. typhi* version of the I-CeuI map within a minute, not knowing that, although thousands of *Salmonella* species have the "*S. typhimurium* type" I-CeuI map, *S. typhi* is an exception. Then, I tried to align the XbaI and BlnI fragments onto the false I-CeuI map (I did not know the I-CeuI map was false). As the reader may have guessed, the previous problem appeared again: locally, the groups of XbaI and BlnI fragments were mutually well-aligned, but they could not be joined into a single DNA circle. My very initial, and curiosity-driven, question was becoming a new one, or an updated version: why is *S. typhi* so different from all other *Salmonella* species, not only in pathogenesis, but also in mapping? It was the third try; my first try was in 1991, ending up with failure; my second try was in 1993, ending up with another failure; the third try, at this point, was in 1995, ending up with what?

Holding the pencil and facing the long printer paper on a very large black table, I was staring at the experimental results, including pen records, ethidium bromide stained PFGE gel pictures, and X-ray films, fully loaded with anxiety, without a single pencil stroke on the long piece of paper for a straight two days again. I needed some coffee and I poured a cup from Donna's coffee maker. Donna prepares a full pot of coffee, first thing when she comes in to work, and everyone in the lab could have a cup or two without having to ask her. I was going to have another sip but found that the cup was empty. I felt dizzy and realized that I had had too much coffee that afternoon. I needed a change. So I changed to tea. I suddenly realized that I had been tackling the *S. typhi* mapping issue by exactly the same way of thinking for all three tries. I needed a change here, too. So I forced all the earlier findings about the *Salmonella* genomes from out of my mind, such as the highly similar genome structures among all known *Salmonella*, the high co-linearity of gene order among bacteria of different genera in the *Enterobacteriaceae* family, *etc*. However, the "one-minute mapping" of I-CeuI cleavage fragments should be no problem, I thought, as this endonuclease cuts within the *rrn* operons and the genomic locations of the *rrn* operons had been evolutionarily so sturdily conserved for hundreds of millions of years. "Do not waste time doubting things that have been facts since the dinosaur era", I was telling myself, with the teacup in my left hand and a pencil in my right hand. I was looking at a PFGE gel run for genomic DNA cleaved by I-CeuI for seven independent wild-type strains of *S. typhi*: all the bandings were so neatly separated and clearly shown. All of a sudden, however, I eyed something extremely extraordinary or simply impossible: two faint bandings of "absolutely impossible" sizes, 648 kb and 180 kb (Fig. 7-5)!

How could they be there? How could these bandings be true?

The reason for my surprise was that, on the I-CeuI maps of *S. typhimurium* and many other *Salmonella* lineages, the seven I-CeuI fragments are arranged on the genome in the order of A, B, C, D, E, F and G, which is why I could make the I-CeuI map of a new *Salmonella* lineage within one minute (I had always thought so, until I knew and understood *S. typhi*), but the seven I-CeuI fragments of *S. typhi* seemed to not be following this order!

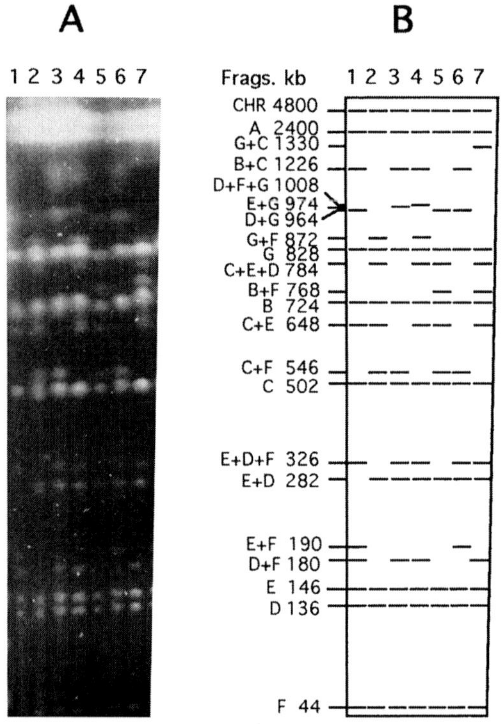

Figure 7-5. I-CeuI cleavage of genomic DNA from seven wild-type *S. typhi* strains. A, PFGE gel; B, illustration and annotation of the bandings on the gel.

I could hardly believe my eyes and almost spilled the tea onto the piece of long printer paper with this startling visual fact. In the first two tries, I sketched all the available data by pencil: the data were correct but fragmentary – they just could not be joined into a single DNA molecule. The "strange" bandings I saw at that moment were absolutely real, true, clear, and white on black, with 648 kb unambiguously indicating the sum of Fragments C+E and 180 kb indicating the sum of Fragments D+F. Such neighboring relationships between C and E and those between D and F were totally different from those of *S. typhimurium* and many other *Salmonella* lineages. Within a minute, I had constructed the real and correct I-CeuI map for *S. typhi* strain Ty2 (Fig. 7-6), one minute on a background of four years, and this *S. typhi* I-CeuI map was to tell an interesting story about the evolution of *S. typhi*.

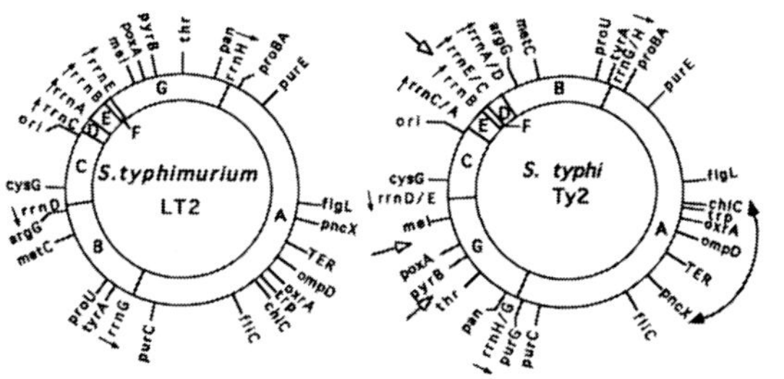

Figure 7-6. The I-CeuI map of *S. typhi* strain Ty2 in comparison with *S. typhimurium* LT2. Compared to the A–G order of the I-CeuI fragments in *S. typhimurium* LT2 (left), the homologous I-CeuI fragments are in the order of A, G, C, E, F, D and B in *S. typhi* Ty2 (right). In addition, there is an inversion around the TER region (double arrowheads, on the right part of the genome, with the two ends of the inversion being close to genes *chlC* and *pncX*, respectively). The hollow arrows on the left side of the Ty2 map indicate the locations of three insertions in the genome of *S. typhi* Ty2.

Using the "genuine" I-CeuI map of *S. typhi* Ty2 as the genomic framework, I aligned all the previously fragmentary data blocks and successfully joined them into a single DNA molecule, finally completing the physical map of *S. typhi* (Fig. 7-7).

In this mapping project, I used another rare cutter, SpeI, to further improve the resolution and accuracy of the map. The Tn*10* sequence does not have a cleavage site for SpeI, so its insertion into a genomic locus will not break the SpeI fragment into two but instead will increase the size of that SpeI fragment, i.e., 9 kb in the wild-type Tn*10* or 4 kb in the mini-Tn*10* transposon (Liu and Sanderson 1995b).

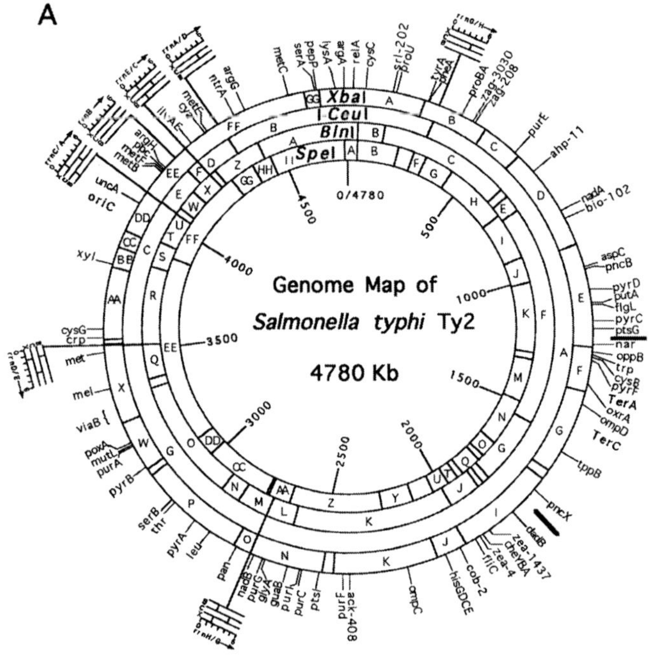

Figure 7-7. A physical map of *S. typhi.*

CHAPTER 8

REARRANGEMENTS OF THE *SALMONELLA* GENOME: HOMOLOGOUS RECOMBINATION AND THE *ORIC* - *TERC* BALANCE

If the queerly altered genome structure of *S. typhi* was associated with the distinct pathogenesis, deciphering the molecular events and mechanisms driving the genomic changes would be a key step toward the elucidation of *S. typhi* speciation to become a particular pathogen. Based on the common knowledge that bacterial genomic DNA replication starts from *oriC*, goes along in both clockwise and counter clockwise directions, and ends at *terC*, it is reasonable to deduce a scenario in which the two halves of newly replicated genomic DNA have to arrive at *terC* simultaneously; that is, the two halves of newly replicated genomic DNA will have to be of the same length. If one half were longer than the other, it would take longer to finish a cycle of DNA replication, slowing down the growth rate of the bacteria and placing the bacteria in a disadvantageous situation in competition for nutrients with bacteria that have a balanced genome. Therefore, I predicted the existence of a fairly large genomic insertion, making one half of the replication fork longer; to counteract the stress of this genomic imbalance caused by the imaginary large insertion, the genome may have to undergo secondary rearrangements of DNA segments to become rebalanced. As such, I conducted genomic comparisons between *S. typhi* and other mapped *Salmonella* lineages and, as predicted, found a very large genomic insertion in *S. typhi* Ty2; this insertion was identified as being a Salmonella Pathogenicity Island (SPI7, 134 kb) in the sequencing project of *S. typhi*

CT18 six years later.

We thus proposed a hypothesis to interpret the co-existence of the large genomic insertion and structural rearrangements in *S. typhi*: genomic rearranging for re-balancing.

The unusual physical map of *S. typhi*: what caused the disrupted *rrnHGDCABE* genomic framework?

The insertion of the 134 kb SPI7 to the genome would disrupt the original 180°-180° genomic balance and lead to a 190°-170° imbalance, which may trigger a series of homologous recombination events to rearrange the physical structure of the genome (Fig. 8-1).

In addition to the rearrangements illustrated in Fig. 8-1, which are all homologous recombination events, there is another inversion within I-CeuI A, which is a rearrangement not involving *rrn* but mediated by other homologous sites, such as pairs of prophages and IS*200* (Liu and Sanderson 1995b; Parkhill, *et al.* 2001).

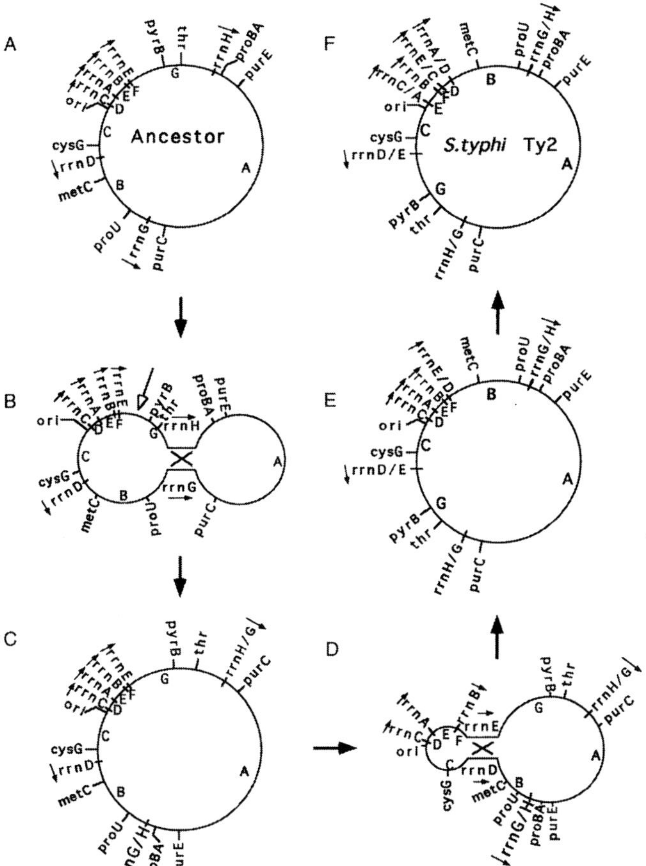

Figure 8-1. Hypothesized DNA recombination events leading to the rearrangements and *oriC-terC* re-balancing of the *S. typhi* genome. A, an imaginary ancestor of *S. typhi*, with the seven I-CeuI fragments ordered as in *S. typhimurium* or many other *Salmonella* lineages, *i.e.*, ABCDEFG; B, insertion of a large DNA segment (here, the 134 kb SPI7, illustrated as a hollow arrow), causing genomic imbalance and triggering homologous recombination events, such as that between *rrnH* and *rrnG*; C, the original *rrnH* and *rrnG* becoming hybrids, i.e., *rrnH/G* and *rrnG/H*, inverting I-CeuI fragment A (about half of the genome); D, by

recombination between *rrnE* and *rrnD*; E, the original *rrnE* and *rrnD* becoming hybrids, i.e., *rrnE/D* and *rrnD/E*, making another inversion across *ori*; F, translocation of I-CeuI fragment D, making a hybrid *rrnE/C* and creating a new hybrid *rrnA/D*. This series of homologous recombination events would bring the imbalanced genome from 190°-170° back to the current better balanced genome structure of *S. typhi*, close to 180°-180°.

The plastic genome of *S. typhi*: rearranging for re-balancing

When I looked at additional wild-type strains of *S. typhi*, I was amazed to find that the genome structure *S. typhi* Ty2 (see Fig. 7-8) was not common to all *S. typhi* strains; in fact, there are many different genome structures among the mapped *S. typhi* isolates (Liu and Sanderson 1996), a phenomenon never reported previously. Based on this rather weird finding, I postulated that the dynamic rearrangements of large DNA segments might not bring the genome back to a precise re-balance; if so, recombination at different homologous sites may lead to rather diverse genome structures, all being better, if not perfectly balanced, than the after-insertion but pre-rearrangement state of the genome. This postulation was supported by analysis of the balance status of mapped genomes among a large number of independent *S. typhi* isolates (Fig. 8-2).

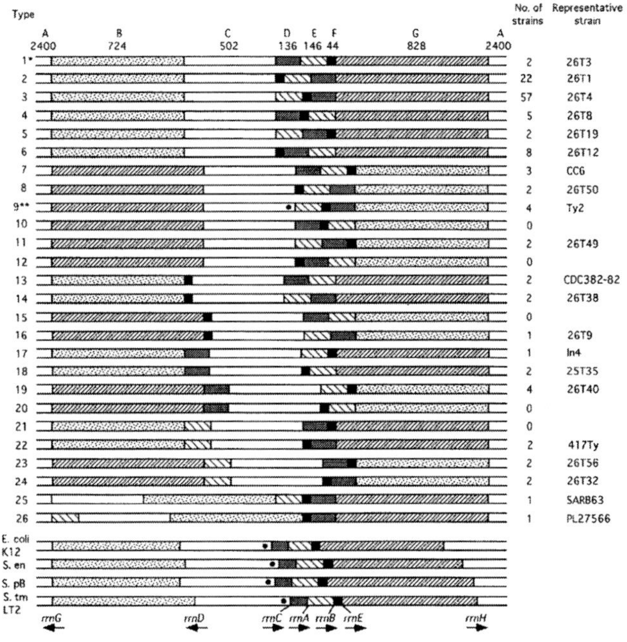

Figure 8-2. Genomic balance status of wild-type strains of *S. typhi*. "Type" on the left side of the figure means a particular genome structure. A-G at the top of the figure indicate I-CeuI cleavage fragments, with only half of A (half genome) and full sizes of B-G shown for conciseness. "No. of strains" means the number of strains having a particular genome structure in the total 127 strains analyzed; 0 strain means that particular genome structure was theoretical but absent in this analysis. The genome structure of a number of other bacterial strains were given at the bottom for comparison, which all have the seven I-CeuI fragments arranged similarly to that of *S. typhimurium* LT2.

I confirmed, based on this analysis, that genomes with better balanced status are associated with larger numbers of representative strains (Table 8-1).

Table 8-1. Associations of genome balance status with the number of representing strains.

Genomic Balance Status of *Salmonella typhi* Genome Types

GT[a]	Representative Strain	*ori* kb	*ter* kb	Balance Status CW/CCW[b]	Degree off Balance	Number of Strains in the Same Sub GT
1a	26T3	3,920	1,545	178/182	2	4
2a	26T5	3,920	1,545	182/178	2	17
2b	26T27	3,920	1,435	174/186	6	3
3a	26T7	3,920	1,545	182/178	2	40
3b	26T4	3,920	1,435	174/186	6	19
4a	26T17	3,920	1,545	182/178	2	2
4b	26T8	3,920	1,435	174/186	2	3
5a	26T19	3,920	1,545	182/178	2	3
6a	26T16	4,000	1,545	179/181	1	6
6b	26T12	3,920	1,435	174/186	6	3
7a	CC6	3,745	1,545	195/165	15	3
8a	26T50	3,825	1,545	192/168	12	2
9a	Ty2	3,750	1,544	194/166	14	4
9b	CT18	3,765	1,435	186/174	6	1
11a	26T49	3,745	1,545	195/165	15	2
13b	CDC382-82	3,970	1,435	170/190	10	2
14b	26T38	3,970	1,435	170/190	10	1
16d	26T9	4,210	1,435	152/208	28	1
17b	In4	4,135	1,435	161/199	19	1
18a	25T35	3,565	1,545	211/149	31	1
18c	ST1	4,075	1,545	165/195	15	1
21b	TYT1668	4,090	1,435	161/199	19	1
22a	417Ty	3,580	1,545	203/157	23	1
22c	3434-73	4,090	1,545	169/191	11	1
23d	9032-85	4,125	1,435	158/202	22	1
24c	26T32	4,125	1,545	166/194	14	1
25a	SARB63	3,215	1,545	235/125	55	1
26a	PL27566	3,375	1,545	223/137	43	1
27a	701Ty	3,225	1,545	234/126	54	1

[a] The main GTs are as previously published (Liu and Sanderson 1996; Kothapalli et al. 2005). Subtypes: a, I-CeuI A being oriented as in Ty2; b, I-CeuI A being oriented as in CT18; c, I-CeuI C being oriented as in Ty2 and CT18 (this fragment takes the same orientation in both Ty2 and CT18); and d, I-CeuI C taking the opposite orientation; see the text for more details.

[b] CW, clockwise on the genome map; CCW, counterclockwise on the genome map.

To further validate such associations, by observing and finding hypothesized instantly rearranging bacterial genomes, I started a culture of *S. typhi* CT18 with a single colony, streaked the culture onto LB plates, randomly picked up 100 colonies and mapped the genomes. Three of the 100 colonies were significantly smaller than average and I predicted that bacteria forming small colonies might have very unbalanced genomes, based on the reasoning that such bacteria would grow more slowly. I mapped the three CT18 derivatives, designated CT18-1, CT18-2, and CT18-3, and found that all three had inversions but at different loci, making the genome more unbalanced even than the wild-type CT18 (Fig. 8-3). Among these three, CT18-3 made very small colonies and its genome was extremely unbalanced (263°/97°).

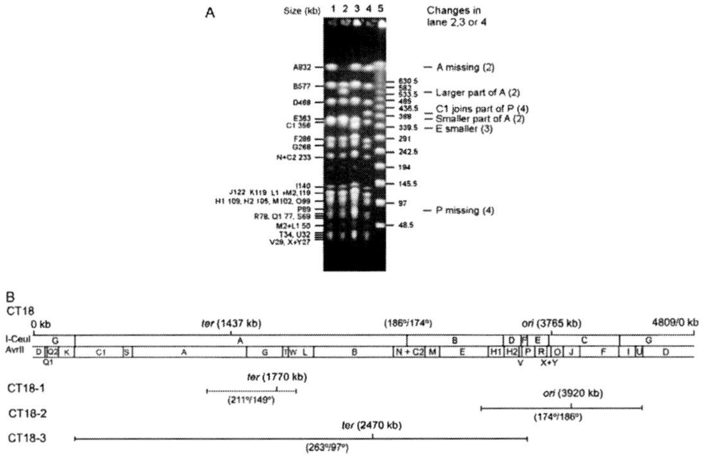

Figure 8-3. Dynamically rearranging genome structure of *S. typhi* CT18. (A) PFGE patterns of AvrII cleaved genomic DNA of CT18 and its derivatives. Lanes: 1, wild-type CT18; 2, CT18-1; 3, CT18-2; 4, CT18-3; 5, λ DNA concatemer as size marker. Changes are indicated on the right side of the PFGE picture. (B) Mapping of the genomic inversions in the three CT18 derivatives. Lines below the maps indicate the range of the inversions. The moved positions of *ori* and *ter* are indicated above the lines and the resulting balance status indicated beneath the lines (degrees clockwise/counterclockwise).

The fact that none of the three rearranged CT18 derivatives had a better balanced genome may explain why they did not become dominant. This fact also nicely supported my previous prediction that, rather than "genomic imbalance triggering genomic rearrangements to regain a physical balance", homologous recombination may happen spontaneously between any pair of genomic loci sharing high sequence similarity, but only the strains with better balanced genomes would have more chance of being selected.

Based on such findings, and starting from this tentative explanation, I further anticipated that a derivative would increase in proportion in the population if it became better balanced. Therefore, minority populations with less balanced genome structures should at least occasionally be detected in *S. typhi* strains at different frequencies, depending on how well the genome in a particular strain is balanced. For example, we did not find any further rearrangement in *S. typhi* strains with genomes that are only 1-2° off balance; on the other hand, rearrangements have been detected at high frequencies in strains with very unbalanced genomes, such as in SARB63, in which the genome is as much as 55° off balance. According to my postulation, subpopulations with better balanced genome structures than the parental SARB63 should be readily detectable.

I thus set out with strain SARB63 to see how easy or how difficult it may be to isolate better balanced derivatives from this legendarily unbalanced strain. The experiments were carefully designed, because some parts of the experiments were expensive. But I did not worry too much, as in that same year I received three national research grants – very unusual – as receiving just one single national research grant in any year for a lab would be a rare event and enough to trigger great euphoria in the whole lab. And I had received three in the same year: from the Natural Sciences and Engineering Research Council of Canada (NSERC), the Medical Research Council of Canada (MRC) and the Canadian Institutes of Health Research (CIHR; *i.e.*, the previous MRC). I had four graduate students, two postdocs, one research assistant, one quarter administrative assistant (one shared by four Principal Investigators) and a couple of undergraduate summer students in the lab. We celebrated by having lunch together on the lawn of the campus on a beautiful sunny day and came back down to earth in the afternoon to begin the project. I could not afford to waste any time and, after all, three national grants together do not come to a billion dollars. So, I had to be extremely careful about every penny.

To accelerate the experiments, we applied a stressed condition, i.e., Caco2 epithelial cell invasion, on *S. typhi* SARB63, hypothesizing that bacteria with a better balanced genome might be more competitive in invading the epithelial cells and thus would have a higher chance to be selected for after the infection experiments. Remarkably, cells of SARB63 that passed the Caco2 monolayer exhibited a great diversity in colony size on LB plates (Fig. 8-4A). SARB63 cells from colonies of different sizes had different genome structures, with those of larger colonies having better balanced genomes (Fig. 8-4B).

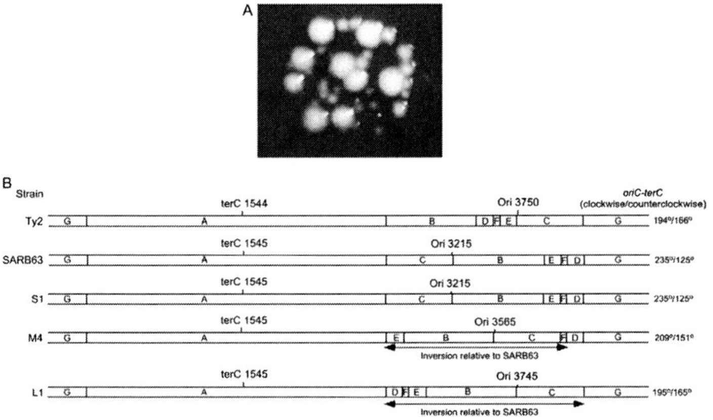

Figure 8-4. Association of colony size with genome structure of *S. typhi* SARB63. A, colonies formed by *S. typhi* cells that passed through the Caco2 monolayer, showing obvious size diversities; B, genome maps from bacteria of representative SARB63 colonies. Note the clear tendency that bacterial cells in large (L1) and medium (M4) sized colonies have better balanced genomes than those in small (S1) colonies and the parental strain.

My explanation is that, among the benefits that balanced genomes could render the bacteria, an optimal time length for DNA replication might be most important, because any level of imbalance would delay replication time in one half of the genome between *ori* and *ter* and growth curve analyses perfectly supported this prediction (Table 8-2).

Table 8-2. Correlation of genomic balance status with generation time.

Strain	Description	Balance Status (CW/CCW)[a]	Degrees off Balance	Generation Time (min)
SARB63	Parental strain of S1, M4, and L1	235/125	55	33.5
S1	Small colony former	235/125	55	33.5
M4	Medium colony former	209/151	29	26.1
L1	Large colony former	195/165	15	25.2
Ty2	Reference strain	194/166	14	24.4

[a] CW, clockwise on the genome map; CCW, counterclockwise on the genome map.

The dynamic genome structure: rearranging toward an optimized balance

Is the dynamic genome structure phenomenon unique to *S. typhi* or a general rule of bacterial genomic evolution? We first looked into this issue by conducting a survey of a broad range of sequenced bacteria and found that there was a general tendency of the genome structure toward a physical balance (Song, *et al.* 2003), not only among bacteria with circular chromosomes but also among those with linear chromosomes, such as the spirochete *Borrelia burgdorferi* (Fig. 8-5).

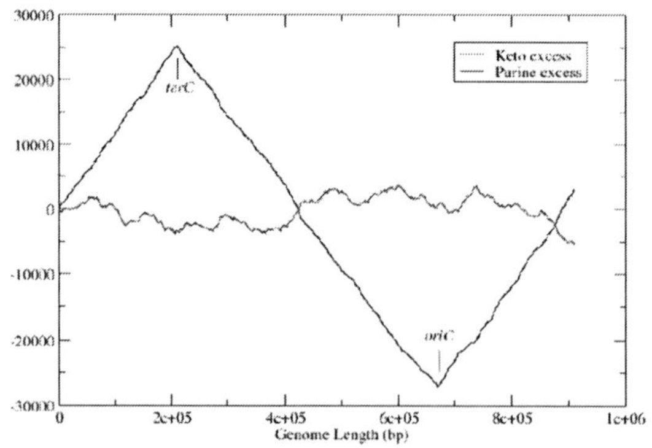

Figure 8-5. Genomic balance status of *Borrelia burgdorferi* inspected by GC Skew data with Wavelet analysis.

In the meantime, we looked at different *Salmonella* lineages and found that host-adapted *Salmonella* species tended to have rearranged or even dynamic genome structures (Fig. 8-6).

In Fig. 8-6, the genome on top is from *S. agona,* with the following order of the I-CeuI fragments A (only one end of A shown here), B, C, D, E, F, G, and A (the other end of A shown here), the same order as in *S. typhimurium*; most other genomes have this order of I-CeuI fragments. However, some host adapted *Salmonella* lineages, e.g., *S. gallinarum* (Ga in Fig. 8-6, adapted to fowl), *S. pullorum* (Pu in Fig. 8-6, adapted to fowl), and *S. paratyphi* C (Pc in Fig. 8-6, adapted to man), in addition to *S. typhi* (Tp in Fig. 8-6, adapted to man), have different orders of the I-CeuI fragments.

There are four *Salmonella* lineages that are adapted to humans, including *S. typhi,* and *S. paratyphi* A, B and C. Typhoid fever, caused by *S. typhi,* and paratyphoid fever, caused by *S. paratyphi* A, B or C, have very similar clinical manifestations, so I was very interested in the genomic features that are common to all of the four typhoid and paratyphoid agents but are absent from the other thousands of *Salmonella* lineages. I first focused on *S. paratyphi* C, which had long been known to have several common features with *S. typhi,* such as the Vi antigen. We obtained three sets of selected *Salmonella* strains representing the most frequently isolated *Salmonella* lineages from Dr. Robert K. Selander, including *Salmonella* Reference A, B and C (Beltran, *et al.* 1991; Boyd, *et al.* 1993), and the *S. paratyphi* C strain we first analyzed was RKS4594 (Liu, *et al.* 2007). I-CeuI cleavage analysis showed a rearranged genome relative to that of *S. typhimurium* LT2 and most other *Salmonella* lineages (Fig. 8-7).

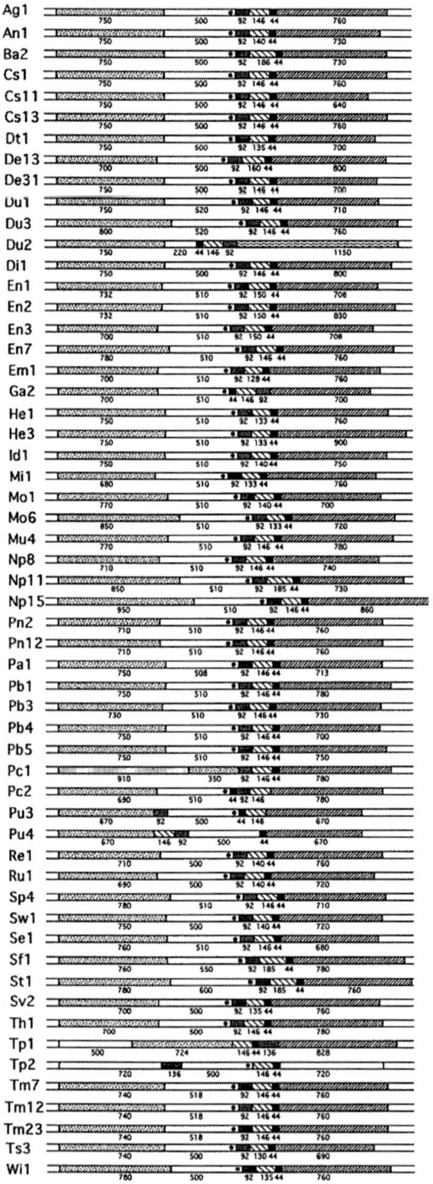

Figure 8-6. I-CeuI maps of a selected set of *Salmonella* lineages. For I-CeuI fragment A, only two ends were shown for conciseness. Ag, *S. agona*; An, *S. anatum*;

Ba, *S. brandenburg*; Cs, *S. choleraesuis*; Dt, *S. decatur*; De, *S. derby*; Du, *S. dublin*; Di, S. *duisburg*; En, S. *enteritidis*; Em, *S. emek*; Ga, *S. gallinarum*; He, *S. heidelberg*; Id, *S. indiana*; Mi, *S. miami*; Mo, *S. montevideo*; Mu, *S. muenchen*; Np, *S. newport*; Pn, *S. panama*; Pa, *S. paratyphi* A; Pb, *S. paratyphi* B; Pc, *S. paratyphi* C; Pu, *S. pullorum*; Re, *S. reading*; Ru, *S. rubislaw*; Sp, *S. saintpaul*; Sw, *S. schwarzengrund*; Se, *S. sendai*; Sf, *S. senftenberg*; St, *S. Stanley*; Sv, *S. Stanleyville*; Th, *S. thompson*; Tp, *S. typhi*; Tm, *S. typhimurium*; Ts, *S. typhisuis*; Wi, *S. wien*.

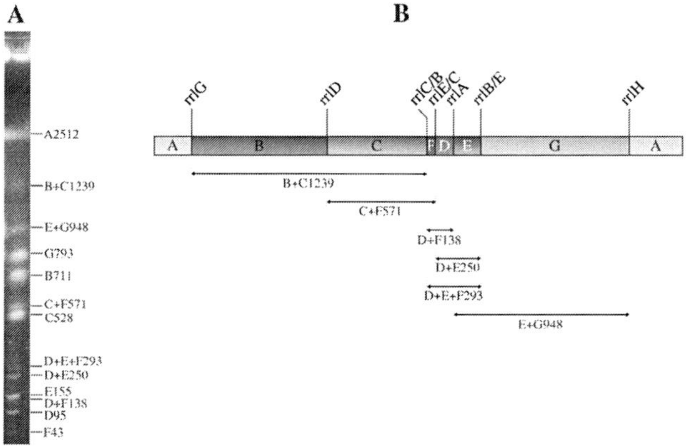

Figure 8-7. I-CeuI mapping of *S. paratyphi* C RKS4594. A, PFGE separation of I-CeuI cleaved genomic DNA, showing both complete and partial cleavage bandings of the genomic DNA; B, I-CeuI cleavage map based on the PFGE pattern in A. Only parts of fragment A (2512 kb) are shown at the ends of the linear map and the remaining six fragments are drawn to scale

When cleavage fragments by XbaI and AvrII (isoenzyme of BlnI, having the same six-base cleavage sequence) were aligned onto the I-CeuI map, we made the genome map (Fig. 8-8). Of great interest is a large insertion, 90 kb, at around 11 o'clock on the map.

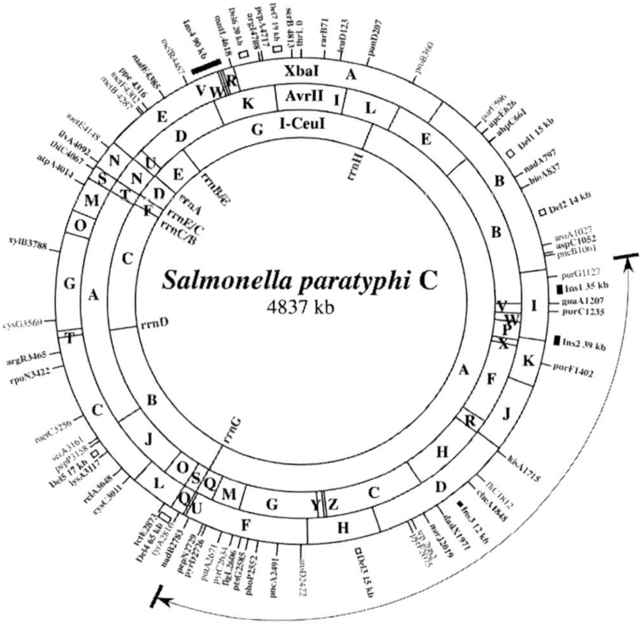

Figure 8-8. Genome map of *S. paratyphi* C RKS4594. Solid rectangles indicate insertions (Ins1–4) and open rectangles indicate deletions (Del1–7), numbered clockwise, relative to *S. typhimurium* LT2. The double-headed arrow, with one end being between *pncB* (at 1061 kb) and *purG* (at 1127 kb) and the other between *pepN* (at 2729 kb) and *nadB* (at 2783 kb), covers the region of inversion with respect to the chromosome of *S. typhimurium* LT2.

We then looked at additional strains of *S. paratyphi* C to discover whether the RKS4594 map could represent *S. paratyphi* C as a whole. I-CeuI cleavage revealed a diversity of genome structures among the wild-type strains of *S. paratyphi* C (Fig. 8-9), reminiscent of the plastic genome structure of *S. typhi*.

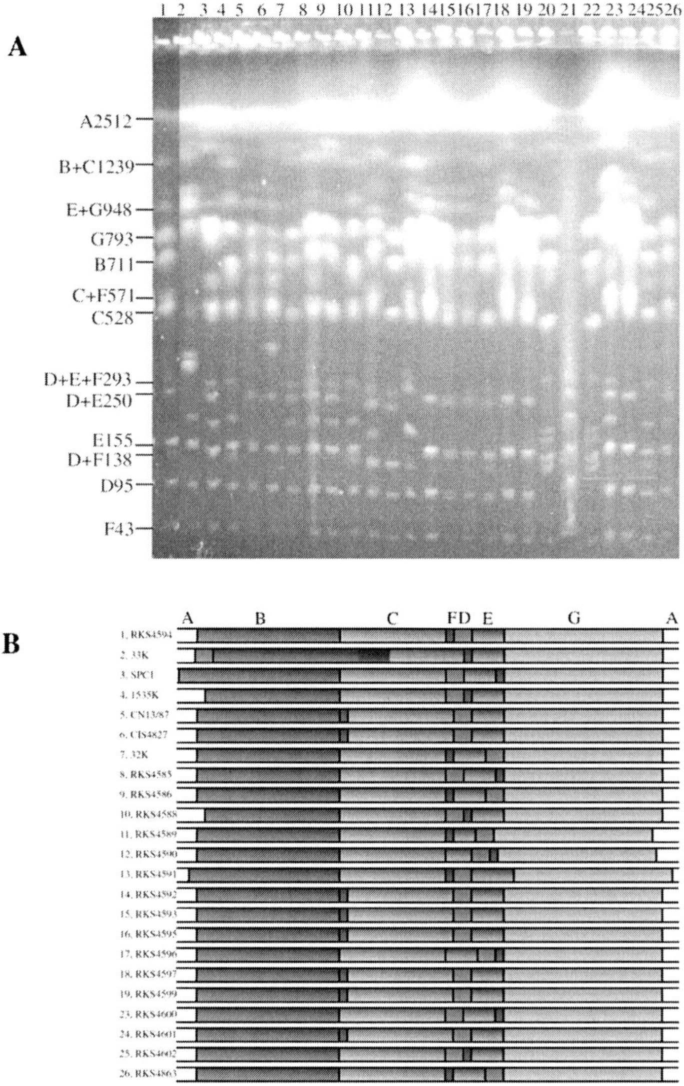

Figure 8-9. Diversity in genome structure among wild-type strains of *S. paratyphi* C. A, PFGE patterns of I-CeuI cleaved genomic DNA from wild-type strains of *S. paratyphi* C. Lanes: 1, RKS4594 (IP2/88); 2, RKS4587 (33K); 3, SPC1;

4, 1535K; 5, CN13/87; 6, CIS4827; 7, 32K; 8, RKS4585; 9, RKS4586; 10, RKS4588; 11, RKS4589; 12, RKS4590; 13, RKS4591; 14, RKS4592; 15, RKS4593; 16, RKS4595; 17, RKS4596; 18, RKS4597; 19, RKS4599; 20, *S. typhi* Ty2 (for comparison); 21, λ DNA concatemer as size marker; 22, *S. typhi* Ty2; 23, RKS4600; 24, RKS4601; 25, RKS4602; 26, SA4863. B, I-CeuI maps of *S. paratyphi* C wild-type strains based on the PFGE data shown in A.

The findings in *S. typhi* and *S. paratyphi* C may suggest similar genomic evolutionary scenarios in *S. paratyphi* A and B also, but they seemed to have quite different stories. As shown in Fig. 8-6 above, *S. paratyphi* A appeared to have a non-rearranged genome structure, with the seven I-CeuI fragments arranged in the order of ABCDEFG, but a higher resolution genome map with cleavage data of XbaI, AvrII and SpeI revealed key information on the possible evolutionary process of the genome: a large insertion and a half genome inversion (Fig. 8-10).

A large insertion of about 100 kb was identified on the genome of *S. paratyphi* A ATCC 9150 between *rrnG/H* and *proB*; very interestingly, a full length inversion of I-CeuI fragment A co-existed with the 100 kb insertion on the genome (Fig. 8-11). Calculations showed that the genome having the large insertion regained a perfect 180°/180° physical balance between *oriC* and *terC* by the inversion. This 180°/180° physical balance was seen in all analyzed wild-type strains of *S. paratyphi* A and all these *S. paratyphi* A strains had the same genome structure as seen in Fig. 8-10 (Liu and Sanderson 1995a).

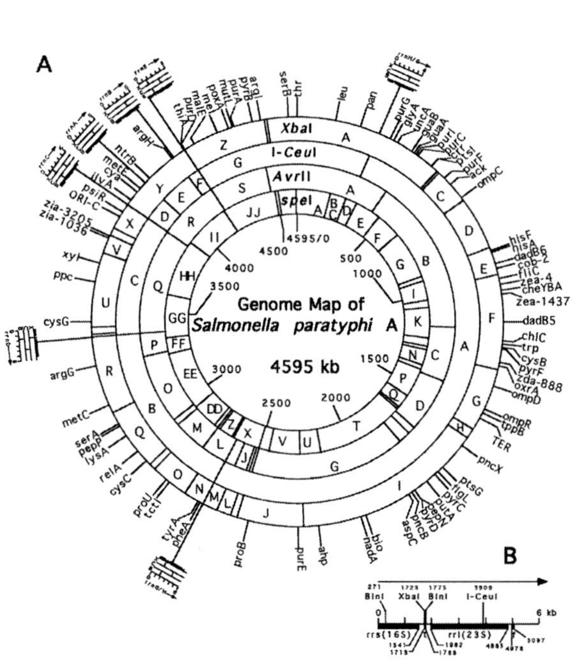

Figure 8-10. High resolution genome map of *S. paratyphi* A strain ATCC 9150. A, Genomic map based on cleavages with XbaI, I-CeuI, BlnI, and SpeI, with genes located by Tn*10* insertion. Note that *rrn* operons at the two ends of I-CeuI A are hybrids of *rrnH/G* and *rrnG/H*. B, Structure of an *rrn* operon, exemplified by *rrnB*.

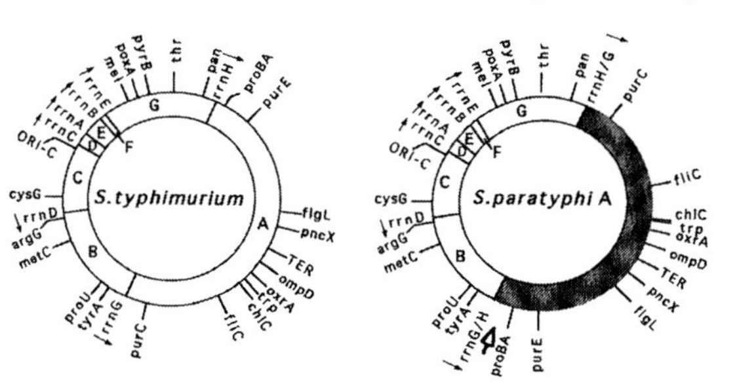

Figure 8-11. Physical structure of *S. paratyphi* A genome in comparison with that of *S. typhimurium*. The open arrowhead indicates the location of an insertion of *ca.* 100 kb. The shaded fragment, I-CeuI-A of *S. paratyphi* A, is inverted compared with that of *S. typhimurium*.

Findings in *S. paratyphi* A have provided additional strong support to the re-arranging for re-balancing hypothesis about bacterial genome evolution. First, large insertions, such as the 134 kb SPI7 in *S. typhi*, the 90 kb mini-SPI7 in *S. paratyphi* C, and the 100 kb insertion in *S. paratyphi* A, all co-existed with rearranged genome structures without exceptions. Second, this hypothesis predicts that if genomic rearrangements could not regain a balance, genome rearranging at different homologous loci may continue, leading to differently structured genome, which we call a plastic genome (Liu, *et al.* 2007); but if a single rearrangement can perfectly rebalance the genome, no further genomic rearrangements would be needed and so the genome may not be plastic. So the scenario of the genomic evolution in *S. paratyphi* A would be: 1, acquisition of a 100 kb insertion; 2, genomic imbalance; 3, genomic inversion, perfectly rebalancing the physical structure. As such, this rearranged but perfectly rebalanced genome structure of *S. paratyphi* A is anticipated to be the only one for all *S. paratyphi* A strains.

But, will it be possible for a bacterial genome to have large insertions but not have to rearrange the genome? Findings in *S. paratyphi* B, another paratyphoid agent, have provided a pointed answer to this question.

The *S. paratyphi* B genome has two large insertions in tandem relative to *S. typhimurium*, but the genome was not rearranged. Analyses revealed that the genomic imbalance caused by the two insertions together, one 68 kb between *pan* and *rrnH* and the other 64 kb between *bio* and *aroA*, could be significantly mitigated by a deletion immediately adjacent to *aroA*, 102 kb between *aroA* and *aspC* (Fig. 8-12). The "net" physical length change, *i.e.*, (68 kb + 64 kb) – 102 kb = 30 kb, is not enough to cause significant genomic imbalance, so will not trigger genomic rearrangements (Kottilil, *et al.* 2003).

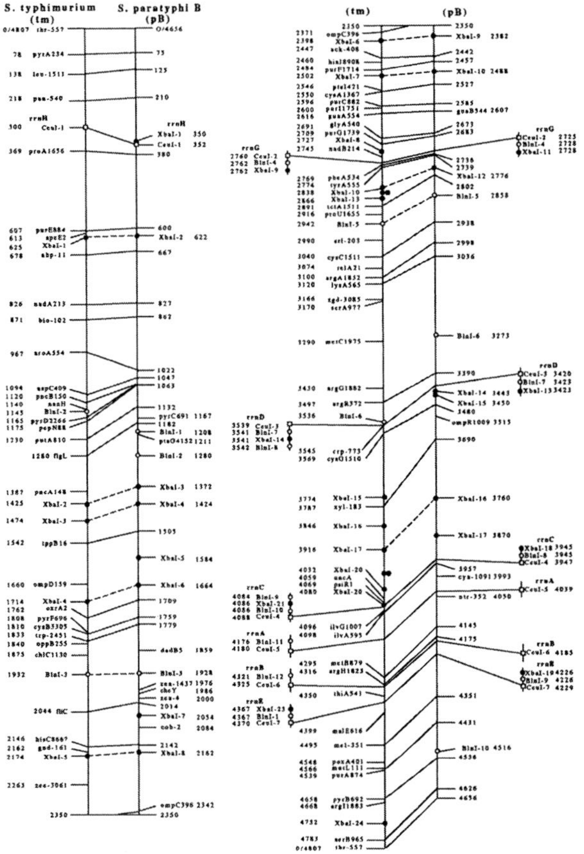

Figure 8-12. Comparison of the genomic cleavage maps of *S. paratyphi* B IP87/87 with *S. typhimurium* LT2.

The genomic rearranging phenomenon was initially documented in *S. typhi* and was interpreted to be a mechanism for rebalancing the physical structure of the genome; this interpretation was later supported by findings in all four paratyphoid agents and also other bacteria (Liu, *et al.* 2002a; Wu, *et al.* 2005). The key point is that, when bacteria acquire a large insertion, such as a pathogenicity island or prophage, the genome will suffer from imbalance and large scale rearrangements, such as inversions, deletions, further insertions, duplications, or translocations from one genomic position to another, may have the physical structure of the genome rebalanced. If the rearrangements lead to a well-balanced genome, such as those in *S. paratyphi* A and B, no further rearrangements would be needed for further rebalancing of the genome; if simple rearrangements of large genomic segments cannot rebalance the genome reasonably well, rearrangement will continue, leading to differently structured genomes, called plastic genomes. All inversions take place between homologous loci, such as *rrn* genes, prophages or ISs and go across *oriC* or *terC*.

I use the term "trigger" to describe the "large insertion leading to genomic inversion" process, just for the sake of simplicity in describing and interpreting the phenomenon. However, in fact, the term "trigger" does not say the truth, because homologous recombination spontaneously takes place during genomic DNA replication. When genomic imbalance occurs, the bacterial cells with the "right" type of rearranged genome regaining the "best" balance among the subpopulations will be selected as the best fit due to their advantage in growth rate for resource competition.

PART III

GENOMIC DIVERGENCE OF THE *SALMONELLA* PATHOGENS: SALTATORY OR GRADUAL?

The over 2700 *Salmonella* lineages are extremely similar in genetics, but radically distinct in pathogenesis. They all originated from a common ancestor and have evolved into different pathogenic lineages. Are the evolutionary processes saltatory or gradual? Many generations of students have pursued this issue with me since the 1990s. In the meantime, international communication and collaboration activities have also greatly facilitated the investigations on bacterial systematics and pathogenesis.

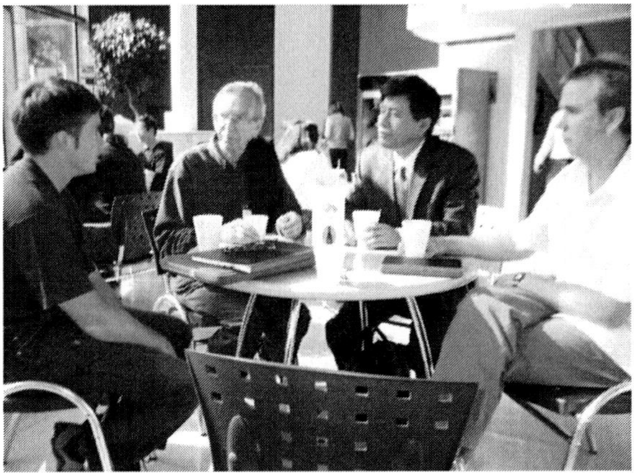

Visiting The Wellcome Trust Sanger Institute

CHAPTER 9

SEQUENCING OF *SALMONELLA* GENOMES WITH THE PHYSICAL MAP AS A FRAMEWORK TO PIN AND LINK CONTIGS

The 1990s witnessed the dawn of the comparative genomics of *Salmonella* exclusively as a result of the physical mapping techniques and analysis strategies. In addition to revealing the highly conserved genome structure in evolution and the diverting genomic events that might have started the speciation process for a *Salmonella* lineage to evolve toward a particular pathogen, the physical maps also played a key role in the sequencing efforts on *Salmonella* by providing a genomic framework for pinning and linking sequence contigs. At the finishing stage of a genome sequencing project, a high resolution physical map was used to close the sequence gaps and check the accuracy of the sequenced genome.

The first *Salmonella* sequence maps were published in the first year of this century (McClelland, *et al.* 2001; Parkhill, *et al.* 2001), requiring extraordinarily huge amounts of budgets, facilities, and human time and labor. To avoid overlapping, or even repetition, of the tedious and extremely expensive sequencing efforts, scientists of the international *Salmonella* research society tried their best to communicate with one another to know what *Salmonella* genome sequencing projects were planned or on-going.

My invited visits to the Genome Research Center of Washington University in the late 1990s and to the Wellcome Trust Sanger Institute in 2005 brought me from the physical mapping to whole genome sequencing platforms.

Genome sequencing of *S. typhimurium* LT2 as the prototype *Salmonella* pathogen for pathogenesis studies

S. typhimurium LT2 was one of the best studied bacterial strains and the very best studied *Salmonella* strain to date. And, it is the first sequenced *Salmonella* strain. The sequencing project of *S. typhimurium* LT2 was initiated in the 1990s at the Genome Research Center of Washington University in St. Louis and the sequencing platform used was the Sanger technology. For this project, I provided a high resolution genome map of *S. typhimurium* LT2 and I flew to St. Louis from Calgary to help with AvrII cleavage and PFGE techniques for the construction of "local genomic DNA sub-libraries", because it was extremely difficult to pin the sequence reads from a random library to a genomic locus.

Dr. Sandra Clifton, who invited me to the Genome Research Center for the collaboration, showed me the pipeline of the sequencing tasks, which was a chain of many labs, one lab a task for a group of people with specific sets of machines, such as PCR apparatus, PFGE machines, *etc*. I was very surprised to see so many PFGE machines in a single place. My *Salmonella* physical mapping work began with a Tyler machine, which ran a tiny gel and could hardly work to separate the rare cutter fragments. After the publication of physical maps on *S. typhimurium, S. enteritidis, S. paratyphi* A and B, and finally *S. typhi*, Dr. Sanderson eventually had the required research achievements to qualify for successfully obtaining grants from national funding sources. So, eventually, he was able to purchase his own PFGE machines and return the Tyler machine back to Dr. Kapoor. First, he bought a BioRad DRII and then a BioRad Mapper, with which I could map many more *Salmonella* genomes with far greater efficiency. And here, at the Genome Research Center of Washington University in St. Louis, the PFGE machines that they had were all Bio-Rads!

Then, Sandra escorted me to a huge hall, where I saw so many sequencers (when I went back to Calgary, I told Dr. Sanderson that I saw a sea, or rather an ocean, of sequencers in St. Louis, and he laughed). Showing me the work environment, she grunted: "the machines run without stop and the staff work 24/7, three turns a day". It was the first time I had heard the English expression "24/7", but I understood immediately that people work there 24 hours a day and seven days a week. At this point, I noted that all the people were working in the labs quite solemnly, walking around or pipetting something very quietly and seriously, without talking to each other. No one was smiling and no one looked up at me, the stranger.

The finished genome of *S. typhimurium* LT2 was published in *Nature* on October 25, 2001 (McClelland, *et al.* 2001). I had joked to Dr. Sanderson before the LT2 genome was completed that if my estimation of the *S. typhimurium* LT2 genome size by physical mapping was very different from the sequenced genome, I would have to find an island unknown to anyone and spend the rest of my life there. He laughed and waited for the LT2 sequencing project to be finished. The genome size is 4857 kb, so my estimated size, 4807 kb, by physical mapping was about 99% accurate. I was very happy. All the genomic details revealed by the physical mapping were confirmed to be correct by the sequencing project.

Genome sequencing of the typhoid agent *S. typhi*

The sequencing of *S. typhi* genomes in strains CT18 and Ty2, conducted at The Wellcome Trust Sanger Institute and the University of Wisconsin, respectively, also confirmed the findings made by our physical mapping (Deng, *et al.* 2003; Parkhill, *et al.* 2001), including the rearrangements and the plastic nature of the genome structure, gene locations, homologous loci, and indels. In addition, genome sequencing provided further details of these findings. First, the large insertion that was uncovered by the physical mapping and hypothesized to be the "trigger" of genomic rearrangement (Liu and Sanderson 1995d) was characterized to be a pathogenicity island, designated SPI7, which carries over a hundred genes including those encoding the Vi antigen. Second, all homologous genomic loci were identified, including *rrn* genes, prophages, and insertion sequences (ISs), which could all provide the sequences for recombination leading to genomic rearrangements. Third, all other insertions and also deletions documented by the physical mapping, relative to *S. typhimurium*, were confirmed and characterized, providing important information for studies of genomic evolution, pathogenicity acquisition, and speciation of the bacteria. The sequencing platforms for both *S. typhi* strains were, as in the case of LT2 sequencing, also based on the Sanger technologies, including ABI3700, ABI3730, *etc*. The throughputs were low and the sequence data amounts would have to be high enough to achieve the full coverage of the whole genome. However, no matter how deep the sequencing might be, full coverage was hardly achievable. So contigs (larger pieces of DNA by combining overlapping sequencing reads) would have to be melded by several methods, including primer walking to join small gaps (genomic regions not sequenced yet), local DNA library by rare cutter fragments (like me producing the AvrII fragments for LT2 sequencing (McClelland, *et al.* 2001)) for large gaps, *etc*. The problem was how to find out the sizes of the gaps, small or large? Although *Salmonella* genomes are known or assumed to be highly linear, indels are real and will considerably affect the gap closing strategies. Such problems were nicely overcome in the early *Salmonella* genome sequencing projects by physical mapping (Deng, *et al.* 2003; Liu 2007; Liu, *et al.* 1993c; Liu and Sanderson 1995a, b; McClelland, *et al.* 2004; McClelland, *et al.* 2001).

Genome sequencing of *S. paratyphi* C, a paratyphoid agent that has a broader host range

The appearance of the second generation sequencing technologies greatly facilitated the comparative studies on *Salmonella*. The Roche 454 appeared in 2005, followed by the Illumina Solexa in 2006 and the ABI SOLiD in 2007. When I was visiting The Wellcome Trust Sanger Institute in September of 2005, Dr. Gordon Dougan told me that they were considering using the 454 platform for the next sequencing projects of *Salmonella* genomes. They had about 100 machines of ABI3700 and ABI3730, which I later heard they had donated to some research institutions the year following my visit, and had switched to the Second Generation platforms, beginning with the Roche 454.

I was invited to visit The Wellcome Trust Sanger Institute in September, 2005, to discuss the next strategies of comparative genomic studies on *Salmonella*, especially a list of *Salmonella* lineages to sequence. After one night in London and one day in Cambridge, a young postdoc came to the hotel and picked me up. Dr. John Wein was waiting for me in front of the Sanger Institute buildings. We spent about half an hour for a mini trip around the buildings and a few departments in the main building. At 9:00 am, we returned to the main hall to have a cup of coffee. Then, several PIs joined us, greeting, drinking coffee and talking about Calgary and *Salmonella*. At 10:00 am, the seminar began. In the one-hour presentation, I made three points. First, the next *Salmonella* lineages to sequence should include *S. paratyphi* C, which, like *S. typhi*, causes a kind of typhoidal disease (called paratyphoid fever, clinically indistinguishable from typhoid fever) in humans but, unlike *S. typhi*, infects not only humans, but also other mammals such as mice; therefore, it was suitable for animal experiments to study the pathogenesis of typhoidal diseases. Second, the phylogenetic or taxonomic status of *Salmonella* lineages should be elucidated by the comparative genomic studies to clarify, for example, whether *S. typhi* and

S. typhimurium should be treated as individual species in their own right, or whether they should be categorized into the same species, or the same subspecies, even though they are totally different pathogens. Third, the *Salmonella* sequencing projects should make good use of physical mapping strategies to facilitate the work and save both time and resources. I then showed the successful use of physical maps in the sequencing projects of *S. typhimurium* LT2, *S. typhi* Ty2, *S. paratyphi* A, *etc*. Many questions were asked, followed by some heated discussions. Dr. Gordon Dougan was especially interested in the history of *S. typhi* nomenclature and agreed with me that *S. typhi* and *S. typhimurium* should have the status of independent species.

The whole day communication activities were extremely effective and fruitful. Then, dinner time was literally a carnival. I do not remember how much beer was consumed but everyone was in very high spirits. One guy, the first author of many Science and Nature papers, told me that they had been sequencing SL1344, a strain of *S. typhimurium*, for comparison with strain LT2, the former being a representative wildtype and highly virulent strain and the latter being a lab and non-virulent strain, to reveal the involved pathways of pathogenesis. "The genome is still linear, and we have tried all methods to circularize the genome, including primer walking and local library cloning, and yet we cannot make the ends meet". Everyone laughed. "I think", he continued, "the SL1344 strain genome has telomeres", which elicited an outburst of even louder laughter. But I was serious and suggested making a physical map and estimating the size of the gap between the "telomeres" in order to make the ends meet. All laughed again, knowing that no *Salmonella* genomes have any telomere-like structures.

They did send me the strain and I mapped it, finding that merely a few more kb would make the ends meet. I sent the mapping results to them, along with the corresponding region in LT2 and possible endonuclease cleavage sites.

I also suggested pairs of PCR primers to close the gap.

While in the Sanger Institute, I demonstrated my plan to sequence *S. paratyphi* C to avoid work overlapping or, worse, repetition among research teams in the *Salmonella* society. As soon as I came back from the Wellcome Trust Sanger Institute trip, I initiated the *S. paratyphi* C sequencing project. I had moved to the Peking University Health Sciences Center and set up a laboratory there. To choose a suitable strain for sequencing, I mapped a large number of wild-type strains of *S. paratyphi* C. *S. paratyphi* C, like *S. typhi*, also had a "plastic" genome (see Fig. 8-9), with large genomic segments rearranged by recombination events in known homologous sites, such as those in the *rrn* operons, and other sites (Liu, *et al.* 2007), which were probably also homologous, such as prophages or ISs, to be known by whole genome sequencing.

We chose one strain, RKS4594 (lane 1 in Fig. 8-9 A and the map on the top of maps in Fig. 8-9 B), to make a detailed physical map for use as a genomic framework in whole genome sequencing. This genome carries several indels relative to *S. typhimurium* LT2, with the one at 11 o'clock being as large as 90 kb (Fig. 9-1). Consistent with the previous findings in other *Salmonella* lineages in which large genomic insertions co-exist with genomic inversions, we saw similar facts in *S. paratyphi* C RKS4594.

We began the sequencing efforts in 2005, using the ABI 3700 platform and had the genome completed in 2009 (Liu, *et al.* 2009). We were intrigued to find that the 90 kb insertion is almost a shorter version of SPI7 (the "full" version in *S. typhi* is 134 kb), lacking many genes present in *S. typhi* SPI7 but containing the Vi genes, and also some other genes, not present in *S. typhi* SPI7. Frequent genomic rearrangements have hybridized several *rrn* genes, e.g., B/E, E/C and C/B in RKS4594 (see Fig. 9-1) and other hybrids in other wild-type strains of *S. paratyphi* C. The large inversion between 3 and 7 o'clock on the physical map shown in Fig. 9-1 was mediated by a pair of phage remnants, Gifsy-1 and Gifsy-2, which contain homologous sequence regions (Fig. 9-2).

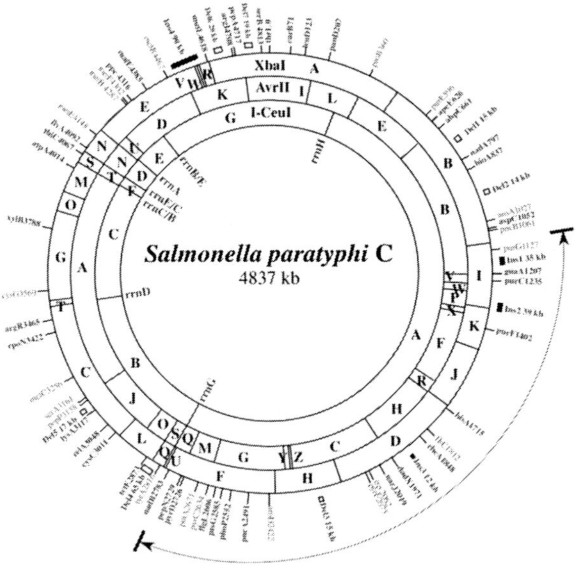

Figure 9-1. A detailed physical map of the *S. paratyphi* C RKS4594 genome. The most significant features of the map include four insertions (solid rectangles, Ins. 1-4), seven deletions (open rectangles, Del. 1-7), and a large inversion (double-headed arrow) relative to *S. typhimurium* LT2.

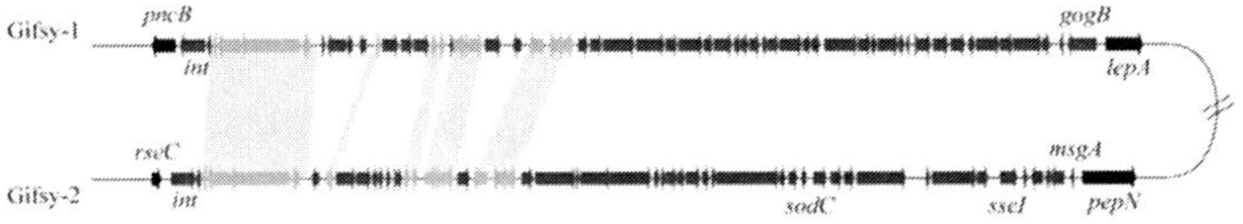

Figure 9-2. Genomic rearrangement mediated by Gifsy-1 and Gifsy-2. Common genes in Gifsy-1 and Gifsy-2 are colored in yellow, with the remaining genes of Gifsy-1 being colored in red and those of Gifsy-2 in green; conserved genes adjacent to Gifsy-1 and 2 are in black. The blue shade indicates a shared identity of >90% between Gifsy-1 and Gifsy-2.

CHAPTER 10

GENETIC SWITCHES MODULATE *SALMONELLA* GENOMIC STABILITY AND MUTABILITY

The physical structure of bacterial genomes could be conserved for multiple millions of years in evolution as evidenced by the collinear genomes of *E. coli* and *Salmonella*. *Salmonella* has branched off to over 2700 distinct lineages each with unique biological properties, such as in host range and pathogenesis, but the genomic collinearity remains among all the lineages. How can the genome be so highly conserved and how can pathogenic divergence be possible if the genomic stability is under strict modulation?

The genome of *S. typhimurium* LT7: real time rearranging

We had a wonderful opportunity to investigate the issue of *Salmonella* genomic stability and mutability.

One day at the end of the last century, I received a call from Prof. Abraham Eisenstark of the University of Missouri. He told me that he had more than twenty thousand *Salmonella* strains stocked at room temperature for over 40 years and wondered if there might be any genomic changes in them. He asked me whether I would be interested in looking into such a pure "curiosity-based" issue with the physical mapping techniques. I was extremely interested, of course, and encouraged him to send me some of the strains, quickly! He soon sent me *S. typhimurium* strain LT7, along with twelve auxotrophic mutants derived from LT7.

By that time, I was already rich enough to have as many as two PFGE machines, thanks to the national grants from NSERC, MRC, CIHR, and also funds from some other sources. Additionally, I was no longer doing the experiments, collecting and analyzing the results, and summarizing the data all by myself. I began to have students and research assistants (Fig. 10-1). The two PFGE machines were producing large amounts of *Salmonella* genomic data every day, 24/7. My students and research assistants were fully energetic and enthusiastic about the LT7 project, from receiving the bacterial strains, growing and stocking them, isolating DNA from them, to conducting PFGE analysis on them.

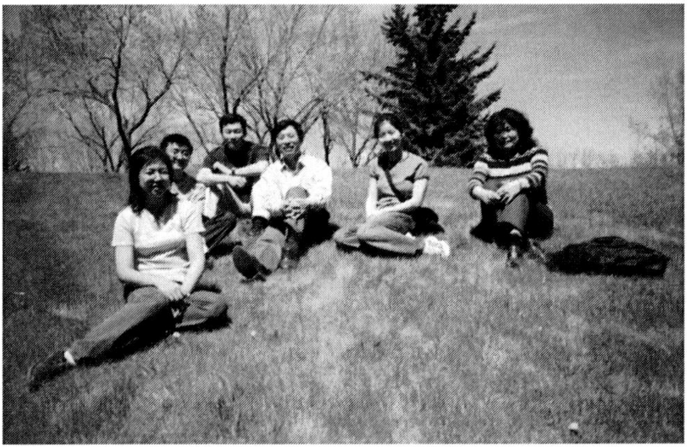

Figure 10-1. The Liu *Salmonella* research team in 2001.

We put the whole contents of the vials that we received from Prof. Eisenstark into a tube of LB broth and cultured the bacteria overnight. Then we assigned stock numbers to the thirteen strains and stocked them under -80°C. As a rule, we would not do single-colony isolation for stocking bacterial strains received from any source, even though the received tube contains mixtures or even contaminations of bacteria, in order to avoid stocking the wrong bacteria and, in the meantime, discarding the right bacteria. But for analysis, we routinely streak the stock and inspect the single colonies to guarantee the purity of the bacteria for use in the analysis. When the colonies exhibit uniform *Salmonella*-like morphology, we would assume that the stock is from a pure culture. Then, from the many identical colonies, we pick up a well isolated one and initiate the experiments. This time, surprisingly, I saw an unbelievable scene: colonies of bacteria from a vial exhibited a great diversity of morphologies and almost no two colonies resembled each other on an LB plate. Bacteria from all thirteen vials had similar situations. Assuming that they were all mixtures of different bacteria, I told my student working on this project to pick up a colony that looked typical for a *Salmonella* colony and streak it to a fresh LB plate. The next day, we saw colonies of various morphologies again.

At this point, I postulated that the genome might be rearranging to produce bacteria that have different efficiencies in DNA replication, cell growth, or nutrient competition due to the different balance status of the physical structure of the genome. To validate this postulation, we compared the prototype LT7, stocked under -80°C, and the LT7 derivatives of Dr. Eisenstark by PFGE analysis and found diverse genomic changes among the derivatives, including translocations, inversions, duplications, and point mutations, as exemplified by the 155 kb DNA duplication in the derivative strain 8117C (Fig. 10-2) and half genome inversion in 8111D323 (Fig. 10-3).

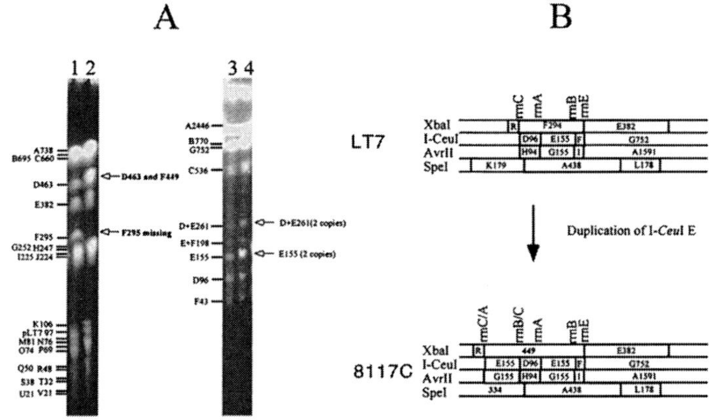

Figure 10-2. Genomic duplication exemplified by strain 8117C (a derivative of LT7). (A) PFGE gels of LT7 and 8117C cleaved by XbaI and I-CeuI (lanes 1, 2, 3, 4, respectively). (B) Local comparison of LT7 and 8117C showing the 155 kb DNA segment (called I-CeuI E) duplication in 8117C, which created two hybrid *rrn* operons, *rrnC/A* and *rrnB/C*.

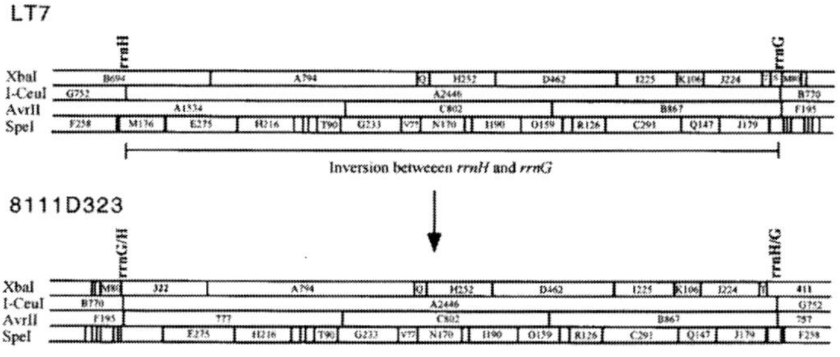

Figure 10-3. Genomic inversion exemplified by strain 8111D323. Local genomic comparison of the prototype LT7 and 8111D323 showing the large inversion between *rrnH* and *rrnG*, which resulted in two hybrid *rrn* operons, *rrnG/H* and *rrnH/G*.

Strain 8111 was one of the derivatives of LT7. The first streaking of 8111 produced very large, large, medium, small, tiny, and iota colonies, which we designated A, B, C, D, E and F by diameter of the colony (>4 mm, 2-4 mm, 1-2 mm, 0.5-1 mm， 0.3- 0.5 mm, and < 0.3 mm, respectively). For repeated streaking after the English capital letter colony "generation", the colony sizes were represented by numerals 1-6, in places of A, B, C, D, E and F, respectively. For example, strain 8111D was a small colony of 8111; in the ensuing experiments, we worked on a medium-sized colony, 8111D3. As 8111, 8111D and 8111D3 all had different genomic rearrangements, we continued analyzing "next and next generations" of 8111D3 including 8111D32, which was a large colony from 8111D3, and 8111D323, which was a medium-sized colony from 8111D32; all 8111, 8111D, 8111D3, 8111D32 and 8111D323 had different genomic rearrangements, and the rearrangements took place in real time, *i.e.*, during growth in the lab (Liu, *et al.* 2003).

Then the question came into my mind: what happened to the genome of LT7 during the forty years under room temperature storage? If the question was answered, we may have a chance to look into the key mystery about the modulation of a balance between genomic stability and mutability in *Salmonella* or, hopefully, bacteria in general.

The MMR genes spontaneously modulate the balance between genomic stability and mutability as genetic switches

My immediate speculation about the mechanism controlling the genomic stability and mutability in *Salmonella*, after seeing the real time genomic changes, was the functionality of the mismatch repair (MMR) system, which had long been known to play a key role in safeguarding the bacterial genome against variations (Harfe and Jinks-Robertson 2000; Kunkel and Erie 2005; LeClerc, *et al.* 1996; Li 2008; Miller 1998; Rayssiguier, *et al.* 1989; Schofield and Hsieh 2003; Sniegowski, et al. 1997). However, the real time genomic changes in LT7 were so queer that it would be really hard to tell whether they might be associated with MMR just by educated reasoning. However, I felt that the elucidation would be extremely interesting. I then assigned the analysis of MMR to a summer student, Wei-Qiao, who had just graduated from senior high school and had been admitted to the University of Calgary. He applied for funding to support his post-senior high and pre-university summer studentship and he was successful. His summer studentship was from the Alberta Heritage Foundation for Health Research. I told him to design and order primers for sequencing *mutL*, *mutS*, and *mutH* genes of the MMR system to see whether they might have any changes. He was excited and began working on this project seriously, because until that time he had been taught to learn the knowns, but for the first time he was to learn the unknowns by hands-on investigations.

One morning, I was working on a manuscript and heard Wei-Qiao running to me, shouting "I found the secret of LT7 genomic diversification!"

I put aside the writing and looked at the sequence result of *mutL*. "Look at the deletion of the hexa-nucleotide sequence. There are three tandem copies in the wild-type gene of LT2 but only two copies in LT7 derivatives…" Yes, he'd got it right. Clearly, both LT2 and the original LT7 kept at -80°C (not that kept at room temperature for four decades by Dr. Eisenstark), had three tandem copies of the hexa-nucleotide sequence GCTGGC but two derivatives of LT7, 9052D1 and 8111F2, had only two copies (Fig. 10-4). We thus designated the defective *mutL* with a Δ and called it 6bpΔ*mutL* (Gong, *et al.* 2007).

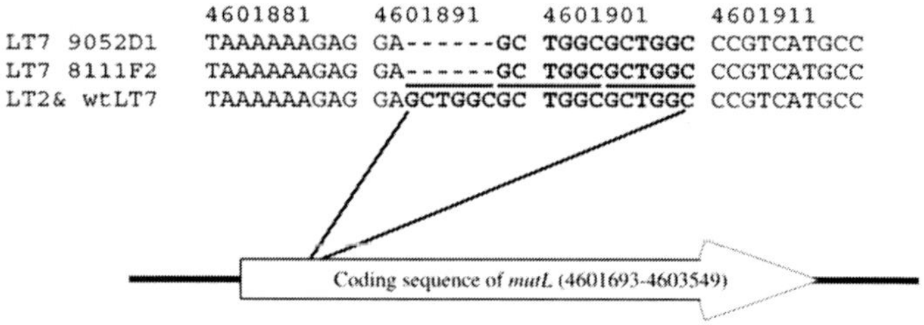

Figure 10-4. One copy deletion of the hexa-nucleotide sequence GCTGGC in *mutL* of LT7 mutants exemplified by 8111F2 and 9052D1. The numbers on top of the sequence show the genomic location of the nucleotides as in the genome of LT2.

To validate the associations of genomic diversification with the 6bpΔ*mutL* genotype, we compared the mutability of 6bpΔ*mutL* and wild-type *mutL* strains and found that the 6bpΔ*mutL* genotype elevated the bacterial mutational frequency by more than a hundred times (Fig. 10-5).

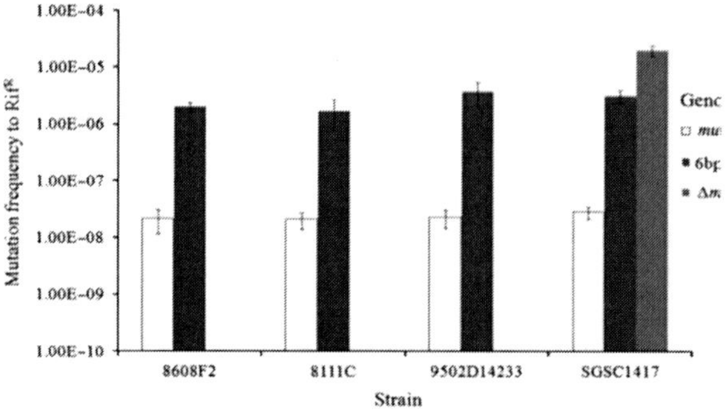

Figure 10-5. Frequency of mutations resistant to rifampicin. The left three pairs of strains are for comparison of mutability between the *mutL* and 6bpΔ*mutL* genotypes. The last group of three bars (on the right side of the figure) was included for a comparison between 6bpΔ*mutL* and Δ*mutL* (*mutL* is completely deleted). There are no significant differences in mutability between 6bpΔ*mutL* and Δ*mutL* genotypes, demonstrating that the defective MutL protein encoded by 6bpΔ*mutL* is entirely nonfunctional.

The behavior of a peculiar strain, 9052D132111, totally surprised me. I initially analyzed a small colony of strain 9052 (9052D) and picked up a very large colony from it, larger than 4 mm in diameter, and I called it 9052D1. From 9052D1, I picked 9052D13 (medium sized colony) and from 9052D13 I picked 9052D132 (large colony). Bacteria from all these differently sized colonies had different genomic rearrangements, so I continued to isolate the next, then the next, and the next generations of 9052D132 for different colony sizes. However, when I got to 9052D1321, all next generation colonies from 9052D1321 were very large, and I designated them 9052D13211 and 9052D132111. Curious, I had their *mutL* gene sequenced and found that they all had three tandem copies of GCTGGC, rather than two copies as in 9052D, 9052D1, 9052D13, or 9052D132, and all the 9052D1321 series, including 9052D1321, 9052D13211 and 9052D132111, had a uniform genome structure as in 9052D1321 without any further genomic variations found. This demonstrated that 9052D1321 somehow regained a copy of GCTGGC, passed it to the next generations, and rendered high genomic stability to the bacteria. These results unambiguously indicate that the high mutability of LT7 derivatives was due to the 6bpΔ*mutL* genotype, which, of remarkable interest, could be spontaneously converted to *mutL*. As tandem repeats of short sequences may readily lose or gain a copy during DNA replication by slippage of the nascent chain from the template chain, we postulated that the conversion between 6bpΔ*mutL* and *mutL* could have taken place by this slippage replication mechanism. If so, such a conversion may be spontaneous and the "product" of the conversion, either 6bpΔ*mutL* or *mutL*, may become dominant for better fitness: 6bpΔ*mutL* may be selected to render appropriate mutability to the bacteria in adapting to the changing environment and *mutL* may be selected to render high genomic stability to the bacteria for their sustainability as a natural species. By the same logic, but viewing the issue from the other side, I hypothesized that the conversion, such as that from *mutL* to 6bpΔ*mutL* as in the case of LT7 (*mutL* in wild-type becoming 6bpΔ*mutL* under storage at room temperature) or that from 6bpΔ*mutL* to *mutL* as in the case of the LT7 derivative 9052 (6bpΔ*mutL* in 9052, 9052D, 9052D1, 9052D13 and 9052D132, suddenly becoming *mutL* in 9052D1321 and remaining as *mutL* in 9052D13211 and 9052D132111) spontaneously modulates the balance between bacterial genomic stability and mutability for better fitness, according to environmental changes.

To test this hypothesis, we disrupted the tandem repeats by substituting a couple of synonymous nucleotides at appropriate places to make each of the tandem repeats a unique sequence, so that strand slippage during DNA replication would not be possible as it was before. Therefore, as a matter of fact, we were to lock the *mutL* or 6bpΔ*mutL* at their *mutL* or 6bpΔ*mutL* status without giving them a chance for mutual conversion. Unbelievably, we obtained results that looked too good to be true: *Salmonella* strains with the *mutL* GCTGGC GCTGGC GCTGGC being converted to GCTTGC CCTGGC GCTGGC (modified bases are underlined) had greatly lower mutability; on the other hand, strains with the 6bpΔ*mutL* GCTGGC GCTGGC being converted to GCTTGC CCTGGC had even higher mutability (Chen, *et al.* 2010a; Chen, et al. 2010b). Note that, after the nucleotide substitutions, the hexa-nucleotide sequence encodes the amino acids LA as before, as the substituted and substituting nucleotides are synonymous. When the locked *mutL* or 6bpΔ*mutL* was unlocked by nucleotide substitutions back to the natural sequences, the higher or lower mutability in *Salmonella* strains with locked 6bpΔ*mutL* or *mutL* came back to the pre-locking levels (Chen, *et al.* 2010a).

These results provided conclusive evidence indicating the association of the LT7 genome diversification phenomenon with the 6bpΔ*mutL* genotype but also raised new questions: how come the locked *mutL* genotype rendered higher genomic stability to the bacteria, or how come the locked 6bpΔ*mutL* genotype rendered even higher genomic mutability to the bacteria, if both locked and wild-type *mutL* three tandem sequences encode LALALA, or both locked and the natural 6bpΔ*mutL* two tandem sequences encode LALA?

My interpretation is that natural bacterial populations with the *mutL* genotype may have basal frequencies of 6bpΔ*mutL* subpopulations, which can promptly and transiently "take over" the whole population to deal with suddenly changed environmental conditions by allowing beneficial genomic changes to play an emergent role for rescue; conversely, the bacterial population with the 6bpΔ*mutL* genotype may have basic frequencies of *mutL* cells, which can safeguard the genome against unnecessary genomic variations and gradually take over the population to rescue the bacterial species. I thus anticipate that very deep genome sequencing will eventually clarify whether such very low frequency subpopulations may exist. We also looked at other MMR genes, such as *mutS*, which may also play a role to balance bacterial genomic stability and mutability (Chen, et al. 2010a). As such, I conclude that the MMR genes spontaneously modulate the balance between genomic stability and mutability as genetic switches.

The genetic switch working in the real world: LALALA motif as part of the ATP binding pocket

How may the 6bpΔ*mutL* genotype demolish the function of the MutL protein? To approach this question, we first did computer simulations, which predicted conformational changes in the defective MutL protein. The GCTGGC hexa-nucleotide sequence is involved in encoding two amino acids, leucine (L) and alanine (A). The LALALA motif, as a part of the ATP-binding pocket in the MutL protein, fits a molecule of ATP, but a defective MutL protein encoded by 6bpΔ*mutL* contains LALA and so will not fit ATP (Fig. 10-6).

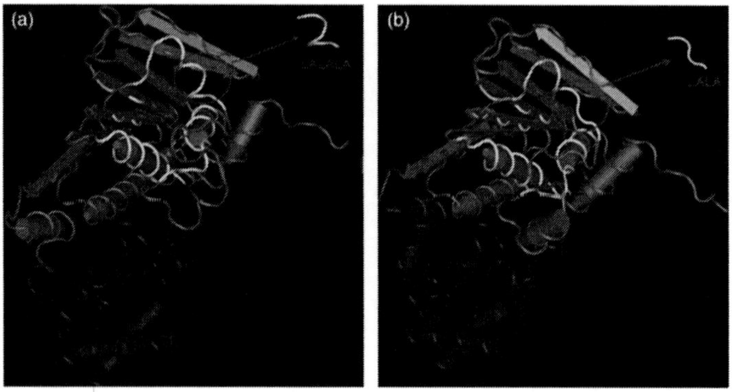

Figure 10-6. Computational modeling of the proteins encoded by *mutL* and 6bpΔ*mutL*. (a) Wild-type MutL protein; (b) mutant MutL protein. The ATP binding pockets are highlighted in yellow. The tandem repeats LALALA or LALA (in red circles) lie in the region that forms the lid of the ATP-binding pocket of the MutL protein.

Our collaborator, Dr. Alba Guarné, at McMaster University experimentally observed the genetic switch working in the real world with a focus on the specific molecular mechanisms. Dr. Guarné and colleagues characterized the defects in the ATP lid of *E. coli* MutL that caused transient hypermutability and found that strains with high mutability could spontaneously arise in bacterial populations under stress, supporting our previous conclusion that MutL plays a key role as the genetic switch spontaneously modulating bacterial mutability for appropriate evolutionary adaptability. Dr. Guarné engineered a series of *E. coli* MutL variants with shorter/longer LA motifs and characterized their ATPase and DNA binding functions. They found that the deletion or insertion of a single LA repeat did not compromise the structural integrity of the protein, nor did it affect MutS- or DNA-binding activities. However, it severely compromised ATP binding and, consequently, the engagement of the N-terminal domains, both being essential for proper DNA mismatch repair (Pillon, *et al.* 2013). The LALALA motif is conserved

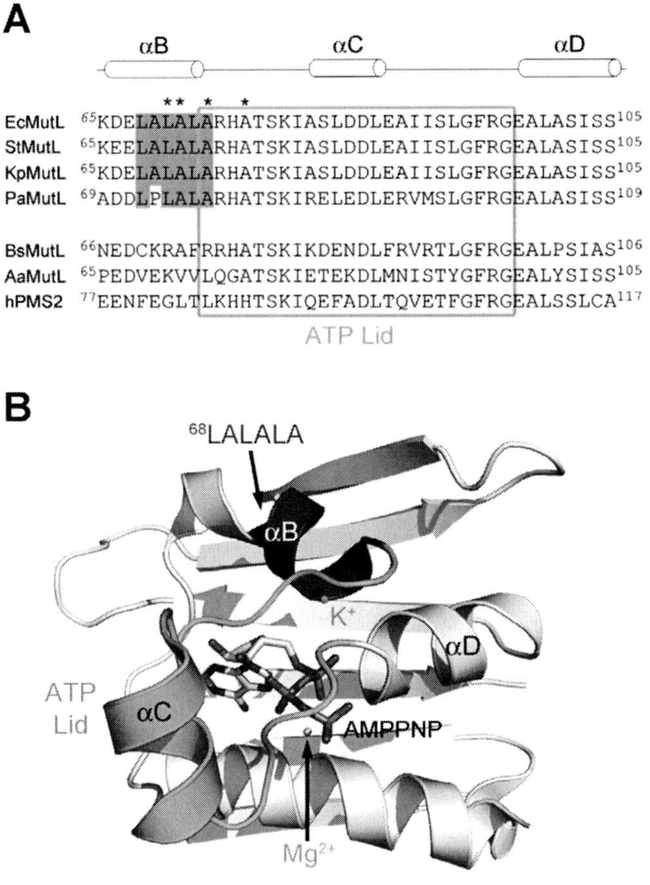

Figure 10-7. The LALALA motif as part of the ATP binding pocket. (A) Sequence alignment of the MutL ATP lid from *E. coli* K12 (Ec), *S. typhimurium* LT7 (St), *Klebsiella pneumoniae* (Kp), *Pseudomonas aeruginosa* (Pa), *Bacillus subtilis* (Bs), *Aquifex aeolicus* (Aa), and human MutL homologue PMS2 (hPMS2). The secondary structure corresponds to the *E. coli* MutL crystal structure (PDB ID 1B63). The lid region is indicated by a blue box and the LALALA motif is highlighted in purple. *E. coli* MutL residues involved in chelating the monovalent

metal ion are indicated by black asterisks. (B) Ribbon diagram of the *E. coli* MutL nucleotide binding pocket (PDB ID 1NHI). The LALALA motif is shown in purple and the ATP lid is in blue. The AMPPNP molecule is shown as color-coded sticks and the Mg2+ and K+ ions are shown as yellow and green spheres, respectively. (For interpretation of the references to color in this figure legend, the reader is referred to the web version of this article (Pillon, *et al.* 2013)).

among the bacteria of *Enterobacteriaceae* and the ATP binding pocket is conserved broadly, from evolutionarily diverse bacteria to man (Fig. 10-7), where in the latter case defects in the MMR DNA repair pathway are associated with high rates of colon cancer development. We may speculate that DNA repair efficiency may in this case also be modulated to low or high levels as cancer cells evolve or metastasize to novel tissue niches, further emulating the behaviours of adapting bacterial species (but this will require more research in the future).

CHAPTER 11

SALMONELLA GENOMIC DIVERGENCE LEADING TO NEW PATHOGENS: DIVERTING AND ADJUSTING

All extant bacteria have their territories (specific ecologic niches), networking and overlapping but not congruent. Formation of such bacterial lineage-specific territories is evolutionarily dynamic, as the physicochemical conditions keep changing – gradually or drastically. As a result, bacterial community compositions will also change, accordingly, and the bacteria will strive to survive by overcoming the selection pressures, becoming fit again by accumulating beneficial genetic traits, or extinct due to the lack of chances to obtain the relevant beneficial genetic traits. Any vacant micro niches would eventually be occupied or invaded by newcomers, which may or may not become adapted to the ecologic conditions. These new bacterial lineages may come from adaptive variants of the original inhabitants by divergent evolution, or from nascent bacterial species arising by acquisition of novel biological traits through convergent evolutionary processes.

S. gallinarum biovars: adapting to the same host but causing distinct diseases

S. gallinarum and *S. pullorum* appeared in the first edition of Bergey's Manual of Systematic Bacteriology in 1984 as *Salmonella* "serovars" but, in the meantime, retained the Latinized binary species names consisting of the name of the genus (*Salmonella*) followed by a specific epithet (*gallinarum* and *pullorum*, respectively) (Le Minor 1984). Later, the two *Salmonella* species were re-classified into the same species, the same subspecies and the same serovar as two separate pathovars or biovars (Le Minor and Popoff 1987; Popoff and Le Minor 2005). Indeed, the two *Salmonella* lineages share very high genetic similarity, including >90% common genes between their genomes and >40% of common genes with zero nucleotide degeneracy (Tang, *et al.* 2013a), and they both infect fowl as the only natural host. However, they cause distinct systemic illnesses, with *S. gallinarum* eliciting typhoid-like fever and *S. pullorum* causing dysentery-like diarrhea. Obviously, *S. gallinarum* and *S. pullorum* have evolved with distinct pathogenic mechanisms. Can the differences in pathogenesis be elucidated by comparative genomic analysis between the two *Salmonella* lineages?

We conducted genomic comparisons between *S. gallinarum* and *S. pullorum* by physical mapping, with the allegedly ancestral lineage *S. enteritidis* as a reference. We found that, like other *Salmonella* lineages, *S. gallinarum*, *S. pullorum* and *S. enteritidis* had a common genomic framework, as reflected by I-CeuI cleavage patterns on PFGE (Fig. 11-1a). However, a genomic distinction among the three *Salmonella* lineages was clearly revealed by XbaI and SpeI cleavages (Fig. 11-1b and c), reflecting sequence degeneracies during evolution, after their divergence.

Sequence analysis showed different laterally acquired DNA segments and differential nucleotide substitution patterns (Tang, *et al.* 2017a; Tang, *et al.* 2017c). These findings provided further support to our early hypothesis on the divergence of *Salmonella* lineages, which stated that laterally acquired genes encoding novel biological traits divert the bacteria in a new evolutionary direction and genomic nucleotide sequence amelioration adjusts codon usage for the bacteria to become better adapted in the divergent evolutionary process (Liu, *et al.* 2002a; Liu and Sanderson 1995d; Tang, *et al.* 2017a).

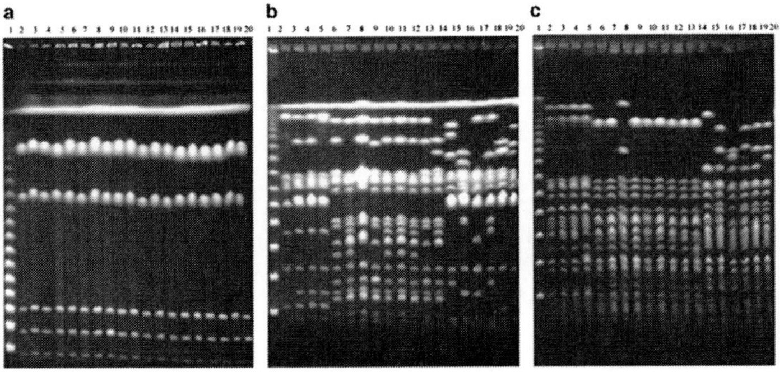

Figure 11-1. Genomic DNA PFGE patterns of strains representing *S. enteritidis*, *S. pullorum* and *S. gallinarum*, cleaved with I-CeuI (a), XbaI (b) and SpeI (c). Lanes: 1, DNA size marker; 2-5, *S. enteritidis* (SE310, SE154, SE301, LK5); 6-14, *S. pullorum* (RKS5078, CDC1983-67, SARB51, 04–6767, NS387, 00–19557, 02–15951, 03–16062, 98–13777); 15–20, *S. gallinarum* (287/91, RKS5021, SGSC2293, 91–29327, 90–5289, 92–7995).

S. paratyphi C: divergence from *S. choleraesuis* and convergence with *S. typhi*

S. paratyphi C is a paratyphoid agent, which causes a febrile disease very similar to typhoid fever caused by *S. typhi*. The very close relatedness between *S. paratyphi* C and *S. choleraesuis* strongly suggests their divergence from a common recent ancestor. Conversely, though pathogenically similar, *S. paratyphi* C and *S. typhi* obviously diverged from different recent ancestors by biologically convergent evolutionary processes (Fig. 11-2).

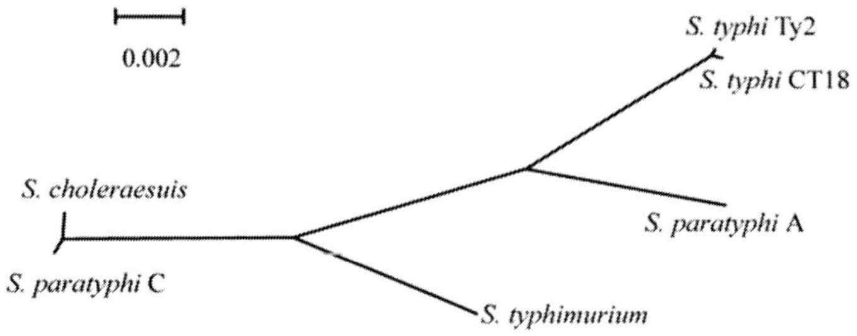

Figure 11-2. Phylogenetic tree for six representative *Salmonella* pathogens. The tree is based on whole-genome sequences, showing the close relatedness of *S. paratyphi* C with *S. choleraesuis*, but not with pathogenically similar *S. typhi*.

We focused on strain KRS4594 of *S. paratyphi* C and sequenced its genome, which consists of a chromosome and a plasmid (Fig. 11-3). A series of indels relative to other *Salmonella* genomes makes *S. paratyphi* C a unique lineage. The 90 kb insertion is a shorter version of SPI7, which is 134 kb in *S. typhi*. The 90 kb and 134 kb SPI7 islands share many core genes, including those encoding the Vi antigen.

Both *S. paratyphi* C and *S. choleraesuis* cause systemic diseases in their host, with *S. paratyphi* C primarily infecting man and *S. choleraesuis* primarily infecting hogs.

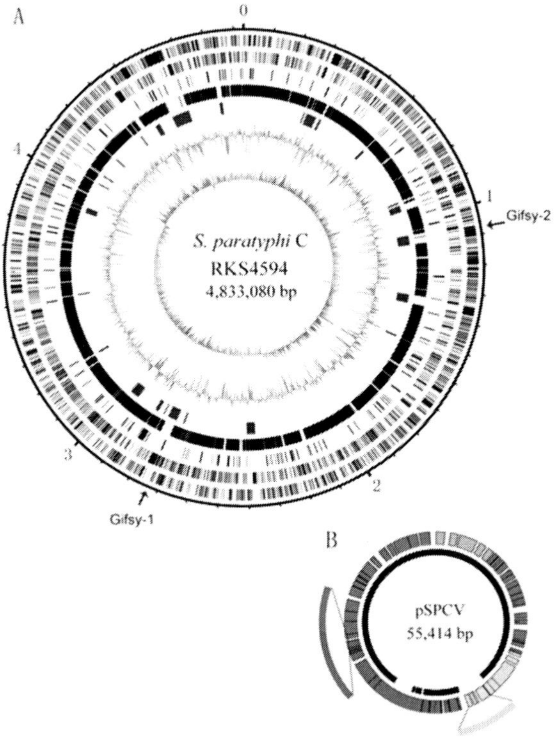

Figure 11-3. The *S. paratyphi* C RKS4594 genome. (A) The chromosome. Circles from 1 (outer circle) to 7 (inner circle): 1 and 2, genes on the forward and reverse strands, respectively; 3, pseudogenes; 4, genes conserved among all six sequenced strains compared in this study; 5, rRNA operons (blue), and prophages and SPIs (brown); 6, G+C content, with values greater than average in green and smaller in red; and 7, GC skew (G2C/G+C), with values greater than zero in green and smaller in red. (B) The virulence plasmid. For more details, see (Liu, *et al*. 2009).

Comparisons among *S. paratyphi* C, *S. typhi* and *S. choleraesuis* provide excellent opportunities for studies of divergent evolution leading to dissimilar pathogens from a common recent ancestor and studies of convergent evolution leading to similar pathogens descended from different ancestors.

Genomic islands and nucleotide sequence amelioration in individual *Salmonella* lineages

To gain insights into the divergent and convergent evolutionary processes that lead to distinct pathogens, we hypothesized the formation of a novel bacterial pathogen with *S. typhi* as a model, stating that the acquisition of a large genomic insertion (*ca.* 100 kb or larger) starts the new pathogen formation process, providing novel pathogenic traits to the bacteria, and adaptive genomic streamlining, including rebalancing of the physical structure of the bacterial chromosome and other genomic variations, makes the nascent pathogen a species (Liu and Sanderson 1995d); we later refer to this hypothetic model as "the Adopt-Adapt Model of bacterial speciation" (Liu, *et al.* 2002a). Here "Adopt" refers to the "adoption" of novel genetic materials by lateral gene transfer and "Adapt" refers to the "adaptation" of the bacteria to retain the acquired "foreign" DNA block by regaining a physical balance of the genome disrupted by the insertion of a large DNA block through genomic rearrangement, and adapting to the new physicochemical and biological conditions of the ecologic niche by accumulating genetic variations. This latter process is referred to as nucleotide amelioration.

All sequenced, or physically mapped, *Salmonella* genomes contain lineage-specific indels relative to other *Salmonella* lineages, such as *S. paratyphi* C (see Fig. 11-3 for the various insertions and deletions specific to *S. paratyphi* C). The Adopt-Adapt Model assumes that one of the laterally acquired DNA blocks initiates the process of novel pathogen formation, but identification of the "initiator" is not easy, as there are many laterally acquired DNA blocks in a *Salmonella* genome. One way to approach this issue would be to identify the "oldest" large insertion that should be present in all strains of the same lineage, but not in any other bacteria of the same genus. For ordering the identified large insertions by their relative "ages", we compared their nucleotide ameliorating levels using the tetranucleotide sequence CTAG as an indicator. This was based on the finding that the CTAG sequence tends to be eliminated by the Very Short Patch repair system in *Salmonella* and other closely related bacterial lineages, such as *E. coli* (Bhagwat and McClelland 1992; Lieb 1983; McClelland and Bhagwat 1992; Tang, *et al.* 2017a; Tang, *et al.* 2017b). As most laterally transferred DNA segments (LTDSs) acquired by *Salmonella* are from sources that are phylogenetically remote from *Salmonella,* and so are assumed to contain statistically average frequencies of the CTAG sequence for an "ordinary" bacterial genome (*i.e.*, not of *E. coli* or *Salmonella*), we postulated that older LTDSs may have much lower frequencies of the CTAG sequence than younger LTDSs. We tested this assumption on two >50 kb insertions in *S. heidelberg* strain SL476 and found that Insertion 1 had a much higher CTAG frequency than Insertion 2. This result is consistent with the hypothesized progressive reduction of CTAG sequences in the LTDSs by the Very Short Patch repair system in *Salmonella.* Interestingly, the amelioration process seems to progress from the two ends of the inserted large DNA segment toward the central part (Fig. 11-4). Whether this particular LTDS actually started the formation of a novel pathogen will, of course, have to be validated by further investigations, including animal experiments.

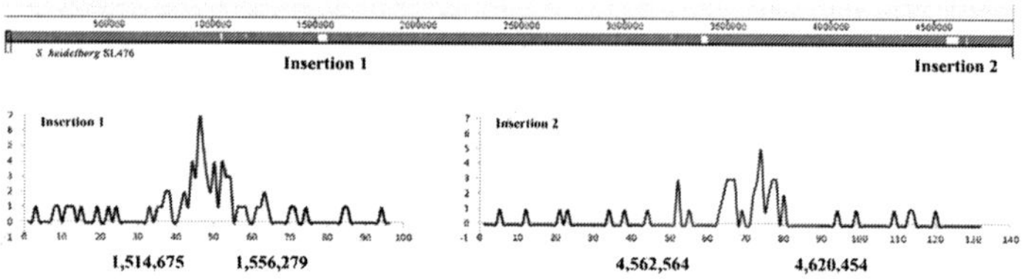

Figure 11-4. Distribution patterns of CTAG inside Insertions 1 and 2 of the *S. heidelberg* SL476 genome. The red color indicates the regions of the insertions, with the start and end positions marked in both insertions, and the black color indicates the up- and down-stream genomic sequences.

Different nucleotide amelioration patterns reflect distinct adaptation mechanisms and non-congruent ecologic conditions between even very closely related bacterial lineages – quite often, they are referred to as belonging to the same bacterial lineage. One example is the relationship between *S. gallinarum* and *S. pullorum*, which both had Latinized scientific species names and had been treated as separate bacterial species. *S. gallinarum* and *S. pullorum*, both being non-flagellated and both infecting only fowl as their natural host, are so similar biologically that they can hardly be unambiguously differentiated by routine microbiological or biochemical assays. Even more strikingly, *S. gallinarum* and *S. pullorum*, both having the same antigenic formula 1:9;12:-:-, are genetically so similar that they were categorized into the same species and the same subspecies, *Salmonella enterica* subspecies *enterica*, as different biovars of the serovar Gallinarum in 1987 (Le Minor and Popoff 1987). However, they cause distinct systemic infections in fowl and have distinct nucleotide amelioration patterns (see Fig. 11-1a). As the result of adaptive selection of codons, distinct nucleotide amelioration patterns clearly demonstrate non-congruent micro niches and clear-cut genetic boundaries between these extraordinarily close relatives.

Another example is the relationship of *S. java* and *S. paratyphi* B (Liu, *et al.* 1994). These two *Salmonella* lineages have drastically different pathogenic properties, with *S. java* having a broad host range and causing gastroenteritis in humans but *S. paratyphi* B infecting only humans and causing paratyphoid fever. *S. java* is often referred to as a tartrate positive variant of *S. paratyphi* B, as routine clinical assays and even serological tests can hardly distinguish them – they have the same antigenic formula 1,4,[5],12:b:1,2 and are extremely similar in genetics and biochemistry. However, they are definitely different in phylogeny, as their genome sequences have distinct ameliorating patterns, which can be intuitively demonstrated by endonuclease cleavage patterns on PFGE gels (Fig. 11-5). Additionally, their genomic distinction unambiguously indicates clear genetic boundaries between the two lineages.

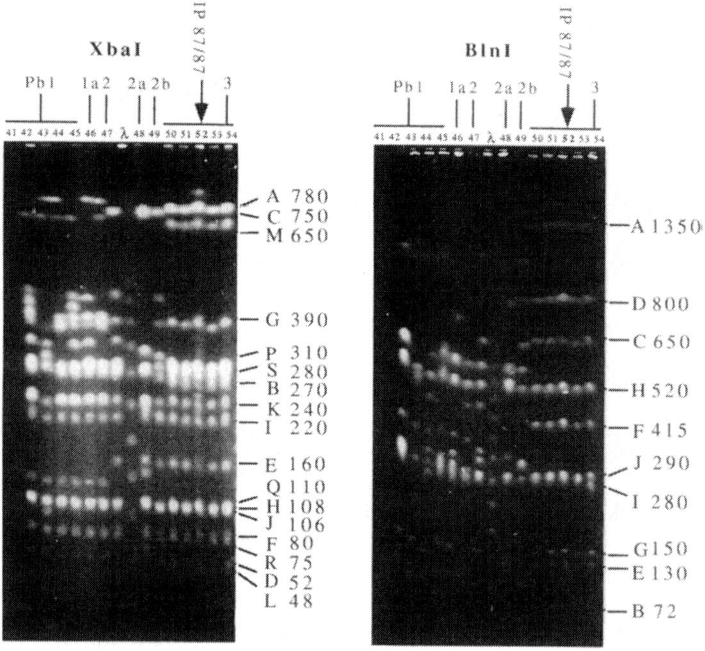

Figure 11-5. XbaI and BlnI cleavage patterns of the *S. paratyphi* B and *S. java* genomes. Lanes: 41 to 47, *S. paratyphi* B strains; 48 to 54, *S. java* strains.

CHAPTER 12

PATHOGENIC BACTERIAL SPECIES: ORIGINS AND EVOLUTION

My pursuit for the origin of pathogenic bacterial species is rooted in a desperate curiosity about whether bacteria exist in discrete phylogenetic units in nature, resembling natural species of mammals like humans or chimpanzees. Over the past decades, in search of suitable bacterial parameters to define the elusive natural species, my students and I have eventually obtained decisive evidence showing that bacteria are indeed clustered into phylogenetic groupings, separated by clear-cut genetic boundaries, and such discrete clusters are equivalent to natural species. New pathogenic bacterial species arise by acquisition of laterally transferred pathogenic traits and ensuing genomic variation events, gradually diverging from the ancestral bacteria. The genomic variation events include structural changes to regain a physical balance and nucleotide substitutions to ameliorate gene sequences toward improved functions for better chances of adaptation to the new ecologic settings. Elucidation of the origins and evolution of pathogenic bacterial species helps develop novel strategies for the control of pathogens. Such knowledge may also elicit novel thinking for developing control measures against other microbial pathogens, such as SARS-CoV-2 that caused the COVID-19 pandemic.

A long journey to define bacterial species: from morphology and biochemistry to genomics

Many bacteriologists are now inclined to believe that bacteria are phylogenetically clustered into discrete groupings, equivalent to natural species. The often asked question is: how to define bacterial species by objective parameters without any arbitrary cutoffs? Historically, investigators have used a large variety of methods to classify bacteria into taxa, from phyla down to species, by a diverse variety of parameters, such as cell shape, Gram-staining, motility, oxygen requirements, biochemical characteristics, or the mode of energy production, but most of the delineating criteria were more or less arbitrarily chosen and the bacterial species so defined often contain multiple natural phylogenetic groups. Gradually, researchers realized that natural species of bacteria should reflect biology, with a focus on ecology and evolution, analogous to the biological species concept (Mayr 1944, 1996), rather than merely phenotypic similarities. Nevertheless, when people attempted to apply the biological species concept in bacteria (Ravin 1960), it became obvious that the criteria used for the biological species definition were suitable only for sexual organisms.

Beginning from the early 1970s, genomic DNA-DNA hybridization has been used for assessing the levels of genomic similarity between bacterial strains and estimating the relatedness among the bacteria (Brenner, *et al.* 1982; Crosa, *et al.* 1973). It was an important first step to approach bacterial taxonomy from a genetic dimension. A 70% level of DNA-DNA re-association rate was set as a minimal criterion to define a group of related bacteria as a single species, and such a standard is currently still in use.

In the late 1970s and early 1980s, Dr. Carl Woese of the University of Illinois at Urbana-Champaign published a series of classic research articles on the use of small subunit ribosomal RNA (rRNA) sequences for phylogenetic studies of all life forms (Fox, *et al.* 1980; Woese 1987; Woese, *et al.* 1990). The rRNA sequences are present in all kinds of organisms, from bacteria to fungi, to protozoa, to vegetables, to trees, to mice and to humans, so they must have originated from a common remote ancestor and are indeed highly conserved during evolution. They all change overtime but very slowly and evenly, like a clock. As such, the sequence differences among bacteria would reflect their phylogenetic relationships. Based on comparative studies of rRNA sequences, Dr. Woese united the four kingdoms of eukaryotic life, *i.e.*, protozoa, fungi, plants and animals, into a higher rank, the Eukarya domain, and divided prokaryotic life into two domains – Bacteria and Archaea. The delineation of life into three rRNA-based phylogenetic domains was a revolutionary event in biology – it comes from the theory of evolution and, in turn, contributes greatly to the theory of evolution.

Ribosomes are subcellular structures for the production of proteins and consist of large and small subunits. Bacterial ribosomes contain 23S, 16S and 5S ribosomal RNA (here "S" represents the sedimentation coefficient). These RNA molecules are all highly conserved in evolution, but only 16S rRNA is used for phylogenetic analysis, because it contains reasonably rich evolutionary information for its relatively small molecule, which is *ca.* 1500 bp. On the other hand, 23S rRNA is about twice as large as 16S rRNA but the effective evolutionary information carried in the molecule is not doubled. In the 1980s-1990s, molecular sequencing was quite expensive, so nobody wanted to spend twice as much money for virtually the same amount of information. In fact, sequencing 23S rRNA was much more than double the expense of sequencing 16S rRNA. 5S rRNA is more than 10 times smaller than 16S rRNA and it carries too little information to be useful for phylogenetic analysis.

Thus, the use of 16S rRNA in bacterial systematics opened a new era of bacterial taxonomic and phylogenetic studies. In view of this, the 1984 edition of Bergey's Manual was radically updated and the book title was also changed from "Determinative" to "Systematic" Bacteriology, which became the foundation of the modern bacterial taxonomic system (Holt 1984; Holt, *et al.* 1994).

Currently, bacterial taxonomy and systematics are essentially 16S rRNA sequence-based, and the 97% 16S rRNA sequence identity and the 70% genomic DNA-DNA re-association rate together remain as the criteria for defining bacterial species (Cohan 2002; DeLong and Pace 2001; Woese 2000; Woese, *et al.* 1990). However, these criteria are not ideal, because both the 16S rRNA sequence similarity and the genomic DNA-DNA re-association rate data are continual among bacteria and, therefore, cannot resolve bacterial clusters into discrete phylogenetic units to be defined as natural species. Therefore, alternative bacterial species concepts have been proposed, such as the genomic-phylogenetic species concept (Staley 2006) and the adaptive divergence species concept (Bennett and Lenski 2007; Vos 2011). But a general consensus has not been reached to date, and the natural bacterial species concept requires truly objective and natural parameters for tests and verification.

Based on my previous work, I proposed three basic requirements for defining natural bacterial species, including close relatedness among all members of the same species, clear-cut genetic boundaries between even highly related species, and common biological features shared only by members of the same species. As the three requirements all start with the letter "C", we call these criteria the triple C (3C) requirements to define bacterial species (Tang and Liu 2012). Information supporting the triple C requirements would ultimately come from the analyses of bacterial genomes.

Natural bacterial species: a phylogenetic cluster of bacteria circumscribed by genetic boundaries

Having proposed the 3C criteria to define natural bacterial species, we would have to provide specific details about the 3Cs. The first C refers to "*close* relatedness among all members of the same species", but how close is close? The second C refers to "*clear-cut* genetic boundaries between even highly related species", but how clear is clear? And finally, the third C refers to "*common biological features* shared only by members of the same species", but since all bacteria have so many biological features, and many of the biological features may be common to phylogenetically diverse or even remote bacteria, then how could we choose the "right" common biological features for defining natural bacterial species? We tackled these 3C issues using *Salmonella* as the experimental models. The main advantages for using *Salmonella* as the models in such studies include the high genetic similarity among the pathogenically distinct lineages and the exceptionally large number of documented lineages with particular pathogenic properties.

We first focused on the first "C" issue, *i.e.*, how *close* the members of a phylogenetic group of bacteria (or a natural species) should be in genetics. We compared the genomes of a representative pair of *Salmonella* lineages, *S. typhi* and *S. typhimurium*, which are distinct pathogens, and found that these two lineages are indeed genetically very close – they share nearly 90% overall genomic similarity. Will this level of genomic similarity be said to be close? Yes, I supposed, but I predicted that, within *S. typhi* or *S. typhimurium*, the level of genomic similarity should be even significantly higher. More importantly, I gathered, there should be a *clear-cut* genetic boundary between bacteria as closely related even as *S. typhi* and *S. typhimurium*, which would lead to the characteristics of the second "C". My PhD student, Le Tang, now an associate professor at Shantou University, was extremely excited about the "how close is close and how clear is clear" issues and was especially obsessed with finding a parameter to unambiguously delineate the pair of *Salmonella* lineages into discrete phylogenetic clusters by *clear-cut* boundaries. She was leading a small team consisting of MSc and undergraduate students to approach this issue by way of wet experiments and genomic analyses (Fig. 12-1).

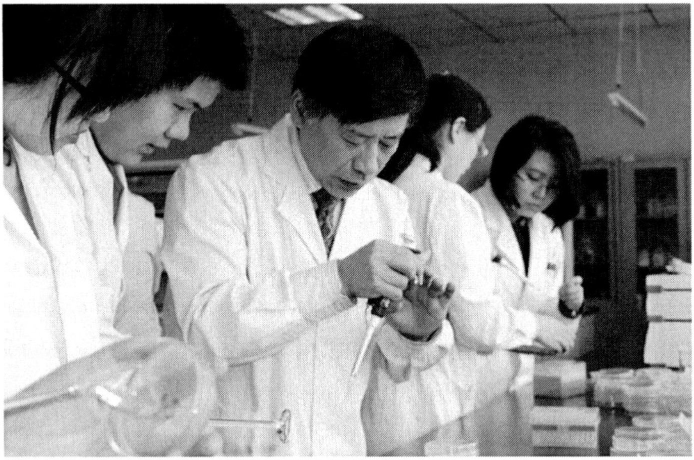

Figure 12-1. Team work to tackle the genetic boundary issue for delineating bacteria into discrete phylogenetic clusters. Dr. Le Tang, first from right.

One morning, Le rushed to my office, shouting "Dr. Liu, I found the genetic boundary!" She then showed me a figure (Fig. 12-2), pointing to the three clusters of columns: "the left and right clusters of high columns represent the *S. typhi* and *S. typhimurium* strains, respectively, and the cluster of low columns in the middle represents the mixture of *S. typhi* and *S. typhimurium* strains. The parameter I used was the ratio of common genes with zero sequence degeneracy among the strains compared". She then showed me the experimental records along with summary figures and tables.

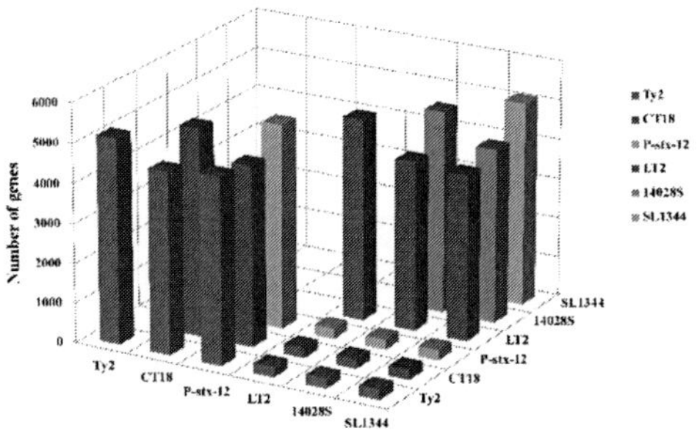

Figure 12-2. Landscape of genomic similarity among the *Salmonella* strains. *S. typhi* and *S. typhimurium* strains form two clusters of organisms with drastic genomic distinction.

I carefully examined the results and found that without doubt they could perfectly describe the first and second "Cs". Although *S. typhi* and *S. typhimurium* are highly close relatives (*e.g.*, they have about 80% of their genes in common), within *S. typhi* and *S. typhimurium*, the relatedness is even closer, with well over 90% of their genes being in common among strains within *S. typhi* or *S. typhimurium*. On the other hand, among the 4833 genes common to the analyzed *S. typhi* strains, 4463 had identical sequences or zero sequence degeneracy, a ratio of 92% (4463/4833); the ratio in *S. typhimurium* is a little lower, being 79% (3631/4616), still pretty high. In sharp contrast, among the 3927 genes common to both *S. typhi* and *S. typhimurium* strains analyzed, only 240 had zero degeneracy, a ratio of only 6%. The radical difference of zero degeneracy ratios between those inside *S. typhi* or *S. typhimurium* and that of mixed *S. typhi* and *S. typhimurium* strains demonstrates a broad window of genetic distinction or genetic boundary between *S. typhi* and *S. typhimurium.* We believe that such a genetic distinction or genetic boundary takes a certain evolutionary time to form due to the niche isolation of the two bacterial lineages (Tang, *et al.* 2013b).

The genetic boundary concept is consistent also with previous findings. For example, when we moved the Tn*10* set of insertion mutants from *S. typhimurium* to other *Salmonella* species for mapping, such as *S. enteritidis* or *S. paratyphi* B (Liu, *et al.* 1994; Liu, *et al.* 1993b), we had to first disrupt the *mutL* gene of the recipients (Liu 2007). Otherwise, P22-mediated general transduction would hardly bring *S. typhimurium* DNA to the other *Salmonella* lineages. We conducted systematic investigations to evaluate the robustness of the genetic boundary in "safeguarding" a bacterial lineage as a species and found that transduction frequencies dropped radically, even between such closely related species as *S. gallinarum* and *S. pullorum* (Fig. 12-3). *S. gallinarum* and *S. pullorum* have extremely high levels of genomic sequence identity and over 40% of their homologous genes have zero nucleotide degeneracy, with most of the remaining 60% common genes between the two *Salmonella* lineages also having greater than 95% sequence identity. Nevertheless, transduction frequencies are low between them, strongly indicating that the robust genetic boundary is formed not merely by genomic sequence differences but is also enhanced by molecular mechanisms to be elucidated (Bao, *et al.* 2014; Tang, *et al.* 2013a).

Based on these findings, I proposed a semi-closed gene pool hypothesis to further delineate the genetic boundary concept, stating that all members of a bacterial species share a common and unique gene pool (not overlapping with any other bacterial species), which, however, is leaky, allowing for limited genetic exchanges between species.

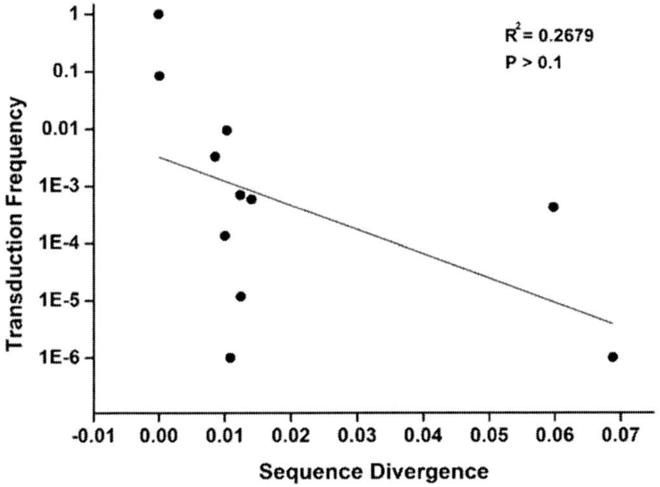

Figure 12-3. Demonstration of the existence of genetic boundaries between bacterial species by a radical drop of DNA exchange efficiencies. This figure shows transduction frequencies against levels of relatedness among the *Salmonella* strains: a subtle drop in sequence similarity would cause a radical drop in transduction frequency.

This kind of genetic boundary has also been detected in other bacteria (Tang, *et al.* 2013a), but its broader applicability needs further work to prove or disprove.

For the last "C", *i.e.*, "*common biological features* shared only by members of the same species", we picked pathogenesis for comparison between *S. typhi* and *S. typhimurium*, both infecting humans, with the former eliciting typhoid fever and the latter causing gastroenteritis. Different bacterial pathogens all have different pathogenic properties. Therefore, even if the first and second "Cs" (close relatedness and clear-cut genetic boundary, respectively) could possibly be generalized for defining natural bacterial species, the last "C" (common biological features) would have to be individualized for the bacteria in question.

Origins of novel bacterial pathogens and evolution of nascent pathogenic species: trigger and adaptive evolution

So, based on the 3Cs criteria, we think it reasonable to define *S. typhi* and *S. typhimurium* as individual natural pathogenic species. Previous findings by other methods, including physical mapping (Liu and Sanderson 1995c, d), multi-locus enzyme electrophoresis (Selander, *et al.* 1986), whole genome sequencing (Cooke, *et al.* 2008; Deng, *et al.* 2003; Holt, *et al.* 2008; McClelland, *et al.* 2001; Parkhill, *et al.* 2001), and pathogenesis studies (Feng, *et al.* 2011; Parry, *et al.* 2002; Roumagnac, *et al.* 2006), also similarly demonstrate tight genetic relatedness among strains within the same *Salmonella* lineages and clear-cut genomic as well as pathogenic distinctions between even very closely related *Salmonella* lineages, such as *S. typhi* and *S. typhimurium*, but, for the first time, the zero degeneracy parameter provides decisive and natural criteria.

We have obtained consistent results and conclusions in many additional *Salmonella* lineages, including *S. paratyphi* A (Liu and Sanderson 1995a; McClelland, *et al.* 2004), *S. paratyphi* C (Liu, *et al.* 2009; Liu, *et al.* 2007), *S. choleraesuis* (Chiu, *et al.* 2005), and *S. gallinarum* (Feng, *et al.* 2013; Thomson, *et al.* 2008; Wu, *et al.* 2005). Representative strains across all eight *Salmonella* subgroups have a common overall genomic framework (Liu, *et al.* 1999), but individual lineages all have unique sets of lineage-specific insertions (laterally acquired DNA) and nucleotide ameliorating patterns (Tang, *et al.* 2014; Tang, *et al.* 2017a; Tang, *et al.* 2017b).

According to the Adopt-Adapt Model of bacterial speciation (Liu, *et al.* 2002a; Liu and Sanderson 1995d), the acquisition of a special set of laterally transferred DNA may divert the bacteria in a new evolutionary direction, possibly initiating the speciation process as a trigger. Such acquired DNA segments carry novel genes that encode particular biological (*e.g.*, pathogenic) functions, which may help the bacteria fit into a potential niche.

However, all genetically distinct bacterial lineages have their unique sets of laterally transferred DNA segments and it is, in most cases, extremely difficult to determine which of them might be the "speciating" DNA set that may eventually have led to the formation of a new bacterial species. We once speculated that the pathogenicity island SPI7 might be the "speciating" DNA insertion of *S. typhi* and many investigators also pay high attention to SPI7 (Liu and Sanderson 1995b, d; Parry, *et al.* 2002). However, we found that many isolates of *S. typhi* do not have SPI7 (Kothapalli, *et al.* 2005). It is not known whether such *S. typhi* isolates never had SPI7 or lost it during the isolation or stock processes. Experimentally evaluating the pathogenic roles of SPI7 in typhoid by using animal models is impossible, as *S. typhi* do not infect any experimental animals. Fortunately, another human typhoidal pathogen, *S. paratyphi* C, carries a shorter version of SPI7 and this human typhoidal *Salmonella* lineage can also infect other animals, such as mice (Zou, *et al.* 2010). Therefore, a simple design of animal experiments, such as infecting inbred mice with *S. paratyphi* C strains, with or without SPI7, may unambiguously determine the role of SPI7 in the infection of a host. However, to be scientifically valid, the pair of *S. paratyphi* C strains for the experiments, one with and one without SPI7, will have to be isogenic. Such a designed experimental investigation is anticipated to provide key information for the elucidation of the origins of pathogenic bacteria. A preliminary work using a prophage, SPC-P1, incorporated into the genome of *S. paratyphi* C as the experimental "speciating" DNA, with the wildtype strain without SPC-P1 as an isogenic control, demonstrated that SPC-P1 significantly elevated the bacterial virulence to mice (Zou, *et al.* 2010). SPC-P1 is an intact phage, which can be readily isolated from a lysogenized *S. paratyphi* C strain and used to infect the *S. paratyphi* C strains that do not carry it. This method could be generalized to other potential speciating DNA segments for evaluating their roles in the pathogenicity of the bacteria.

If the incorporated new genes bring in novel pathogenic traits and, in the meantime, stay stably in the bacterial genome, rather than hit and run, it would be very possible that the bacteria would move to a new niche, such as becoming a nascent pathogen to dwell in a new ecological environment, broadening the host range or causing different infections (at different ecologic or anatomic sites). If so, the bacteria carrying the newly acquired genes will inevitably be under different selection pressures and may have different spontaneous variations accumulated over time for better fitness. And, it is the accumulation of the spontaneous variations that makes the offspring genetically distinct from the ancestor and such distinction is natural and digitally documentable. There are two excellent examples to illustrate such postulated evolutionary scenarios.

The first is the divergent evolution of *S. paratyphi* C and *S. choleraesuis*, two very closely related *Salmonella* lineages (Fig. 12-4), with the former causing paratyphoid fever in humans and the latter eliciting systemic infection in hogs. They diverged from a common ancestor not long ago but have accumulated more than a thousand nucleotide substitutions, demonstrating the necessity of genomic variations for a nascent bacterial pathogen to become fit during the struggle for adaptation to a new niche (Liu, *et al.* 2009).

The second, and very well-known example, comes from the comparison of *S. gallinarum* and *S. pullorum*, which are both adapted to fowl but cause different systemic infections, with the former causing typhoid-like disease and the latter causing dysentery-like disease. This pair of *Salmonella* pathogens have often been treated as different biovars, or pathovars, of the same serotype （1,9,12： -： -）, although they have accumulated distinct nucleotide variations, as reflected by the different CTAG tetranucleotide decaying patterns (Tang, *et al.* 2014; Tang, *et al.* 2017a; Tang, *et al.* 2017b).

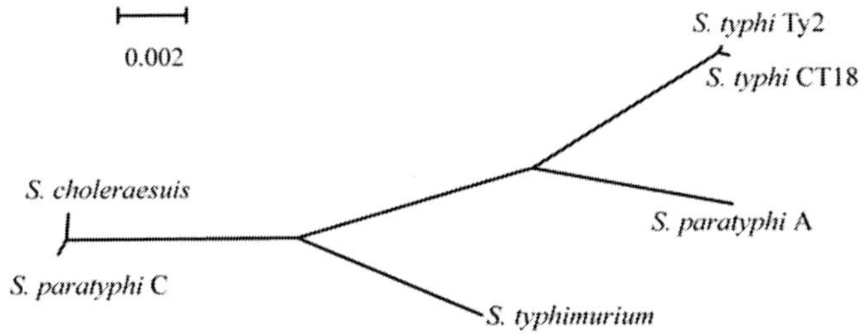

Figure 12-4. Phylogenetic tree for the representative *Salmonella* lineages. This tree is based on whole-genome sequences. *S. paratyphi* C and *S. choleraesuis* have diverged even more recently than *S. typhi* and *S. paratyphi* A, the latter pair of *Salmonella* pathogens being well known for their fairly recent divergence and genomic relatedness.

Undoubtedly, different nucleotide variations or amelioration patterns are the result of bacterial adaptation following their divergence from a common ancestor, reflecting the differential advantages of different codon choices for better fitness. Once a set of selected nucleotide variations bring in adaptive advantages, however obvious or subtle they might be, they will be retained by the bacteria; bacterial cells with such advantages will increase in population size and eventually outcompete other members of the same species to become dominant. Therefore, systematic analysis of nucleotide differences between *S. paratyphi* C and *S. choleraesuis*, as well as between *S. gallinarum* and *S. pullorum*, by molecular and animal experiments, in addition to bioinformatics predictions, is expected to give revealing insights into the genomic streamlining process of bacterial pathogenic speciation.

AFTERWORD

All lines of evidence from previous studies support a general scenario of pathogenic bacterial emergence and evolution – originating from lateral acquisition of pathogenic traits and speciating by adaptive genomic variations. The main genomic variations include structural rearrangements for rebalancing and nucleotide sequence amelioration for better fitness.

During the whole process of pursuing the origins of pathogenic bacterial species, I have never thought pathogenic bacteria to be life and death enemies. They are natural creatures and have an equal right to life like the author and readers of this book. Eliciting diseases in us is not their intention – they just strive for a better life, such as richer nutritious resources or safer shelters. When bacteria, with or without pathogenic traits, encounter mankind for the first time, conflicts may hardly be avoidable, which may eventually lead to one of three consequences: 1, harmony and co-evolution, like most of the extant bacteria in the human intestinal microbiota; 2, peaceful avoidance, and no further direct contact, like Cyanobacteria, which are important for life on Earth but do not need humans as a shelter, nor are they needed by humans for physiology; and 3, invasion and anti-invasion head-on confrontations, like the pathogenic bacteria that we face nowadays, which are innocently trying to explore the human body for a new habitat without purposely intending to hurt the human host. Eventually, the third consequence may be transformed to docility or the domestication of the pathogenic bacteria by the human body, but also, possibly, to everlasting invasion and anti-invasion battles between humans and the pathogenic bacteria. In the latter case, an arms race between the two parties may keep increasing in intensity until one side is defeated, and the defeated side is often the human host, such as in cases of antibiotic abuse leading to multidrug resistance.

Therefore, pathogenic bacteria should not be regarded as life or death enemies in the first place but, rather, they should be made less pathogenic or minimally infectious, which can be achieved by a simple kitchen endeavor – more food materials rich in lignans for your next meals. This simple kitchen endeavor is based on *the concept of elevating relative infectious doses of pathogens by harnessing the intestinal microbiota*.

All infectious agents have a natural infectious dose, or size of inoculum (*i. e.*, the number of microbial cells or particles entering the host body), below which a pathogen is hardly capable of establishing infections in its host. For example, if *S. typhi* needs an inoculum of ten thousand cells to elicit typhoid fever in the human host, an intake of a hundred *S. typhi* cells is far from enough to establish an infection and will readily be conquered by the host. Microbial infectious doses are the consequences of human-pathogen interactions over long evolutionary periods. However, the minimal sizes of such naturally formed infectious doses could be raised by elevating the overall anti-infection resistance of the host. Such overall resistance includes, but is not limited to, immunity, as many other factors are also very important. It is a well-known fact that neuro-humoral factors such as mental stress prior to an unprepared for exam, and lower functionality of other systems, may significantly weaken the general resistance against microbial infections – the student may have exaggeratedly swollen gums with unbearable toothache during the pre- and post-exam periods due to an infection of the gum by some normally not so aggressive bacteria. Conversely, good mood, sufficient nutrition, normal digestion and metabolism of food, healthy cardiovascular and renal system functions, *etc.*, can all greatly enhance anti-infection resistance. However, among so many factors influencing human resistance against microbial infections, intestinal microbiota plays a key and outstanding role. Our recent work demonstrates that dietary lignans can effectively ameliorate the population structure and functionality of the intestinal microbiota, which, in turn, would significantly enhance human resistance against infectious and malignant diseases (Wu, *et al.* 2021). In animal experiments, mice receiving dietary lignans had higher resistance by two orders of magnitude against *Salmonella* infection than the control mice (Liu team, unpublished work).

We anticipate the generalization of the concept of elevating relative infectious doses of pathogens also to a broader range of microbes such as viruses. SARS-CoV-2 is highly transmissible and extremely infectious, but people exposed to the COVID-19 agent may not necessarily be infected by the virus. Many factors may contribute to the high resistance of these uninfected people, but our work indicates that the intestinal microbiota status is highly relevant. Patients with various malignancies have serious intestinal microbiota dysbiosis (Zhuang, *et al.* 2019), which can be ameliorated by ceasing antimicrobial abuses and ingesting lignan-rich diets. The practice of harnessing microbiota through increased lignan ingestion, by most members of the public, may significantly elevate the general resistance of the community to microbial infections and form effective herd-resistance against pandemics.

I sincerely wish that a life and death arms race between mankind and microbes may be minimized in the future. Instead, avoidance of potentially pathogenic microbes should be maximized by minimizing unnecessary contact and elevating herd resistance through well harnessed intestinal microbiota, so that our children will live safer and happier lives.

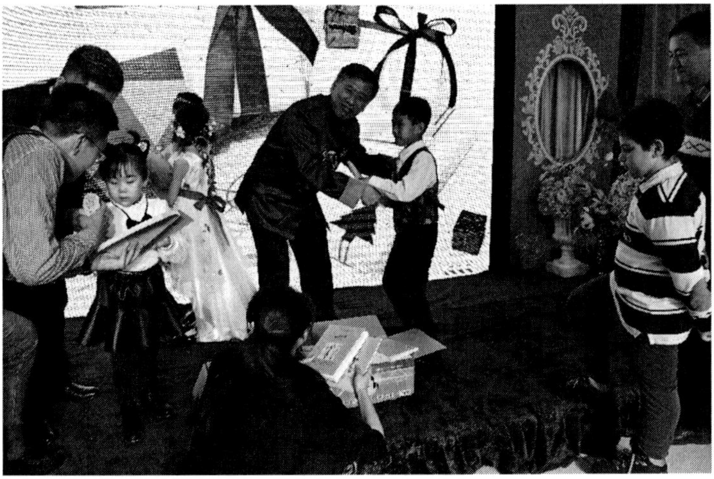

Annual New Year Party to distribute tale books to children as gifts

BIBLIOGRAPHY

The author is affiliated with Harbin Medical University, China, and University of Calgary, Canada. His career with microbes began in 1971 at the clinical laboratory of Fujin Central Hospital. In 1978, he was admitted to Harbin Medical University and graduated with a medical degree in 1982. He conducted PhD studies from 1985 to 1990 at Gifu University, Japan. After graduation, he moved to University of Calgary to work, initially as a postdoctoral fellow and then as a PI. Remaining associated with University of Calgary, he worked at Peking University from 2002 to 2008 and at Harbin Medical University since 2008. His publications include 160 original papers and 16 books or book chapters in English, Chinese or Japanese. His research is mostly on microbes, with *Salmonella* as primary models for genomic evolution and pathogenesis studies. He advocates non-killing measures to control microbial pathogens. His current research is focused on intestinal microbiota.

The following 81 pages are the first pages of representative papers.

INFECTION AND IMMUNITY, Aug. 1988, p. 1967–1973 Vol. 56, No. 8
0019-9567/88/081967-07$02.00/0
Copyright © 1988, American Society for Microbiology

Intact Motility as a *Salmonella typhi* Invasion-Related Factor

SHU-LIN LIU, TAKAYUKI EZAKI,* HIROAKI MIURA, KOUJI MATSUI, AND EIKO YABUUCHI
Department of Microbiology, Gifu University School of Medicine, 40 Tsukasa-machi, Gifu 500, Japan

Received 6 February 1988/Accepted 12 April 1988

Invasiveness of *Salmonella typhi* was investigated. At first, we introduced Tn*5* into the chromosome of a wild-type *S. typhi* strain, GIFU 10007, and screened the independent Tn*5* insertion mutants for noninvasive (Inv^-) strains. During the first half of this work, we obtained 4 Inv^- strains from 1,338 independent Tn*5* mutants. The four were either nonflagellate (Fla^-), nonmotile (Mot^-), or nonchemotactic (Che^-). We then isolated more Fla^-, Mot^-, or Che^- mutants and examined the invasiveness of these mutants. Sixty-three spontaneous or Tn*5* insertion motility mutants, i.e., Fla^-, Mot^-, or Che^-, were independently isolated from the wild-type strain GIFU 10007; all of them were noninvasive. Motile revertants isolated from some of these mutants showed the same invasiveness as the parent strain. P22-mediated transductional crosses were carried out between some of the motility mutants (as the recipients) and the Fla^- reference strains of *S. typhimurium* with known deletion sites on the genome (as the donors). The mutational sites of the *S. typhi* mutants were assigned almost evenly to the three flagellar gene regions (regions I, II, and III) of *S. typhimurium*. The invasiveness of the motile recombinants obtained from the transduction assays was examined. The restoration of intact motility resulted in the restoration of invasiveness. Thus, we conclude that intact motility is an invasion-related factor of *S. typhi*. The relationship of Vi antigen to the invasiveness of *S. typhi* was also studied. Vi-negative mutants with intact motility remained invasive, whereas all 63 Inv^- spontaneous or Tn*5* mutants were Vi positive. Therefore, Vi antigen was not related to the invasiveness of *S. typhi*.

One crucial step in the pathogenesis of enteroinvasive bacteria is the ability of the bacteria to penetrate the epithelial cell border of the intestinal mucosa and multiply within the epithelial cells. Extensive studies have been made employing cell culture techniques to approach the invasiveness of enteroinvasive bacteria such as *Shigella* spp. (10, 14, 15, 19, 27, 29, 30), *Salmonella* spp. (11–13, 18, 21), invasive *Escherichia coli* (2, 4, 24, 28), and *Yersinia enterocolitica* (34); a strong correlation between in vivo virulence and invasiveness in HeLa or HEp-2 cell cultures has been revealed. The invasiveness of most of the bacteria studied to date is suggested to be associated with plasmids.

The invasive mechanism of bacteria without plasmids, such as *Salmonella typhi*, on the other hand, has been poorly documented. *S. typhi* is so peculiar that among the ca. 2,000 genetically closely related serovars in the genus *Salmonella* (26), only *S. typhi* and a few others (e.g., *S. paratyphi* A, etc.) have the ability to elicit typhoid fever in human beings by invading the epithelial cells of the intestine. Vi antigen has been thought to be an important factor in the pathogenicity of *S. typhi*. In our previous (35) and present studies, however, this factor was shown to have nothing to do with the invasiveness of *S. typhi*. To identify the invasive factor(s) of *S. typhi*, we introduced Tn*5* into the chromosome of *S. typhi* and screened independent Tn*5* insertion mutants for noninvasive (Inv^-) strains. The first half of this work told us that invasiveness was somehow related to intact motility of the bacteria. So we isolated more motility mutants, i.e., nonflagellate (Fla^-), nonmotile (Mot^-), or nonchemotactic (Che^-) mutants, and investigated the relationship between the invasiveness and the intact motility of these mutants. The results presented in this report demonstrate that intact motility is an invasion-related factor of *S. typhi*. The mutational sites of some of the Inv^- mutants were mapped; they were almost evenly distributed over all of the three regions containing the flagellar genes of *Salmonella typhimurium*.

* Corresponding author.

MATERIALS AND METHODS

Bacterial and bacteriophage strains. The clinical isolates and NCTC strains and their Vi-antigen negative (Vi^-) derivatives of *S. typhi* used in this study and the deletion strains of *S. typhimurium* used for gene mapping are listed in Table 1. SJW 7371 and SJW1518 have deletions which together cover region I of *S. typhimurium* flagellar genes; deletions of SJW 1399 and SJW 1368 and deletions of SJW 1411, SJW 1572, and SJW 1556 cover regions II and III, respectively. The flagellotropic bacteriophage χ (25) was used to select Fla^- or Mot^- strains. Bacteriophage P22 was used in transduction experiments.

Media. Bacteria were grown in heart infusion (HI) broth (Difco Laboratories, Detroit, Mich.), in L broth (5 g of NaCl, 10 g of Bacto-Peptone [Difco], 5 g of yeast extract, and 1 g of glucose for 1 liter), on HI agar (Difco), or on MacConkey agar (Eiken Chemical Co., Tokyo). When required, media were supplemented with kanamycin, (50 μg/ml), nalidixic acid (50 μg/ml), or ampicillin (100 μg/ml). For the isolation and identification of Fla^-, Mot^-, and Che^- mutants, plates of Gard semisolid agar (9) or soft nutrient gelatin agar (NGA) (36) were employed.

Cell lines. HeLa S3 (ATCC certified cell line 2.2) or Intestine 407 (ATCC certified cell line 6) cells were obtained from Dainippon Seiyaku Co., Osaka, and cultured in Dulbecco modified Eagle medium (DMEM; Nissui Seiyaku Co., Tokyo) supplemented with 10% fetal calf serum (Hyclone Laboratories, Logan, Utah) and 2 mM L-glutamine. Dulbecco phosphate-buffered saline without calcium chloride and magnesium chloride (Nissui Seiyaku Co., Tokyo) was used to wash the cells.

Transpositional mutagenesis. GIFU 10793, a Nal^r derivative of GIFU 10007 containing the plasmid pCHR81*rep*(Ts)::Tn*5* (31) (Table 1), was streaked onto a MacConkey agar plate containing kanamycin (KM-MacConkey) and incubated at

JOURNAL OF BACTERIOLOGY, Mar. 1992, p. 1662–1672 Vol. 174, No. 5
0021-9193/92/051662-11$02.00/0
Copyright © 1992, American Society for Microbiology

A Physical Map of the *Salmonella typhimurium* LT2 Genome Made by Using *Xba*I Analysis

SHU-LIN LIU AND KENNETH E. SANDERSON*

Salmonella Genetic Stock Centre, Department of Biological Sciences, University of Calgary, Calgary, Alberta, Canada T2N 1N4

Received 28 October 1991/Accepted 20 December 1991

XbaI digestion and pulsed-field gel electrophoresis of the genome of *Salmonella typhimurium* LT2 yields 24 fragments: 23 fragments (total size, 4,807 kb) are from the chromosome, and one fragment (90 kb) is from the virulence plasmid pSLT. Some of the 23 fragments from the chromosome were located on the linkage map by the use of cloned genes as probes and by analysis of strains which gain an *Xba*I site from the insertion of Tn*10*. Twenty-one of the fragments were arranged as a circular physical map by the use of linking probes from a set of 41 lysogens in which Mu*d*-P22 was stably inserted at different sites of the chromosome; fragment W (6.6 kb) and fragment X (6.4 kb) were not located on the physical map. *Xba*I digestion of strains with Tn*10* insertions allowed the physical locations of specific genes along the chromosome to be determined on the basis of analysis of new-fragment sizes. There is good agreement between the order of genes on the linkage map, which is based primarily on P22 joint transduction and F-mediated conjugation, and the physical map, but there are frequently differences in the length of the interval from the two methods. These analyses allowed the measurement of the amount of DNA packaged in phage P22 heads by Mu*d*-P22 lysogens following induction; this varies from ca. 100 kb (2 min) to 240 kb (5 min) in different parts of the chromosome.

The genus *Salmonella* belongs to the large, medically important eubacterial family *Enterobacteriaceae*. It is closely related to *Escherichia coli* (21, 24), but in *E. coli*, most strains are harmless commensals of mammals, whereas the salmonellae are ubiquitous pathogens of both warm-blooded and cold-blooded vertebrates. Classified originally by somatic and flagellar antigens into many serotypes by the Kauffmann-White schemes, salmonellae have recently been separated by electrophoretic type into numerous clones (4, 33). Extensive studies of *Salmonella typhimurium* done since the 1950s have yielded much genetic, biochemical, and physiologic data, summarized recently in the volumes edited by Neidhardt et al. (20). The seventh edition of the linkage map located 680 genes on a circular map (31).

Pulsed-field gel electrophoresis (PFGE) is a well-established procedure for the analysis of large DNA fragments. Its use led to the establishment of physical maps for the chromosomes of *E. coli* K-12 (34, 35) and several other bacteria. PFGE resolves the restriction fragments from the chromosome, and the sum of the sizes reveals the size of the genome. Several methods have been used to arrange these fragments into a physical map, which is usually circular. In some cases, as in *E. coli* K-12, an extensive linkage map based on genetic data was already available (2), in which case probing with known cloned genes, analysis of strains with prophages or transposons at known locations, or analysis of strains with known chromosomal rearrangements has been used (34). But the linkage map may be rudimentary or completely unknown, in which case other methods are needed. Two-dimensional pulsed-field gels, including the use of partial digests, resolved the 780-kb map of *Mycoplasma mobile* (3) and the 5.9-Mb map of *Pseudomonas aeruginosa* (25). The 1,900-kb map of *Haemophilus influenzae* was resolved by probing fragments from restriction with one enzyme with fragments from another enzyme isolated following PFGE (15). Similar methods, as well as analysis of strains with transposon insertions, were used by Chen et al. (8) to construct the 9.5-Mb map of *Myxococcus xanthus*.

Since a physical map of the genome of *S. typhimurium* LT2 to test and to extend the utility of the linkage map has not been reported, we undertook a study using PFGE. Previous PFGE data estimated the genome as ca. 5 Mb (11). *Not*I and *Spe*I digest the chromosome of *S. typhimurium* LT2 into ca. 30 and 50 fragments, respectively—too many for convenient analysis (11, 22). According to our data, the chromosome comprises 23 *Xba*I fragments of an estimated size of 4,807 kb plus a 90-kb fragment representing plasmid pSLT. Some of the chromosomal fragments were arranged into a physical map by methods dependent on the linkage map; the locations of known Tn*10* insertions were identifiable because Tn*10* has an *Xba*I site, and cloned genes were used to probe *Xba*I digests. The entire set of fragments was arranged in a circular restriction map by using linking probes from the Mu*d*-P22 "locked-in" prophages developed by Youderian et al. (45) and assembled as a set by Benson and Goldman (6). In addition, we mapped the site of Tn*10* insertions along a restriction fragment through analysis of the size of *Xba*I fragments. An accompanying paper (43) gives a *Bln*I map of the *S. typhimurium* LT2 genome, and another paper describes the set of Mu*d*-P22 lysogens and their use in genetic mapping (6).

MATERIALS AND METHODS

Bacterial strains, phages, plasmids, and cultivation conditions. The strains of *S. typhimurium* LT2 and the plasmids used in the study were obtained from numerous sources and are maintained in the Salmonella Genetic Stock Centre (SGSC). Most of the strains used are listed in Tables 2 and 3. The reference wild-type LT2 was obtained from J. Lederberg as part of a set of the 22 *S. typhimurium* strains isolated by Lilleengen (16) and used by Zinder and Lederberg (46) in their transduction studies. Luria-Bertani (LB) medium (10 g

* Corresponding author.

Proc. Natl. Acad. Sci. USA
Vol. 90, pp. 6874–6878, July 1993
Genetics

Genomic mapping with I-*Ceu* I, an intron-encoded endonuclease specific for genes for ribosomal RNA, in *Salmonella* spp., *Escherichia coli*, and other bacteria

SHU-LIN LIU, ANDREW HESSEL, AND KENNETH E. SANDERSON

Salmonella Genetic Stock Centre, Department of Biological Sciences, University of Calgary, Calgary, AB, Canada T2N 1N4

Communicated by John R. Roth, February 23, 1993 (received for review December 1, 1992)

ABSTRACT Construction of physical maps of genomes by pulsed-field gel electrophoresis requires enzymes which cut the genome into an analyzable number of fragments; most produce too many fragments. The enzyme I-*Ceu* I, encoded by a mobile intron in the chloroplast 23S ribosomal RNA (*rrl*) gene of *Chlamydomonas eugametos*, cuts a 26-bp site in the *rrl* gene. This enzyme digests DNA of *Salmonella typhimurium* at seven sites, each corresponding to one of the *rrl* genes of the *rrn* operons, but at no other site. These seven fragments were located on the previously determined *Xba* I physical map, and the I-*Ceu* I sites, and thus the *rrn* genes of *S. typhimurium*, were mapped on the 4800-kb chromosome. *Escherichia coli* K-12 also yields seven fragments of sizes similar to those of *S. typhimurium*, indicating conservation of *rrn* genes and their location, and a chromosome size of 4600 kb. The sizes of the *E. coli* fragments are close to the size predicted from restriction maps and nucleotide sequence. The I-*Ceu* I maps of *Salmonella enteritidis*, *Salmonella paratyphi* A, B, C, and *Salmonella typhi* were deduced after digesting genomic DNA with I-*Ceu* I and probing with DNA of *S. typhimurium*; the data indicated strong conservation of *rrn* gene number and position and genome sizes up to 4950 kb. Digestion of DNA of other bacteria (species of *Haemophilus*, *Neisseria*, *Proteus*, and *Pasteurella*) suggested that only *rrn* genes are cut in all these species. I-*Ceu* I digestion followed by pulsed-field gel electrophoresis is a powerful tool for determining genome structure and evolution.

Pulsed-field gel electrophoresis (PFGE) has had a dramatic impact on analysis of physical maps of genomes. In bacteria the circular genetic elements must be cut into linear fragments for physical analysis. Most restriction enzymes with 6-bp specificity have many sites and cut the chromosome into too many fragments for analysis. The sequence CTAG is infrequent in the enteric bacteria (1), and the following restriction enzymes which have this sequence in a 6-bp site have been used in genome analysis: *Xba* I (TCTAGA) in *Escherichia coli* (2) and *Salmonella typhimurium* (3); *Bln* I (= *Avr* II) (CCTAGG) in *E. coli* (2, 4) and *S. typhimurium* (5); *Nhe* I (GCTAGC) in *Neisseria gonorrhoeae* (6); and *Spe* I (ACTAGT) in *Myxococcus xanthus* (7). In our search for other suitable enzymes we tested the enzyme I-*Ceu* I, which is a double-strand endonuclease encoded by a group I intron in the large subunit rRNA gene of *Chlamydomonas eugametos* (8, 9); the intron is called CeLSU.5, and the enzyme is designated I-*Ceu* I (the "I" refers to intron). The endonuclease cuts DNA in the 26-bp sequence

↓
TAACTATAACGGTCCTAAGGTAGCGA
ATTGATATTGCCAGGATTCCATCGCT
↑

at the points marked by arrows, leaving a 3′ overhang. The minimum number of bases required in the site is not known, but it is less than 26 bp (9). Since rRNA-determining genes are very highly conserved (10), the enzyme would be expected to cleave the DNA of a wide range of organisms in the rRNA genes. *E. coli* cells carrying a plasmid expressing the I-*Ceu* I protein had reduced growth rate; since the I-*Ceu* I site is present in known sequence in the *rrnB* gene of *E. coli*, Gauthier *et al.* (8) recognized that the *rrn* genes might be cut by I-*Ceu* I.

We show that I-*Ceu* I (hereafter called *Ceu* I) cuts the DNA of enteric bacteria such as *S. typhimurium*, *E. coli* K-12, and other serovars of *Salmonella* at seven sites. The locations of these sites are consistent with the conclusion that a site in each rRNA gene, and no other site, is cleaved. DNA of other species of Gram-negative bacteria is cleaved in a similar fashion. Because of conservation of numbers and locations of *Ceu* I sites, based on conservation of numbers and locations of rRNA genes in the genomes of bacterial species, analysis with *Ceu* I will be valuable for genome comparisons and for comparing genes for rRNA synthesis.

MATERIALS AND METHODS

Bacterial Strains, Phages, Plasmids, and Cultivation Conditions. *S. typhimurium* LT2 and the plasmids were from numerous sources and are maintained at the Salmonella Genetic Stock Centre (SGSC) at the University of Calgary. The following, some described earlier (11), were from R. K. Selander (Pennsylvania State University, University Park): *Salmonella dublin* (RKS 4699); *Salmonella gallinarum* (RKS 4994); *Salmonella enteritidis* (RKS 53); *Salmonella paratyphi* A (RKS 4993); *S. paratyphi* B (RKS 3605); and *S. paratyphi* C (RKS 4587). *Salmonella typhi* (Ty 514), from B. A. D. Stocker (Stanford University, CA), is an *aroA* Δ407 derivative of *S. typhi* Ty2 (12). *Neisseria meningitidis* B16B6, *Haemophilus influenzae* b13, and *Pasteurella haemolytica* h186 were from Anthony Schryvers (University of Calgary). *Proteus morganii* and *Proteus rettgeri* were obtained from Helen Ross (University of Calgary).

The plasmids carrying genes of *S. typhimurium* which were used as probes for *Ceu* I fragments were *Ceu* I-A, pSX62 (from Eric Vimr, University of Illinois, Urbana); *Ceu* I-B, pGS137 (*metC*); *Ceu* I-D, pGS41 (*metE*); *Ceu* I-E (*metBJ*); and *Ceu* I-G (*metH*) (the last four probes were from G. Stauffer, University of Iowa, Iowa City).

Luria–Bertani (LB) medium (10 g of tryptone, 5 g of yeast extract, 10 g of NaCl, 3.5 ml of 1 M NaOH) was used for cultivation of all strains; solid medium also contained 1.5% agar. Tetracycline, ampicillin, and chloramphenicol were used at 20, 100, and 40 μg/ml, respectively. Strains were maintained in 15% (vol/vol) glycerol at −70°C, and a single colony was isolated prior to use.

The publication costs of this article were defrayed in part by page charge payment. This article must therefore be hereby marked "*advertisement*" in accordance with 18 U.S.C. §1734 solely to indicate this fact.

Abbreviation: PFGE, pulsed-field gel electrophoresis.

JOURNAL OF BACTERIOLOGY, July 1993, p. 4104–4120 Vol. 175, No. 13
0021-9193/93/134104-17$02.00/0
Copyright © 1993, American Society for Microbiology

The *Xba*I-*Bln*I-*Ceu*I Genomic Cleavage Map of *Salmonella typhimurium* LT2 Determined by Double Digestion, End Labelling, and Pulsed-Field Gel Electrophoresis

SHU-LIN LIU, ANDREW HESSEL, AND KENNETH E. SANDERSON*

Department of Biological Sciences, University of Calgary, Calgary, Alberta, Canada T2N 1N4

Received 10 February 1993/Accepted 25 April 1993

Endonuclease digestion of the 4,800-kb chromosome of *Salmonella typhimurium* LT2 yielded 24 *Xba*I fragments, 12 *Bln*I fragments, and 7 *Ceu*I fragments, which were separated by pulsed-field gel electrophoresis. The 90-kb plasmid pSLT has one *Xba*I site and one *Bln*I site. The locations of the fragments around the circular chromosome and of the digestion sites of the different endonucleases with respect to each other were determined by excision of agarose blocks containing fragments from single digestion, redigestion with a second enzyme, end labelling with ^{32}P by using T7 DNA polymerase, reelectrophoresis, and autoradiography. Forty-three cleavage sites were established on the chromosome, and the fragments and cleavage sites were designated in alphabetical order and numerical order, respectively, around the chromosome. One hundred nine independent Tn*10* insertions previously mapped by genetic means were located by pulsed-field gel electrophoresis on the basis of the presence of *Xba*I and *Bln*I sites in Tn*10*. The genomic cleavage map was divided into 100 units called centisomes; the endonuclease cleavage sites and the genes defined by the positions of Tn*10* insertions were located by centisome around the map. There is very good agreement between the genomic cleavage map, defined in centisomes, and the linkage map, defined in minutes. All seven rRNA genes were located on the map; all have the *Ceu*I digestion site, all four with the tRNA gene for glutamate have the *Xba*I and the *Bln*I sites, but only four of the seven have the *Bln*I site in the 16S rRNA (*rrs*) gene. Their inferred orientation of transcription is the same as in *Escherichia coli*. A rearrangement of the *rrnB* and *rrnD* genes with respect to the arrangement in *E. coli*, observed earlier by others, has been confirmed. The sites for all three enzymes in the *rrn* genes are strongly conserved compared with those in *E. coli*, but the *Xba*I and *Bln*I sites outside the *rrn* genes show very little conservation.

The introduction of pulsed-field gel electrophoresis (PFGE) techniques for separating large DNA molecules has had a large impact on the study of genetics of both prokaryotic and eukaryotic organisms. PFGE overcomes the size limitations of conventional electrophoresis by forcing DNA molecules to reorient periodically from one electric field direction to another (51). Physical maps have been established for the chromosomes of several bacteria, and the methods are also being used in studying eukaryotic chromosomes. In studies of the covalently closed circular genomes of bacteria, genomic DNA embedded in agarose is digested with an endonuclease which cuts the chromosome into a limited number of fragments, and then these fragments are separated by PFGE.

Several methods have been used to arrange these fragments into a physical map. For *Escherichia coli* K-12, for which an extensive linkage map was already known (1), the restriction map was based on probing with known cloned genes, analysis of strains with prophages or transposons at known locations, partial digestion and DNA probing, and analyses of strains with chromosomal rearrangements (52). When a linkage map was not available, other methods were used. Two-dimensional pulsed-field gels were used for *Mycoplasma mobile* (2) and *Pseudomonas aeruginosa* (39). Probing fragments from digestion with one enzyme with fragments from another enzyme, isolated following PFGE, was used to derive the maps of *Haemophilus influenzae* (20) and of *Myxococcus xanthus* (9).

The genus *Salmonella* belongs to the large eubacterial family *Enterobacteriaceae*. It was originally classified into many serotypes by use of somatic and flagellar antigens to develope the Kauffmann-White classification, but more recently all strains have been proven to belong to the same DNA reassociation group, representing one or a very small number of species (10, 24). The salmonellae have recently been separated by electrophoretic typing into numerous clones (47). Studies on the cellular and molecular biology of *Salmonella typhimurium* have been summarized in volumes edited by Neidhardt et al. (33). The use of the name *Salmonella enterica* serovar typhimurium rather than the name *S. typhimurium* is gaining wide acceptance and is a better indicator of relationships within this group, but we use the traditional name *S. typhimurium* in this report. Linkage maps of *S. typhimurium* have reported 680 genes on a circular linkage map (46). Physical maps of the *S. typhimurium* LT2 chromosome have been determined for *Xba*I (27, 28), for *Bln*I (=*Avr*II) (57), and for I-*Ceu*I (26). The fragments were arranged on a circular map by using cloned genes as probes, using transposon Tn*10* inserted at known sites to add a restriction site, and using "linking probes" derived from induction of lysogens for Mu*d*-P22 (3, 59). Further locations on the genome have been determined with Tn*5* derivatives (58).

An important task in construction of the physical map of a genome for more than one enzyme is to determine the exact locations of restriction sites for a second enzyme on the

* Corresponding author. Electronic mail address: kesander@acs.ucalgary.ca.

Molecular Microbiology (1993) **10**(3), 655–664

The *XbaI–BlnI–CeuI* genomic cleavage map of *Salmonella enteritidis* shows an inversion relative to *Salmonella typhimurium* LT2

Shu-Lin Liu, Andrew Hessel and Kenneth E. Sanderson*
Department of Biological Sciences, University of Calgary, Calgary, Alberta, Canada T2N 1N4.

Summary

We have established the genomic cleavage map of *Salmonella enteritidis* strain SSU7998 using pulsed-field gel electrophoresis. The chromosome of 4600 kb was analysed by *XbaI* (16 fragments), I-*CeuI* (7 fragments) and *BlnI* (12 fragments); the genome also contains a plasmid of 60 kb. Cleavage sites of I-*CeuI*, in the large subunit ribosomal RNA gene, are conserved from *Salmonella typhimurium* and *Escherichia coli* K-12, and the *XbaI* and *BlnI* sites in glt-tRNA are also conserved, but other sites are less conserved. Transposon Tn*10*, located at 60 different positions in the chromosome of *S. typhimurium*, was transduced by bacteriophage P22 into *S. enteritidis* and the insertion mapped using the *XbaI* and *BlnI* sites on Tn*10*. Gene order in *S. enteritidis* is identical to *S. typhimurium* LT2 and similar to *E. coli* K-12 except for an inversion of 815 kb, which covers the terminus region including T1 and T2. Endpoints are in the NDZs, or non-divisible zones, in which inversion endpoints were not detected in experiments in *E. coli* K-12 and *S. typhimurium* LT2. This inversion resembles the inversion between *S. typhimurium* and *E. coli*, but is longer at both ends.

Introduction

Salmonellae are important invasive enteropathogens of humans and animals (Finlay and Falkow, 1989; Groisman and Saier, 1990). Recently, the incidence of salmonellosis, especially that caused by *Salmonella enteritidis*, has been increasing rapidly (Cooke, 1990); in developed countries this corresponds with the centralization of food production and processing (Cooke, 1990; Todd, 1990). Ovarian infection in chickens results in contamination of whole shell eggs (Goodnough and Johnson, 1991; St. Louis *et al.*, 1988). *S. enteritidis* infection in humans is primarily caused by ingestion of contaminated eggs, while infection with other *Salmonella* spp. is caused by other foods (St. Louis *et al.*, 1988). Genetic studies in *S. enteritidis* should help the development of DNA probes to detect *Salmonella* in food and in the environment.

Salmonella was classified into many serotypes using the somatic and flagellar antigens of the Kauffmann–White scheme, in which these serotypes were called species, but now all strains have been proved to belong to the same DNA reassociation group (Crosa *et al.*, 1973; Le Minor, 1984). In this report we continue to use the classical species names to refer to serotypes.

S. enteritidis (1,9,12:g,m:-) is in subspecies I of Le Minor (1984), closely related to *Salmonella typhimurium*. The wild-type strain SSU7998 used in this study belongs to the globally predominant clone (En1) determined by multilocus enzyme electrophoresis (MLEE) (E. F. Boyd *et al.*, submitted). The En1 electrophoretic type is a close relative of non-motile strains such as *Salmonella gallinarum* and *Salmonella pullorum*, according to Li *et al.* (1993).

The cellular and molecular biology (Neidhardt *et al.*, 1987) and the linkage maps (Sanderson and Roth, 1988) of *S. typhimurium* have been intensively studied. Recently, genomic cleavage maps of *S. typhimurium* LT2 were established with the enzymes *XbaI*, *BlnI* (=*AvrII*), and I-*CeuI* (hereafter referred to as *CeuI*) (Liu *et al.*, 1993a,b; Liu and Sanderson, 1992; Wong and McClelland, 1992). Some of these studies used double digestion to determine the relationship of the *XbaI*, *BlnI*, and *CeuI* sites, and analysis of 109 independent strains with Tn*10* insertions in genes, which could be mapped through the *XbaI* and *BlnI* sites in the Tn*10*.

In this report we show that the genomic cleavage map of *S. enteritidis* strain SSU7998 for the endonucleases *XbaI* (16 fragments), *CeuI* (7 fragments), and *BlnI* (12 fragments) represents a circular chromosome of 4600 kb and a plasmid of 60 kb. We report cleavage sites on the chromosome in kb and in centisomes (CS, units representing 1% of the physical genome)(Rudd, 1992; Rudd *et al.*, 1992); in *S. enteritidis* each CS is equal to about 46 kb. We have established a genetic map for 60 genes by transducing Tn*10*s at known locations on the map of *S. typhimurium* into *S. enteritidis*, then locating the new *XbaI*

Received 7 June, 1993; revised 28 July, 1993; accepted 29 July, 1993.
*For correspondence. Tel. (403) 220 6792; Fax (403) 289 9311; E-mail kesander@acs.ucalgary.ca.

Journal of Bacteriology, Feb. 1994, p. 1014–1024 Vol. 176, No. 4
0021-9193/94/$04.00+0
Copyright © 1994, American Society for Microbiology

The *Xba*I-*Bln*I-*Ceu*I Genomic Cleavage Map of *Salmonella paratyphi* B

SHU-LIN LIU, ANDREW HESSEL, HAI-YING MARY CHENG, AND KENNETH E. SANDERSON*
Salmonella Genetic Stock Centre, Department of Biological Sciences, University of Calgary, Calgary, Alberta, Canada T2N 1N4

Received 8 September 1993/Accepted 5 December 1993

The genomic cleavage map of *Salmonella paratyphi* B was determined through digestion with endonucleases and separation of the fragments by pulsed-field gel electrophoresis. The chromosome has 19 *Xba*I sites, 10 *Bln*I sites, and 7 *Ceu*I sites. The fragments were arranged in order through excision of fragments from the gel, redigestion with a second enzyme, end labelling with ^{32}P, and reelectrophoresis. Tn*10* transposons inserted in 61 different genes of *S. typhimurium* LT2 were transduced by use of bacteriophage P22 into *S. paratyphi* B. The locations of Tn*10* insertions on the chromosome of *S. paratyphi* B were determined by use of *Xba*I and *Bln*I sites in Tn*10*, revealing the positions of genes with Tn*10* insertions in *S. paratyphi* B. All seven *Ceu*I sites (in *rrl* genes for 23S rRNA) and most of the *Xba*I and *Bln*I sites in *rrn* genes for Glt-tRNA are conserved, but only about half of the *Xba*I and *Bln*I sites outside *rrn* genes are conserved. Gene order is identical in the 68 genes that we could compare between *S. paratyphi* B and *S. typhimurium* LT2, and the lengths of intervals between the genes are often the same, but there are several instances of differences in interval lengths, indicating that insertions or deletions of DNA have occurred during the evolutionary divergence of these bacteria.

The linkage maps of *Salmonella typhimurium* (39) and *Escherichia coli* K-12 (2) and the physical maps of the genomes, based on either genomic cleavage maps or nucleotide sequences (21–23, 25, 30, 35, 36, 43), reveal that the overall chromosome structure and the gene order are strongly conserved between the two genera (37). However, the nucleotide sequences of homologous genes in the two genera have diverged significantly; for example, divergence in proline permease (*putP*) sequences between *S. typhimurium* and *E. coli* is 16.3%, whereas different serovars of the same genus differ by only 0.5 and 2.4% for members of the genera *Salmonella* and *Escherichia*, respectively (28). High (usually greater than 80%) levels of DNA-DNA reassociation and low ΔT_{m_e} values for DNAs within the genera but much lower levels of DNA reassociation and higher ΔT_{m_e} values between the genera (9) also indicate substantial nucleotide sequence divergence between the genera. (ΔT_{m_e} is the thermal elution midpoint, i.e., the temperature at which 50% of the DNA bound to hydroxyapatite is eluted.) Thus, it has been widely believed that nucleotide sequence changes rather than chromosomal rearrangements explain the evolution of these genera. However, both large and small genomic rearrangements have occurred in the evolution of different genera of enteric bacteria. An example of a large rearrangement is the inversion of about 315 kb (22) in the terminal region of the chromosomes (8, 38) of *S. typhimurium* and *E. coli*. In addition, small insertions or deletions distinguish the linkage maps of *E. coli* and *S. typhimurium* (15, 33, 34). For example, *E. coli* ferments lactose, while *S. typhimurium* is Lac$^-$; loops of DNA which carry several genes, including *lac*, are present in *E. coli* but missing from *S. typhimurium* (7, 16). More data are needed to clarify the relative roles of sequence divergence in homologous genes and chromosomal rearrangements in the evolution of different genera. The objective of this study was to use methods of physical genome analysis to determine whether the chromosomal rearrangements of the types found between different genera are also found in different strains which are members of the same genus, *Salmonella*.

We have studied *S. paratyphi* B because it is closely related to but distinct from *S. typhimurium* and because it includes serious human pathogens. *Salmonellae* of serotype 1,4,(5),12: b:(1,2) are generally known as *S. paratyphi* B; the name *S. schottmuelleri* has been used (18), but most workers, including clinicians, use the name *S. paratyphi* B. We continue to use species designations such as *S. paratyphi* B rather than designations such as *S. enterica* serovar paratyphi B because of their historical use, although we recognize that members of this genus, especially those belonging to the same subgenus, are members of a single species, as defined by DNA-DNA reassociation (9, 19, 31). *S. paratyphi* B was initially described as the causal agent of typhoidlike enteric fever in humans. Later, it was recognized that some strains of this serotype do not cause enteric fever but instead produce an acute but mild gastroenteritis. Isolates which cause enteric fevers usually do not ferment *d*-tartrate but form an extracellular slime layer, whereas isolates which cause gastroenteritis are usually able to utilize *d*-tartrate but are deficient in the slime layer. Kauffmann (14) concluded that there are two species of identical serotype, and he proposed the name *S. java* for the *d*-tartrate-positive form and the name *S. paratyphi* B for the *d*-tartrate-negative form. Le Minor et al. (20) proposed that the name *S. java* be dropped and that these strains be considered a biovar of *S. paratyphi* B; we have adopted this usage, as have others (3, 41).

We report here the genomic cleavage map of *S. paratyphi* B IP87/87 for the enzymes I-*Ceu*I, *Xba*I, and *Bln*I (the designation "I" in enzyme I-*Ceu*I indicates that the enzyme is encoded by a class I intron; I-*Ceu*I will be called *Ceu*I in this report). Strain IP87/87 is of the tartrate-positive type and is electrophoretic type Pb3; it would have been called *S. java* by Kauffmann (14). We transduced Tn*10* transposons located in genes of *S. typhimurium* LT2 into *S. paratyphi* B and established the locations of these genes by locating the new *Xba*I and *Bln*I sites in Tn*10*. Gene order is identical in the 68 genes

* Corresponding author. Mailing address: Department of Biological Sciences, University of Calgary, Calgary, Alberta, Canada T2N 1N4. Phone: (403) 220-6792. Fax: (403) 289-9311. Electronic mail address: kesander@acs.ucalgary.ca.

Proc. Natl. Acad. Sci. USA
Vol. 92, pp. 1018–1022, February 1995
Genetics

Rearrangements in the genome of the bacterium *Salmonella typhi*

SHU-LIN LIU AND KENNETH E. SANDERSON

Department of Biological Sciences, University of Calgary, Calgary, AB, Canada T2N 1N4

Communicated by John R. Roth, University of Utah, Salt Lake City, UT, October 20, 1994 (received for review August 9, 1994)

ABSTRACT We have determined the genomic map of the bacterium *Salmonella typhi* Ty2, the causal organism of typhoid fever, by using pulsed-field gel electrophoresis. Digestion of the Ty2 genome with endonucleases *Xba* I, *Bln* I, and *Ceu* I yielded 33, 26, and 7 fragments, respectively, that were placed in order on a circular chromosome of 4780 kb. Transposon Tn*10* was inserted in specific genes of *Salmonella typhimurium* and transduced into *S. typhi*, and thus, the positions of 37 *S. typhi* genes were located through the *Xba* I and *Bln* I sites of the Tn*10*. Gene order on chromosomes of *Escherichia coli* K-12 and *S. typhimurium* LT2 is remarkably conserved; however, the gene order in *S. typhi* Ty2 is different, suggesting it has undergone major genomic rearrangements during its evolution. These rearrangements include inversions and transpositions in the 7 DNA fragments between the seven *rrn* operons for rRNA (postulated to be due to homologous recombination in these *rrn* genes), another inversion that covers the replication terminus region (resembling inversions found in other enteric bacteria), and at least three insertions, one as large as 118 kb. Partial digestion of genomic DNA with the intron-encoded endonuclease I-*Ceu* I, which cuts only in *rrn* genes, shows chromosomal rearrangements, apparently due to homologous recombination in the *rrn* genes, that were detected in all wild-type strains of *S. typhi* tested. These rearrangements may have been selected to compensate for the insertions that otherwise would have altered the locations of genes with respect to the origin and terminus of replication. These observations are relevant to our view of the evolution of the bacterial genome and may be significant in the virulence of *S. typhi*.

Preservation of the gross genomic organization of enteric bacterial chromosomes is a striking example of evolutionary conservation. The genetic maps of *Escherichia coli* K-12 and *Salmonella typhimurium* LT2, which diverged >100 million years ago (1), are very similar (2, 3) as are the recently determined physical maps of the genomes of *E. coli* (4–7), *S. typhimurium* (8), *Salmonella enteritidis* (9), and *Salmonella paratyphi* B (10). In contrast to the stability of these chromosomes during evolution, chromosomes of cultured enteric bacterial cells frequently rearrange. Duplications of segments of the chromosome occur at high frequencies (10^{-2} to 10^{-5}) (11–13), and deletions are also frequent. In contrast, inversions may be less common; at some sites they occur at low frequency and at other sites they were undetectable (14–16). However, inversions with endpoints in the seven copies of the *rrn* (rRNA) operons are fairly common in *E. coli* (17). This high frequency of rearrangements, combined with the stability of the chromosome through evolution, indicates that significant pressures must exist to maintain the order of genes. In this report we show that *Salmonella typhi* is an exception to the conservation of chromosomal gene order seen in other enteric bacteria, because its chromosome shows major rearrangements in gene order in wild-type strains.

S. typhi is the causal organism of typhoid fever, which is a major public health problem in less-developed areas of the world: 13 million cases per year are estimated, exclusive of China (18). Typhoid fever is a severe prolonged disease with a high rate of complications (19). Some vaccines are available, but considerable work is still needed (20). *S. typhi* has been studied much less than *S. typhimurium*; detailed genomic information of *S. typhi* will be important for developing improved vaccines and for determining the basis for pathogenicity.

MATERIALS AND METHODS

Bacterial Strains, Phages, Plasmids, and Cultivation Conditions. *S. typhi* H251.1 was derived from wild-type strain Ty2 and carries an *aroC* mutation that reduces pathogenicity; it was provided by David Hone (University of Maryland School of Medicine, Baltimore) (21). *S. typhi* 25T-40, 9032-85, and 3137-73 are independent wild-type strains of *S. typhi*, obtained from Laboratory Centers for Disease Control, Ottawa, and Centers for Disease Control and Prevention, Atlanta. Cells were routinely grown in LB broth (8) or on LB agar (with 1.5% agar added). Modified Davis minimal medium (8) was used as a defined medium. For growth of H251.1 in defined medium, the following supplements were added (each to 100 μg/ml): tryptophan, tyrosine, phenylalanine, *p*-aminobenzoic acid, and 2,3-dihydroxybenzoic acid. For growth on L-agar, only 2,3-dihydroxybenzoic acid was added.

Phage P22HT105/*int* was propagated in strains of *S. typhimurium* that have transposon Tn*10* insertions at known locations on the genetic and genomic cleavage maps. These lysates were used to transduce *S. typhi* H251.1 to Tn*10*$^+$, by using selection for tetracycline resistance. The frequency of transduction was low, as observed (22, 23). DNA transferred from *S. typhimurium* was normally inserted by homologous recombination into the homologous gene of *S. typhi*, because the recipient acquired the phenotype of the donor strain (e.g., a donor strain that required threonine for growth, because of a Tn*10* insertion into a cysteine synthesis gene, resulted in a transductant with the same growth requirement). In a few cases the transductant did not have the appropriate phenotype; these strains were not used in this analysis. In some of the strains used here, the phenotype was not testable. The location of the Tn*10* insertion was mapped by *Xba* I and *Bln* I digestion, as described in refs. 8–10.

Enzymes and Chemicals. Endonucleases were from New England Biolabs and from Boehringer Mannheim. I-*Ceu* I [an intron-encoded endonuclease derived from a class I mobile intron from *Chlamydomonas eugamatos* (hereafter called *Ceu* I)] cleaves at a 19-bp sequence (24) present only in the seven *rrn* operons of enteric bacteria (25). [^{32}P]dCTP was from New England Nuclear. Most other chemicals, including agarose, were from Sigma.

Techniques Used in Pulsed-Field Gel Electrophoresis (PFGE). Preparation and digestion of high molecular weight genomic DNA, digestion of DNA in agarose blocks, and separation of DNA by PFGE, were as reported (8–10, 25).

The publication costs of this article were defrayed in part by page charge payment. This article must therefore be hereby marked "*advertisement*" in accordance with 18 U.S.C. §1734 solely to indicate this fact.

Abbreviation: PFGE, pulsed-field gel electrophoresis.

JOURNAL OF BACTERIOLOGY, June 1995, p. 3355–3357 Vol. 177, No. 11
0021-9193/95/$04.00+0
Copyright © 1995, American Society for Microbiology

I-*Ceu*I Reveals Conservation of the Genome of Independent Strains of *Salmonella typhimurium*

SHU-LIN LIU AND KENNETH E. SANDERSON*

Department of Biological Sciences, University of Calgary, Calgary, Alberta, Canada T2N 1N4

Received 23 November 1994/Accepted 27 March 1995

The enzyme I-*Ceu*I, encoded by a class I mobile intron inserted in the gene for 23S rRNA in *Chlamydomonas eugamatos*, cleaves a specific 19-bp sequence in this gene. This sequence is present only in the seven genes for rRNA in *Salmonella typhimurium* and *Escherichia coli*. Partial digestion with I-*Ceu*I of DNA from 17 wild-type strains of *S. typhimurium* indicates that the chromosome of these strains is strongly conserved, for the digestion products closely resemble those of strain LT2. The lengths and order of chromosomal segments are conserved in 15 of the strains; 2 show some rearrangements. *Xba*I digestion indicated heterogeneity without revealing the genomic structure. Because of conservation of I-*Ceu*I sites in genes for rRNA and conservation of the number and locations of these genes, I-*Ceu*I provides an excellent tool for the rapid examination of the chromosomes of related species of bacteria; differences in the fingerprints indicate the occurrence of chromosomal rearrangements such as insertions or inversions.

The use of type II restriction endonucleases has revolutionized the study of molecular biology; the intron-encoded endonucleases (3) are beginning to have an impact on the field. I-*Ceu*I (5, 7, 17) is a representative of this kind of endonuclease. Many others have also been reported, and some are commercially available, including I-*Ppo*I (18), I-*Sce*I (3), I-*Sce*II (4), I-*Tev*I and I-*Tev*II (1), and I-*Cre*I (6).

I-*Ceu*I is encoded by a class I mobile intron which is inserted into the *rrl* gene for the large-subunit rRNA (23S rRNA) in the chloroplast DNA of *Chlamydomonas eugamatos*. I-*Ceu*I is specific for and cuts in a 19-bp sequence in the *rrl* gene. Because rRNA sequences are strongly conserved, this 19-bp sequence is present in the genomes of many enteric bacteria (12, 13, 16) and in *Rhizobium meliloti* (9), as well as in chloroplasts and mitochondria of eukaryotes. Because I-*Ceu*I cleaves only *rrn* genes and because the number and locations of these genes are highly conserved in enteric bacteria (10), related wild-type strains yield similar I-*Ceu*I fingerprints which give valuable genomic information on DNA insertions or rearrangements; fingerprints with *Xba*I, a type II restriction endonuclease with a 6-bp site, are much more variable, providing little direct genomic information. Some investigators have reported difficulties in working with I-*Ceu*I, and so in this report we present our protocol for its use.

Salmonella typhimurium LT2, which was obtained from Joshua Lederberg (20), was originally isolated by Lilleengen (11). The strains designated SARA2 to SARA18 were obtained from Robert Selander (2) as part of *Salmonella* reference collection A (SARA), a reference set of electrophoretic types established by using multilocus enzyme electrophoresis; strain LT2 is designated SARA2. Luria-Bertani (LB) medium (10 g of tryptone, 5 g of yeast extract, 10 g of NaCl, 3.5 ml of 1 M NaOH) was used for cultivation of all strains; solid medium also contained 1.5% agar and 0.2% glucose. Strains were maintained in 15% glycerol at −76°C, and a single colony was isolated prior to use. Endonucleases used were I-*Ceu*I from New England Biolabs and *Xba*I from Boehringer Mannheim. Most other chemicals, including agarose, were from Sigma Chemical Co.

Higher-quality DNA is needed for I-*Ceu*I than for other endonucleases, and so we modified our techniques as follows. Bacterial cells were grown overnight with shaking in LB broth, and then 3-ml volumes were centrifuged in 15-ml plastic tubes, resuspended in 0.5 ml of cell suspension solution (10 mM Tris-HCl [pH 7.2], 20 mM NaCl, 100 mM EDTA), warmed to 70°C in a water bath, and mixed with 0.5 ml of 1.2% agarose (regular, not low melting point) which had been boiled and then held at 70°C. The mixture was then immediately drawn into a tuberculin syringe from which the needle adapter had been cut. When the agarose rod had hardened after a 20-min incubation at room temperature, it was sliced into 1-mm-thick discs which were then put into 3 ml of lysing solution (10 mM Tris-HCl [pH 7.2], 50 mM NaCl, 100 mM EDTA, 0.2% sodium dodecyl sulfate, 0.5% *N*-laurylsarcosine) and gently shaken at 70°C for 90 min. The discs were drained, washed once in wash solution (20 mM Tris-HCl [pH 8.0], 50 mM EDTA), and then treated with 3 ml of proteinase K solution (1 mg of proteinase K per ml, 100 mM EDTA, 0.2% sodium dodecyl sulfate, 1% *N*-laurylsarcosine) at 42°C for 18 h. The discs were washed in wash solution and treated with PMSF solution (1 mM phenylmethylsulfonyl fluoride in wash solution) for 1 h at room temperature with gentle shaking to remove the activity of proteinase K. After two washes in wash solution and one in storage solution (10-times-diluted wash solution), the discs were ready for either digestion with endonucleases or storage (in storage solution at 4 to 8°C). This method regularly yields DNA which digests well with I-*Ceu*I and with other enzymes. There are several changes from the methods reported earlier (14), including elimination of the use of lysozyme, but the most important modification is lysis at 70°C rather than at 37°C; this precludes the use of low-melting-point agarose. Enzyme preparations should be titrated prior to use, since digestion with a high concentration of enzyme or digestion for extended times resulted in smears in the gel.

For pulsed-field gel electrophoresis (PFGE), a Bio-Rad CHEF-DRII apparatus was used. Fragment separation is optimal if a pulse time of about 1 s for each 10 kb of fragment is used; thus, a group of DNA fragments sized from 250 to 350 kb requires a pulse time of around 30 s. Timing of the pulses is

* Corresponding author. Phone: (403) 220-6792. Fax: (403) 289-9311. Electronic mail address: kesander@acs.ucalgary.ca.

JOURNAL OF BACTERIOLOGY, Sept. 1995, p. 5099–5107
0021-9193/95/$04.00+0
Copyright © 1995, American Society for Microbiology
Vol. 177, No. 17

Genomic Cleavage Map of *Salmonella typhi* Ty2

SHU-LIN LIU AND KENNETH E. SANDERSON*

Salmonella Genetic Stock Centre, Department of Biological Sciences, University of Calgary, Calgary, Alberta, Canada T2N 1N4

Received 18 April 1995/Accepted 25 June 1995

The genomic cleavage map of *Salmonella typhi* Ty2, 4,780 kb in size, was determined through digestion of the genomic DNA with endonucleases and separation of the fragments by pulsed-field gel electrophoresis. The chromosome has 33, 26, 7, and 35 sites for the enzymes *Xba*I, *Bln*I, I-*Ceu*I, and *Spe*I, respectively. The fragments were arranged around the chromosome through excision of fragments from the gel, redigestion with a second enzyme, end labelling with ^{32}P, and reelectrophoresis and named in alphabetical order. Tn*10* transposons inserted in 82 different genes of *Salmonella typhimurium* were transduced by phage P22 into *S. typhi*, and the location of Tn*10*, and thus of the gene, was mapped through the *Xba*I and *Bln*I sites of Tn*10*. All seven I-*Ceu*I sites (in *rrl* genes for 23S rRNA) were conserved, and the gene order within the I-*Ceu*I fragments resembles that of *S. typhimurium* LT2, but the order of I-*Ceu*I fragments is rearranged from ABCDEFG in *S. typhimurium* LT2 to AGCEFDB in *S. typhi*. In addition, there is a 500-kb inversion which covers the terminus region. Comparisons of lengths of segments between genes showed that *S. typhi* has segments which differ in size from those in *S. typhimurium*. The *viaB* locus, for synthesis of the Vi antigen of *S. typhi*, was shown to be within a 118-kb loop (a segment of DNA with no homolog in most other *Salmonella* species) between *mel* and *poxA* on the chromosome.

Of the more than 2,300 closely related *Salmonella* serovars recognized, *Salmonella typhi* is the only one that grows exclusively in humans and causes typhoid enteric fever (9, 20, 39). Typhoid fever is a major public health problem in many parts of the world; 13 million cases per year are estimated, exclusive of China (9). Because of its importance as a human pathogen, *S. typhi* has been the target of extensive investigation (16, 35, 37, 48), including studies of its invasiveness of human epithelial cells (11, 13, 23).

The division of the genus *Salmonella* into many serovars is based on the somatic and flagellar antigens; these serovars have been called species (19), and *S. typhi* is one of the species. Molecular genetic evidence indicates close relationships of all of these serovars (8), and some researchers use a single species designation (21); in this report, we retain the use of different species names.

A few other *Salmonella* species, including *S. paratyphi* A, B, and C and *S. sendai*, are also human-adapted pathogens which cause similar but milder diseases, called paratyphoid fever. Reeves et al. (40), by using multilocus enzyme electrophoresis to measure the genetic distances within the seven *Salmonella* DNA hybridization subgroups, showed that *S. typhi* strains constitute a single clone which is widely separated from the other species in subgroup I. Selander et al. (47) also concluded that *S. typhi* is a relatively homogeneous group, with no close phylogenetic relationships to the paratyphoid agents.

Genetic changes which occur during evolution of bacteria can be classified into three types: (i) base pair changes, probably due primarily to replication errors, (ii) genomic rearrangements (inversions, translocations, and duplications) involving large blocks of DNA, and (iii) lateral transfer, which results in addition of new genetic material from an external source. Which of these is the most significant in the evolution of species of *Salmonella*? High levels of DNA reassociation and low thermal elution midpoint values in studies with different species of the same genus indicate that base pair changes in homologous genes are infrequent (8). In addition, nucleotide sequencing of homologous genes of different species within subgenus I of *Salmonella* (which includes all of the human-pathogenic species usually studied) indicates low divergence (5), except in highly polymorphic genes, such as *rfb* (41), *fliC*, and *fljB* (22). Genomic rearrangements occur rarely in the genus *Salmonella*; *S. typhimurium* (27), *S. paratyphi* B (24), and *S. enteritidis* (26) have very similar genomic maps. Lateral transfer has resulted in species-specific loops of DNA: the *nanH* gene of *S. typhimurium* LT2 is absent from all other species of subgenus I (17); some *Escherichia coli* serovars have unique blocks of DNA called "pathogenicity islands" (4).

The objective of this study was to examine the ways *S. typhi* differs genetically from other *Salmonella* spp. We previously constructed genomic cleavage maps of *S. typhimurium* LT2 (27, 28), *S. enteritidis* (26), and *S. paratyphi* B (24); comparisons of these maps and that of *E. coli* (2, 38) show that these enteric bacteria share a common basic genomic structure, with some differences specific to individual bacteria. However, we recently reported that the *Xba*I, *Bln*I, and I-*Ceu*I genomic maps of strains of *S. typhi* show major rearrangements, including inversions and translocations due to homologous recombination in the *rrn* genes for rRNA (30). Here we present a detailed analysis of the genomic structure of *S. typhi*, including a *Spe*I map. Comparison with the genome of *S. typhimurium* shows several regions with excess DNA (loops of DNA) which are missing from most species of *Salmonella*. One of these loops is up to 118 kb long, contains the *viaB* locus for Vi antigen synthesis, and is not present in most other *Salmonella* species.

MATERIALS AND METHODS

Bacterial strains, phage, and cultivation conditions. H251.1, a derivative of *S. typhi* Ty2 which carries the mutation Δ*aroC1019*, was obtained from D. M. Hone (15) and was the wild-type strain used to generate the endonuclease cleavage maps and to make Tn*10* insertion mutants. Independent *S. typhi* wild-type strains were obtained from several sources: 382-82, 9032-85, 1707-81, 1196-74, 3434-73, 3137-73, 9228-77, 3185-73, and Ty21a were from the Centers for Disease Control and Prevention, Atlanta, Ga. (40); SA4828 was from the Provincial Laboratory of

* Corresponding author. Phone: (403) 220-6792. Fax: (403) 289-9311. Electronic mail address: kesander@acs.ucalgary.ca.

JOURNAL OF BACTERIOLOGY, Nov. 1995, p. 6585–6592
0021-9193/95/$04.00+0
Copyright © 1995, American Society for Microbiology
Vol. 177, No. 22

The Chromosome of *Salmonella paratyphi* A Is Inverted by Recombination between *rrnH* and *rrnG*

SHU-LIN LIU AND KENNETH E. SANDERSON*

Department of Biological Sciences, Salmonella Genetic Stock Centre, University of Calgary, Calgary, Alberta, Canada T2N 1N4

Received 26 June 1995/Accepted 10 September 1995

***Salmonella paratyphi* A, a human-adapted bacterial pathogen, causes paratyphoid enteric fever. We established the genome map of strain ATCC 9150 by the use of four endonucleases, *Xba*I, I-*Ceu*I, *Avr*II (= *Bln*I), and *Spe*I, which generated 27, 7, 19, and 38 fragments, respectively; the sum of the fragments in each case indicates a genome size of ca. 4,600 kb. With phage P22, we transduced Tn*10* insertions in known genes from *Salmonella typhimurium* LT2 to *S. paratyphi* A ATCC 9150 and located these insertions on the *S. paratyphi* A chromosome through the *Xba*I and *Avr*II sites in Tn*10* and through the increased size of the *Spe*I fragment bearing a Tn*10*. Compared with the maps of other *Salmonella* species, the *S. paratyphi* A genomic map showed two major differences: (i) an insertion of about 100 kb of DNA between *rrnH*/*G* and *proB* and (ii) an inversion of half the genome between *rrnH* and *rrnG*, postulated to be due to homologous recombination between the *rrn* genes. We propose that during the evolution of *S. paratyphi* A, the first rearrangement event was the 100-kb insertion, which disrupted the chromosomal balance between *oriC* and the termination of replication, forcing the *rrnH*/*G* inversion to restore the balance. The insertion and the inversion are both present in all 10 independent wild-type *S. paratyphi* A strains tested.**

There are over 2,300 serovars of *Salmonella*, which are distinguished on the basis of their somatic and flagellar antigens in the Kauffmann-White scheme of classification. Only a few serovars are exclusively or primarily restricted to growth in humans. One of these is *Salmonella paratyphi* A, which causes paratyphoid enteric fever, a disease also caused by *Salmonella paratyphi* B and C and *Salmonella sendai*. *Salmonella typhi* causes typhoid fever, the most-studied enteric fever, which is a severe, prolonged disease with a high rate of complications. The clinical features of paratyphoid fever resemble typhoid fever, but it is a milder illness (12). In this report we construct and analyze a genomic cleavage map of the chromosome of *S. paratyphi* A.

S. paratyphi A has the same flagellar antigens as *S. sendai* (though the phase 2 antigens are frequently not expressed in *S. paratyphi* A), but it is a member of somatic O group A while *S. sendai* is a member of O group D1. Analysis by multilocus enzyme electrophoresis shows that most electrophoretic types of *S. paratyphi* A are closely related to *S. sendai* and not closely related to other species which cause enteric fevers (34).

The division of the genus *Salmonella* into many serovars is based on the somatic and flagellar antigens; these serovars have been called species (13), e.g., *Salmonella typhimurium*. Molecular genetic evidence indicates close relationships of all these serovars (6), and some investigators now use a single species designation (15); in this report we retain the use of different species names.

The general structure of the chromosome and the order of genes on the chromosome of enteric bacteria are usually strongly conserved. The genetic maps of *S. typhimurium* LT2 (17, 20), *Escherichia coli* K-12 (30), *Salmonella enteritidis* (19), and *S. paratyphi* B (16) are very similar; they sometimes differ by an inversion in the termination of replication (TER) region, by insertions of nonhomologous DNA (loops), and by the presence or absence of a plasmid. In addition, about 20 independent wild-type strains of *S. typhimurium* have very similar chromosomes (21). Although the chromosomes of these species have been stable during the evolution of these species, their chromosomes frequently rearrange in culture: spontaneous duplications produced by recombination between *rrn* operons occur at frequencies of 10^{-4} to 10^{-3} (1, 7), deletions occur frequently (10), and inversions with endpoints in the seven copies of the *rrn* (rRNA) operons are common in *S. typhimurium* (1) and *E. coli* (11) while inversions at other sites vary from low frequency to undetectable (24). The occurrence of rearrangements in culture, yet the observed stability of the chromosome during evolution of species, indicates that cells with rearrangements are strongly selected against during evolution and do not survive to form species. In contrast, we recently reported that *S. typhi* does not display this conservative chromosome structure, because inversions and transpositions of the chromosome segments between the *rrn* genes are common; none of the 20 wild-type strains examined had the same order of these segments as that found in *S. typhimurium* and *E. coli* (22, 23). The order of genes on the individual chromosome segments between the *rrn* genes is very similar in *S. typhi* and *S. typhimurium*, but these segments are postulated to be rearranged because of homologous recombinations between the *rrn* genes.

We have constructed a genomic cleavage map of the chromosome of *S. paratyphi* A for the endonucleases *Xba*I, *Avr*II (= *Bln*I), I-*Ceu*I, and *Spe*I. This map reveals that the chromosome of this strain has an inversion of about 50% of the chromosome compared with that of *S. typhimurium*, postulated to be due to a homologous recombination between the *rrnH* and *rrnG* genes. All 10 *S. paratyphi* A strains which were studied have the same inversion.

MATERIALS AND METHODS

Bacterial strains, phage, and cultivation conditions. The wild-type strain of *S. paratyphi* A used for detailed genomic analysis was strain ATCC 9150, ob-

* Corresponding author. Phone: (403) 220-6792. Fax: (403) 289-9311. Electronic mail address: ksander@acs.ucalgary.ca.

JOURNAL OF BACTERIOLOGY, Sept. 1996, p. 5323–5326 Vol. 178, No. 17
0021-9193/96/$04.00+0
Copyright © 1996, American Society for Microbiology

Salmonella typhi Contains Identical Intervening Sequences in All Seven *rrl* Genes

NEIL R. MATTATALL,* DAYLE A. DAINES,† SHU-LIN LIU, AND KENNETH E. SANDERSON

Salmonella Genetic Stock Centre, Department of Biological Sciences, University of Calgary, Calgary, Alberta, Canada T2N 1N4

Received 15 April 1996/Accepted 18 June 1996

***Salmonella typhi* Ty2 *rrl* genes contain intervening sequences (IVSs) in helix-25 but not in helix-45 on the basis of observed 23S rRNA fragmentation caused by IVS excision. We have confirmed this and shown all seven IVSs to be identical by isolating genomic DNA fragments containing each of the seven *rrl* genes from *S. typhi* Ty2 by use of pulsed-field gel electrophoresis; each *rrl* gene was amplified by PCR in the helix-25 and helix-45 regions and cycle sequenced. Thirty independent wild-type *S. typhi* strains, tested by genomic PCR and *Dra*I restriction, also have seven *rrl* genes with helix-25 IVSs and no helix-45 IVSs. We propose that IVS homogeneity in *S. typhi* occurs because gene conversion drives IVS sequence maintenance and because adaptation to human hosts results in limited clonal diversity.**

Several *Salmonella* species (considered serovars by some authors) possess intervening sequences (IVSs) of 90 to 110 bp in some or all of the seven *rrl* (23S rRNA) genes at base pair 550 and base pair 1170 (*Escherichia coli rrl* numbering [15]) (3, 8, 9, 14, 19, 20). These sites correspond to helix-25 and helix-45, respectively, in the proposed secondary structure of the *E. coli* 23S rRNA. IVSs replace these small helices, in part, with an extended stem and loop. Following *rrn* operon transcription, IVSs are cut by RNase III in the stem region, and this cutting causes 23S rRNA to fragment into two or more pieces without any apparent loss in functionality (3).

Salmonella typhimurium LT2 possesses three unique IVSs: two are extensions of helix-25, and one is an extension of helix-45 (14). The two helix-25 IVSs occur in *rrlG* and *rrlH* and are only 56% identical, while the helix-45 IVS is 100% identical in *rrlA*, *rrlB*, *rrlC*, *rrlD*, *rrlE*, and *rrlH*. This distribution of IVSs among the seven *rrl* genes determines 23S rRNA fragmentation stoichiometry (see Fig. 1). The *rrlH* helix-25 IVS was 94% identical to the nucleotide sequence of the helix-25 IVS from *Salmonella arizonae* (3). Similarly, the helix-45 IVS was 100% identical to IVSs from two other *S. typhimurium* strains (3, 19) and was strongly related to IVSs from *S. arizonae* (3) and *Yersinia enterocolitica* (19). We have suggested that these three unique IVSs entered *S. typhimurium* LT2 through lateral transfer and that the helix-45 IVS was distributed to and maintained in the same sequence in six of the seven *rrl* genes through the mechanism of gene conversion (14).

Salmonella typhi is the only *Salmonella* species that grows exclusively in humans and causes typhoid enteric fever. Many studies have shown that independent *S. typhi* strains from different geographic regions are very similar, indicating that their origin is clonal in nature, with no significant recombination with other *Salmonella* species and limited divergence by mutation. For example, by using multilocus enzyme electrophoresis, Reeves et al. (16) showed that *S. typhi* strains constitute a single clone, while Selander et al. (18) found two clones, but both groups propose that *S. typhi* is a relatively homogeneous group widely separated from the other species in *Salmonella* subgenus I. Envelope protein profiles also reveal homogeneity of strains (5). The objective of this report is to examine the homogeneity of IVS possession and nucleotide sequence in *S. typhi*.

23S rRNA fragmentation in *S. typhi* Ty2. *S. typhi* Ty2 line H251.1 (which is derived from wild-type strain Ty2 and which carries an *aroC* deletion that reduces pathogenicity [7]) does not contain intact 23S rRNA (2.9 kb) as detected for *E. coli* K-12; instead, 2.4- and 0.5-kb rRNA fragments (in addition to 16S rRNA) were observed (Fig. 1A). This fragmentation pattern is consistent with the presence of helix-25 IVSs in all seven *rrl* genes, since RNase III cutting at the helix-25 site would generate the fragments observed (Fig. 1B). *S. typhi* Ty2 RNA does not contain 1.7-, 1.2-, or 0.7-kb fragments, which supports the conclusion that *S. typhi* Ty2 does not possess helix-45 IVSs; fragments of these sizes are seen in *S. typhimurium* RNA, as expected (Fig. 1) (14).

Isolation and sequencing of the seven *rrl* genes of *S. typhi* Ty2. *S. typhi* Ty2 *rrl* genes were separated by pulsed-field gel electrophoresis (PFGE) on the basis of the genomic cleavage map for *S. typhi* Ty2 (13) by methods described previously (12). Genomic fragments digested with I-*Ceu*I (New England Biolabs) allowed for isolation of *rrlA*, *rrlB*, *rrlE*, *rrlG*, and *rrlH*; *rrlC* and *rrlD* were copurified on a single I-*Ceu*I fragment that was excised in agarose, restricted with *Spe*I (Boehringer Mannheim), and electrophoresed (by PFGE) to yield two fragments, each containing one *rrl* gene (Table 1). All fragments were purified by GlassMAX (GIBCO BRL) and used as a template for PCR to generate amplicons A and B for each *rrl* gene (Fig. 2). PCRs were performed on a Techne Gene "E" thermal cycler under conditions recommended by the *Taq* polymerase supplier (GIBCO BRL). Agarose gel electrophoresis of amplicon A from all seven *S. typhi* Ty2 *rrl* genes showed that all amplicons were the same size, about 110 bp larger than the amplicon from *E. coli* whole genomic template (data not shown). This indicates that all *S. typhi* Ty2 *rrl* genes contain helix-25 IVSs, as predicted by the RNA fragmentation data (Fig. 1A). Amplicon B from all *rrl* genes was the same size as amplicon B from *E. coli* (data not shown), indicating, as predicted by RNA data (Fig. 1A), that none of the *rrl* genes of *S. typhi* Ty2 possesses helix-45 IVSs.

* Corresponding author. Phone: (403) 220-3572. Fax: (403) 289-9311. Electronic mail address: nmattata@acs.ucalgary.ca.

† Present address: Department of Microbiology and Immunology, University of Rochester Medical Centre, Rochester, NY 14642.

Proc. Natl. Acad. Sci. USA
Vol. 93, pp. 10303–10308, September 1996
Genetics

Highly plastic chromosomal organization in *Salmonella typhi*

SHU-LIN LIU AND KENNETH E. SANDERSON*

Salmonella Genetic Stock Centre, Department of Biological Sciences, University of Calgary, Calgary, AB, Canada T2N 1N4

Communicated by John R. Roth, University of Utah, Salt Lake City, UT, June 20, 1996 (received for review March 8, 1996)

ABSTRACT **Gene order in the chromosomes of *Escherichia coli* K-12 and *Salmonella typhimurium* LT2, and in many other species of *Salmonella*, is strongly conserved, even though the genera diverged about 160 million years ago. However, partial digestion of chromosomal DNA of *Salmonella typhi*, the causal organism of typhoid fever, with the endonuclease I-*Ceu*I followed by separation of the DNA fragments by pulsed-field gel electrophoresis showed that the chromosomes of independent wild-type isolates of *S. typhi* are rearranged due to homologous recombination between the seven *rrn* genes that code for ribosomal RNA. The order of genes within the I-*Ceu*I fragments is largely conserved, but the order of the fragments on the chromosome is rearranged. Twenty-one different orders of the I-*Ceu*I fragments were detected among the 127 wild-type strains we examined. Duplications and deletions were not found, but transpositions and inversions were common. Transpositions of I-*Ceu*I fragments into sites that do not change their distance from the origin of replication (*oriC*) are frequently detected among the wild-type strains, but transpositions that move the fragments much further from *oriC* were rare. This supports the gene dosage hypothesis that genes at different distances from *oriC* have different gene dosages and, hence, different gene expression, and that during evolution genes become adapted to their specific location; thus, cells with changes in gene location due to transpositions may be less fit. Therefore, gene dosage may be one of the forces that conserves gene order, although its effects seem less strong in *S. typhi* than in other enteric bacteria. However, both the gene dosage and the genomic balance hypotheses, the latter of which states that the origin (*oriC*) and terminus (TER) of replication must be separated by 180°C, need further investigation.**

The general structure and the order of genes on the chromosomes of different enteric bacteria are usually strongly conserved (1, 2). The genetic and physical genome maps of *Salmonella typhimurium* LT2 (3–5) (Fig. 1), *Escherichia coli* K-12 (9, 10), *Salmonella enteritidis* (11), and *Salmonella paratyphi* B (12) are very similar in the order of genes, although they sometimes differ by an inversion in the TER region (for termination of replication), by insertions of nonhomologous DNA ("loops"), and by the presence or absence of a plasmid. In addition, 17 independent wild-type strains of *S. typhimurium* have very similar chromosomes (13). Although the chromosomes of these species are very stable during evolution, the chromosomes frequently rearrange when the cells are grown in culture. Spontaneous duplications produced by recombination between *rrn* (rRNA) operons occur at frequencies of 10^{-3} to 10^{-4} (14, 15), and deletions are also frequent (16). Inversions with endpoints in the seven copies of the *rrn* operons are common in *S. typhimurium* (15) and *E. coli* (17); the frequency of inversions at other sites varies from low to undetectable (18). This high frequency of rearrangements in culture, combined with the stability of the chromosome through evolution, indicates that cells with rearrangements are strongly selected

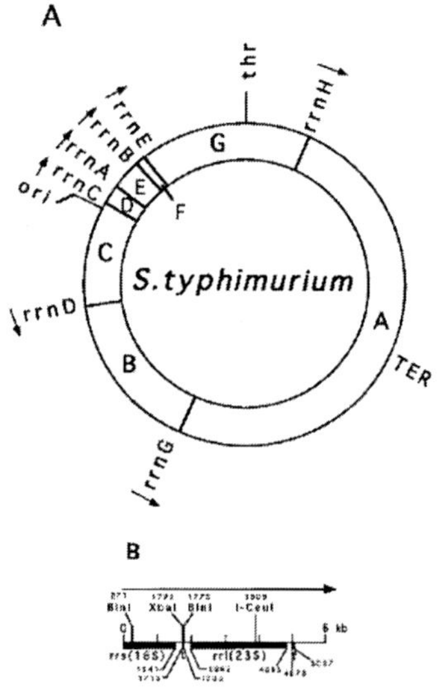

FIG. 1. (*A*) The location and orientation of transcription of the seven *rrn* genes for ribosomal RNA of *S. typhimurium* LT2 (3), each of which has a cleavage site for the endonuclease I-*Ceu*I (6, 7). The seven I-*Ceu*I fragments are in the order ABCDEFG. *oriC* is the site of initiation of bidirectional replication of DNA; TER is the site of termination of replication. Order of *rrn* genes is the same in *Escherichia coli* K-12 (1). (*B*) The structure of the *rrnB* operon for ribosomal RNA of *E. coli* K-12 (8). *rrs*, *rrl*, and *f* are the genes for 16S, 23S, and 5S rRNA. The beginning and end of each gene in base pairs is shown under the genes, and the positions in base pairs of sites for digestion by the endonucleases *Bln*I, *Xba*I, and I-*Ceu*I are also shown (3).

against during evolution and, therefore, do not survive. For example, no *rrn*-mediated rearrangements have been detected in wild-type strains of either *S. typhimurium* or *E. coli*, in spite of the high frequency of rearrangements observed in culture. However, we found that the genome of *Salmonella typhi* is less conservative, for rearrangements of the chromosome segments between the *rrn* genes were detected in strain Ty2 and in a few other wild-type strains (19, 20). The order of genes on the chromosome segments between *rrn* genes is relatively conserved between *S. typhi* and *S. typhimurium*, but these segments were rearranged in *S. typhi*, postulated due to homologous recombination between the *rrn* operons.

The publication costs of this article were defrayed in part by page charge payment. This article must therefore be hereby marked "*advertisement*" in accordance with 18 U.S.C. §1734 solely to indicate this fact.

Abbreviation: PFGE, pulsed-field gel electrophoresis.

*To whom reprint requests should be addressed. e-mail: kesander@acs.ucalgary.ca.

ELSEVIER

FEMS Microbiology Letters 164 (1998) 275–281

FEMS MICROBIOLOGY LETTERS

Homologous recombination between *rrn* operons rearranges the chromosome in host-specialized species of *Salmonella*

Shu-Lin Liu [1], Kenneth E. Sanderson *

Salmonella Genetic Stock Centre, Department of Biological Sciences, University of Calgary, Calgary, Alberta, T2N 1N4, Canada

Received 18 March 1998; revised 6 May 1998; accepted 11 May 1998

Abstract

Partial digestion with I-*Ceu*I, which digests bacterial DNA at the gene coding for the large subunit rRNA, established the *rrn* genomic skeleton (the distance in kb between rRNA operons) in 56 strains of *Salmonella*, from Salmonella Reference B (SARB) set. All had seven I-*Ceu*I sites, indicating seven *rrn* operons. The order of I-*Ceu*I fragments was ABCDEFG in *S. typhimurium* LT2 and in 31 other species, mostly host-generalists; in *S. typhi*, *S. paratyphi* C, *S. gallinarum*, and *S. pullorum* (host-specialized species), these fragments are rearranged, due to homologous recombination between the *rrn* operons. Rearrangements, such as inversions and translocations not involving the *rrn* operons, are rare. I-*Ceu*I fragments of some species are larger than the norm, suggesting the insertion of unique blocks of DNA by lateral transfer from other species. © 1998 Federation of European Microbiological Societies. Published by Elsevier Science B.V. All rights reserved.

Keywords: Salmonella; Chromosome; I-*Ceu*I; Pulsed-field gel electrophoresis

1. Introduction

The gene order in the chromosomes of enteric bacteria such as *E. coli* K-12 and *S. typhimurium* LT2 is strongly conserved [1,2]. This is surprising, because rearrangements occur during culture; duplications are frequent (10^{-3} to 10^{-5}) [3,4], as well as inversions and translocations [3,5]. This stability indicates that forces select against cells with rearrangements.

Pulsed-field gel electrophoresis (PFGE) permits rapid construction of genomic maps especially using the endonuclease I-*Ceu*I [6] to make the '*rrn* skeleton' showing the number and locations of the *rrn* genes for rRNA [7]. I-*Ceu*I is encoded by a class I mobile intron in the *rrl* gene for the large subunit rRNA (23S) in the chloroplast DNA of *Chlamydomonas eugamatos* [8]. I-*Ceu*I recognizes a 19 bp sequence in the *rrl* gene [9], this site is present in all seven *rrl* genes of enteric bacteria, but at no other locations [6]. The order of I-*Ceu*I fragments for *S. typhimurium* LT2, in Fig. 1A, is the same in *E. coli* K-12. Because I-*Ceu*I cleaves only *rrn* operons and because the *rrn* skeleton is highly conserved in enteric bacteria, related wild-type strains usually yield identical fingerprints; for example, 17 independent wild-type *S. typhimurium* strains gave very similar I-*Ceu*I digests, indicating chromosome conservation [7].

However, in *S. typhi* Ty2 the order of I-*Ceu*I frag-

* Corresponding author. Tel.: +1 (403) 220 6792; Fax: +1 (403) 289 9311; E-mail: kesander@acs.ucalgary.ca

[1] Present address: Department of Medical Biochemistry, University of Calgary, Calgary, Alberta, Canada T2N 1N4.

0378-1097/98/$19.00 © 1998 Federation of European Microbiological Societies. Published by Elsevier Science B.V. All rights reserved.
PII: S0378-1097(98)00225-0

JOURNAL OF BACTERIOLOGY, Nov. 1999, p. 6747–6755 Vol. 181, No. 21
0021-9193/99/$04.00+0
Copyright © 1999, American Society for Microbiology. All Rights Reserved.

Bacterial Phylogenetic Clusters Revealed by Genome Structure

SHU-LIN LIU,[1]* ANTHONY B. SCHRYVERS,[1] KENNETH E. SANDERSON,[2] AND RANDAL N. JOHNSTON[3]

Department of Microbiology and Infectious Diseases,[1] Department of Biological Sciences,[2] and Department of Biochemistry and Molecular Biology,[3] University of Calgary, Calgary, Alberta T2N 4N1, Canada

Received 13 April 1999/Accepted 19 August 1999

Current bacterial taxonomy is mostly based on phenotypic criteria, which may yield misleading interpretations in classification and identification. As a result, bacteria not closely related may be grouped together as a genus or species. For pathogenic bacteria, incorrect classification or misidentification could be disastrous. There is therefore an urgent need for appropriate methodologies to classify bacteria according to phylogeny and corresponding new approaches that permit their rapid and accurate identification. For this purpose, we have devised a strategy enabling us to resolve phylogenetic clusters of bacteria by comparing their genome structures. These structures were revealed by cleaving genomic DNA with the endonuclease I-*CeuI*, which cuts within the 23S ribosomal DNA (rDNA) sequences, and by mapping the resulting large DNA fragments with pulsed-field gel electrophoresis. We tested this experimental system on two representative bacterial genera: *Salmonella* and *Pasteurella*. Among *Salmonella* spp., I-*CeuI* mapping revealed virtually indistinguishable genome structures, demonstrating a high degree of structural conservation. Consistent with this, 16S rDNA sequences are also highly conserved among the *Salmonella* spp. In marked contrast, the *Pasteurella* strains have very different genome structures among and even within individual species. The divergence of *Pasteurella* was also reflected in 16S rDNA sequences and far exceeded that seen between *Escherichia* and *Salmonella*. Based on this diversity, the *Pasteurella haemolytica* strains we analyzed could be divided into 14 phylogenetic groups and the *Pasteurella multocida* strains could be divided into 9 groups. If criteria for defining bacterial species or genera similar to those used for *Salmonella* and *Escherichia coli* were applied, the striking phylogenetic diversity would allow bacteria in the currently recognized species of *P. multocida* and *P. haemolytica* to be divided into different species, genera, or even higher ranks. On the other hand, strains of *Pasteurella ureae* and *Pasteurella pneumotropica* are very similar to those of *P. multocida* in both genome structure and 16S rDNA sequence and should be regarded as strains within this species. We conclude that large-scale genome structure can be a sensitive indicator of phylogenetic relationships and that, therefore, I-*CeuI*-based genomic mapping is an efficient tool for probing the phylogenetic status of bacteria.

Bacterial genera or species, as defined by current taxonomic approaches (18, 44), may include bacteria that in fact are not closely related phylogenetically. For example, the DNA G+C content of accepted *Bacillus* species varies from 32 to 69 mol% (8), although species of a genus are not normally expected to differ from one another by more than 10 mol%. This situation results largely from the lack of appropriate methodologies for classifying bacteria on a phylogenetic basis. Consequent errors in bacterial identification could be quite misleading both in basic research and in practical applications. Therefore, the ability to efficiently distinguish phylogenetic groups of bacteria within an apparent taxonomic species is desirable, especially for the correct diagnosis and timely treatment of infectious diseases caused by bacterial pathogens. Molecular techniques such as RNA and DNA or protein sequencing have been extremely useful in establishing the phylogenetic relationships among organisms and in discriminating bacteria by phylogeny. However, such sequence analyses provide information for only a tiny (though important) portion of the genome, and different choices of sequences for analysis can lead to remarkably variable conclusions (10, 21). Furthermore, it can be difficult to distinguish recently diverged bacteria solely on the basis of limited DNA or RNA sequence analysis. For example, 16S rRNA (or ribosomal DNA [rDNA]) sequencing (16), currently the most frequently used technique for phylogenetic studies of bacteria, is efficient only in resolving genera and higher taxa; for ranks lower than genus it loses resolution.

The physical structure of bacterial genomes as revealed by endonuclease mapping, on the other hand, could provide an alternative parameter to be employed in phylogenetic studies (26, 29). The mapping approach involves the use of endonucleases such as I-*CeuI* (17), *XbaI*, *AvrII*, et al. (24, 25). The genomic DNA fragments generated are then separated according to size by pulsed-field gel electrophoresis (PFGE). The maps thus established reveal the size and geometry of the genome, the copy number and genomic distribution of *rrn* operons, and major genomic events, e.g., insertions, duplications, deletions, inversions, and translocations of DNA segments (29–31). Closely related bacteria can have highly similar genome structures; the similarity decreases and eventually vanishes as the phylogenetic relationship becomes more distant.

In this study, we examine the relatedness of bacterial populations within taxonomic species by revealing and comparing their genome structures. We focus on two genera of pathogenic bacteria: *Salmonella*, which consists of more than 2,300 known species, or serovars (38, 39), that display a highly conserved genetic background (9, 19, 22, 23), and *Pasteurella*, which consists of about 25 species of both genetically and biologically more diverse bacteria (3, 7, 11, 36, 40). Our data indicate that the analysis of genome structure readily provides information useful to the elucidation and identification of phylogenetic clusters.

* Corresponding author. Mailing address: Department of Microbiology and Infectious Diseases, University of Calgary, 3330 Hospital Dr., NW, Calgary, AB T2N 4N1, Canada. Phone: 403-220-3799. Fax: 403-283-8727. E-mail: slliu@ucalgary.ca.

JOURNAL OF BACTERIOLOGY, May 2002, p. 2626–2633 Vol. 184, No. 10
0021-9193/02/$04.00+0 DOI: 10.1128/JB.184.10.2626–2633.2002
Copyright © 2002, American Society for Microbiology. All Rights Reserved.

The Evolving Genome of *Salmonella enterica* Serovar Pullorum

Gui-Rong Liu,[1,2] Andrea Rahn,[3]† Wei-Qiao Liu,[3] Kenneth E. Sanderson,[3] Randal N. Johnston,[4] and Shu-Lin Liu[1,2]*

Department of Microbiology and Infectious Diseases,[1] Department of Biological Sciences,[3] and Department of Biochemistry and Molecular Biology,[4] University of Calgary, Calgary, Alberta T2N 4N1, Canada, and Department of Pathogenic Biology, Peking University Health Science Center, 100083 Beijing, China[2]

Received 20 December 2001/Accepted 15 February 2002

Salmonella enterica **serovar Pullorum is a fowl-adapted bacterial pathogen that causes dysentery (pullorum disease). Host adaptation and special pathogenesis make *S. enterica* serovar Pullorum an exceptionally good system for studies of bacterial evolution and speciation, especially regarding pathogen-host interactions and the acquisition of pathogenicity. We constructed a genome map of *S. enterica* serovar Pullorum RKS5078, using I-*Ceu*I, *Xba*I, *Avr*II, and *Spe*I and Tn*10* insertions. Pulsed-field gel electrophoresis was employed to separate the large DNA fragments generated by the endonucleases. The genome is 4,930 kb, which is similar to most salmonellas . However, the genome of *S. enterica* serovar Pullorum RKS5078 is organized very differently from the majority of salmonellas, with three major inversions and one translocation. This extraordinary genome structure was seen in most *S. enterica* serovar Pullorum strains examined, with different structures in a minority of *S. enterica* serovar Pullorum strains. We describe the coexistence of different genome structures among the same bacteria as genomic plasticity. Through comparisons with *S. enterica* serovar Typhimurium, we resolved seven putative insertions and eight deletions ranging in size from 12 to 157 kb. The genomic plasticity seen among *S. enterica* serovar Pullorum strains supported our hypothesis about its association with bacterial evolution: a large genomic insertion (157 kb in this case) disrupted the genomic balance, and rebalancing by independent recombination events in individual lineages resulted in diverse genome structures. As far as the structural plasticity exists, the *S. enterica* serovar Pullorum genome will continue evolving to reach a further streamlined and balanced structure.**

The bacterial genus *Salmonella* consists of more than 2,400 documented species, many of which are important pathogens in humans or animals (4, 14, 16, 41, 42, 44, 45). Selander and colleagues have assembled three sets of reference strains for representative *Salmonella* species (5, 7, 8). The *Salmonella* species are very closely related to one another, as judged by genomic DNA reassociation rates (9, 15), which could be higher than 90%. Despite such close relatedness, different *Salmonella* species may have drastically different biological properties, especially in host range and the nature of diseases they cause. For example, *S. enterica* serovar Typhimurium infects many host species, including humans, mice, and fowl, but *S. enterica* serovar Typhi, a close relative of *S. enterica* serovar Typhimurium , is strictly limited to humans. *S. enterica* serovar Pullorum and *S. enterica* serovar Gallinarum, on the other hand, are both specific to fowl, but they cause distinct diseases, with *S. enterica* serovar Pullorum causing dysentery (pullorum disease) and *S. enterica* serovar Gallinarum causing typhoid fever (45, 46). Our long-term goal is, through genomic comparisons among representative *Salmonella* species, to explore the mechanisms of genomic divergence and evolution that have brought about the genetic differences and made each of the *Salmonella* species unique.

Representative strains of two *Salmonella* serovars have been completely sequenced, *S. enterica* serovar Typhimurium LT2 (33) and *S. enterica* serovar Typhi CT18 (39). Base-to-base comparisons of these sequenced *Salmonella* genomes would surely resolve all the genetic differences between them and provide new insights into the mechanisms of phylogenetic divergence and evolution of these bacteria. However, there are more than 2,400 *Salmonella* serovars, each of which is unique. Sequencing all of them is out of the question. Based on the great genetic similarity among all *Salmonella* species, we suggest and are testing a complementary approach to comparative genomics of salmonellas: determining the overall genome structure and locating genomic differences by physical mapping. This can be done on a very large number of selected *Salmonella* species within a relatively short time. Once insertions are located, they can be further analyzed by sequencing and functional studies. Deletions can be defined through comparisons with the genomic sequence of *S. enterica* serovar Typhimurium. Inversions and translocations can be very efficiently resolved by physical mapping. Previously, we have mapped large-scale genomic insertions, inversions, and translocations in a number of *Salmonella* species (18, 20, 22–24). We have now optimized the techniques to greater accuracy and higher efficiency for systematic comparisons among *Salmonella* spp.

S. enterica serovar Pullorum is highly adapted to fowl, although *S. enterica* serovar Pullorum infections in primates have been reported (36). However, because of the high specificity of *S. enterica* serovar Pullorum for fowl, *S. enterica* serovar Pullorum infections in mammals are extremely rare and therefore have not been a serious public health issue.

* Corresponding author. Mailing address: Department of Microbiology and Infectious Diseases, University of Calgary, 3330 Hospital Dr. NW, Calgary, Alberta, T2N 4N1, Canada. Phone: (403) 220-3799. Fax: (403) 270-0834. E-mail: slliu@ucalgary.ca.
† Present address: Department of Microbiology, University of Guelph, Guelph, Ontario N1G 2W1, Canada.

北 京 大 学 学 报（医 学 版）
JOURNAL OF PEKING UNIVERSITY(HEALTH SCIENCES) Vol. 34 No. 5 Oct. 2002 · 457 ·

·引进人才园地·

Bacterial genome structure: a molecular marker to reveal phylogenetic clusters

LIU Shu-Lin[1,2 △], LIU Gui-Rong[1,2], LI Shao-Xian[3], LIU Wei-Qiao[4], ZHENG Jun-Fang[2], ZHU Wan-Fu[2], GU Hong-Xi[3], GUO Xiao-Kui[3], MA Jia-Yu[3], Kenneth E. Sanderson[4], ZHOU Yu-Guang[5], Randal N. Johnston[6]

(1. Department of Microbiology and Infectious Diseases, 4. Department of Biological Sciences, 6. Department of Biochemistry and Molecular Biology, University of Calgary, Calgary, AB, Canada; 2. Department of Microbiology, Peking University School of Basic Medical Sciences; 3. Department of Microbiology, Harbin Medical University; 5. Institute of Microbiology, Chinese Academy of Sciences)

KEY WORDS Genome structure; Phylogenetic cluster; I-*Ceu* I

Bacteria form phylogenetic clusters, reflecting common ancestry. The genus *Salmonella*, for example, contains more than 2 400 known species, or serovars[1-3], all of which are closely related: (1) genomic DNA/DNA re-association is mostly over 70% and could be as high as more than 90%[2,4]; and (2) 16 S rRNA sequence identity is 98% or higher (Liu Shu-Lin, unpublished data). Suitable molecular markers need be found to reveal the phylogenetic clusters of bacteria for categorizing these microorganisms according to their natural relationships. The use of 16 S or 23 S rRNA sequences has revolutionized bacterial phylogenetic studies during the past two decades[5,6], but the small information contents of the rRNA sequences limited their usage, especially for taxonomic ranks of genus and below. As a result, the current classification system of bacteria is still based on phenotypic features that do not necessarily reflect phylogeny and many bacterial taxa contain phylogenetically diverse bacteria. We have been evaluating some global features of the entire genome to extract the phylogenetic information. The physical structure, among other parameters, of the bacterial genome, for instance, is one of the candidates to be tested for its usefulness in phylogenetic studies.

The first line of evidence suggesting that the physical structure of the bacterial genome may be highly conservative in evolution and thus may reflect the bacterial phylogeny comes from the comparison of the genetic maps of *Escherichia coli* and *Salmonella typhimurium*[7], bacteria of two related genera that have diverged for over 100 million years[8-10] but still have strikingly similar genome structures. Some evolutionary events, including base pair substitutions, horizontal gene transfers, genomic deletions, and rearrangements, are the known factors causing the bacteria to diverge from their ancestors and, eventually, to adapt into new niches as new species; all of these events have the potential to make substantial changes on the physical structure of the genome. One key issue here is how to resolve the bacterial genome structure and detect such changes in order to reveal the phylogenetic clusters of bacteria according to their genomic similarities and differences.

Currently, the most commonly used technologies for revealing the genome structures are sequencing and physical mapping. Genomic sequencing has the highest resolution of analysis and provides a complete set of information about the whole organism. Since the completion of the whole genome sequencing of *Haemophilus influenzae* Rd in 1995[11], hundreds of bacterial genomes have been or are being sequenced. However, because large numbers of bacterial strains have

Fund Project: Supported by an operating grant from the Medical Research Council of Canada (MRC, Grant # GOP 38106) to Liu Shu-Lin, an operating grant from the Natural Sciences and Engineering Research Council of Canada (NSERC, Grant # 216912-00) to Liu Shu-Lin, an operating grant from the Canadian Institutes for Health Research (CIHR, Grant # MOP-47817) to Liu Shu-Lin, a "985 Plan" grant from Peking University Health Science Center to Liu Shu-Lin, an NSERC operating grant to Sanderson KE, and an MRC operating grant to Johnston RN. Liu Shu-Lin was also supported by Alberta Cancer Board. Liu Wei-Qiao is a summer student of Sanderson KE supported by Alberta Heritage Foundation for Medical Research

△ Corresponding author email: sllin@ucalgary.ca

?1994-2015 China Academic Journal Electronic Publishing House. All rights reserved. http://www.cnki.net

JOURNAL OF BACTERIOLOGY, Nov. 2002, p. 6190–6197 Vol. 184, No. 22
0021-9193/02/$04.00+0 DOI: 10.1128/JB.184.22.6190–6197.2002
Copyright © 2002, American Society for Microbiology. All Rights Reserved.

Inversions over the Terminus Region in *Salmonella* and *Escherichia coli*: IS*200*s as the Sites of Homologous Recombination Inverting the Chromosome of *Salmonella enterica* Serovar Typhi

Suneetha Alokam,[1] Shu-Lin Liu,[2] Kamal Said,[1] and Kenneth E. Sanderson[1]*

Departments of Biological Sciences[1] and Microbiology and Infectious Diseases,[2] University of Calgary, Calgary, Alberta T2N 1N4, Canada

Received 25 April 2002/Accepted 19 August 2002

Genomic rearrangements (duplications and inversions) in enteric bacteria such as *Salmonella enterica* serovar Typhimurium LT2 and *Escherichia coli* K12 are frequent (10^{-3} to 10^{-5}) in culture, but in wild-type strains these genomic rearrangements seldom survive. However, inversions commonly survive in the terminus of replication (TER) region, where bidirectional DNA replication terminates; nucleotide sequences from *S. enterica* serovar Typhimurium LT2, *S. enterica* serovar Typhi CT18, *E. coli* K12, and *E. coli* O157:H7 revealed genomic inversions spanning the TER region. Assuming that *S. enterica* serovar Typhimurium LT2 represents the ancestral genome structure, we found an inversion of 556 kb in serovar Typhi CT18 between two of the 25 IS*200* elements and an inversion of about 700 kb in *E. coli* K12 and *E. coli* O157:H7. In addition, there is another inversion of 500 kb in *E. coli* O157:H7 compared with *E. coli* K12. PCR analysis confirmed that all *S. enterica* serovar Typhi strains tested, but not strains of other *Salmonella* serovars, have an inversion at the exact site of the IS*200* insertions. We conclude that inversions of the TER region survive because they do not significantly change replication balance or because they are part of the compensating mechanisms to regain chromosome balance after it is disrupted by insertions, deletions, or other inversions.

The order of orthologous genes on the chromosomes of enteric bacteria such as *Escherichia coli* K12 and *Salmonella enterica* serovar Typhimurium LT2 was shown by classical genetic exchange methods to be strongly conserved (24, 37), and this has now been confirmed by nucleotide sequence data (6, 30). This conservation was retained even after the genera diverged over 100 million years ago (32) and in spite of base pair divergence of orthologues, which averages about 15%. In addition, lateral genetic transfer has inserted nonorthologous genes that comprise about 30% of the total genetic structure, resulting in mosaic chromosomes. This conservation is surprising, because during growth in culture, chromosome rearrangements such as duplications occur at high frequencies (10^{-3} to 10^{-5}) (3, 19) and some inversions and translocations, especially those with end points in the *rrn* operons, are common (36). These rearrangement types must have been selected against in evolution, because they are rarely detected in wild-type strains from nature. In contrast to this conservation within the enteric bacteria, gene order in most bacteria is not conserved during evolution (10, 21, 31), though species of *Chlamydia* also show striking conservation (35).

However, even in the enteric bacteria, two types of genomic rearrangements are often observed. Firstly, inversions and translocations due to homologous recombination between the seven *rrn* operons are common in species such as *Salmonella enterica* serovar Typhi; among 127 wild-type strains there were 21 different genome types, based on differences in order of the fragments between the *rrn* operons (28). Rearrangements were also found in some other serovars, such as *S. enterica* serovar Pullorum and *S. enterica* serovar Gallinarum, which are "host specialized," but most species, especially those that are "host generalists," do not show these types of rearrangements (29). Secondly, some wild-type strains show inversions which cover the terminus of replication (TER) region; this was first detected by genetic analysis as an inversion between *E. coli* K12 and *S. enterica* serovar Typhimurium LT2 (11, 38). This inversion was confirmed using pulsed-field gel electrophoresis (PFGE); the same technique detected inversions in the TER region involving *S. enterica* serovar Typhimurium, *S. enterica* serovar Enteritidis, and *S. enterica* serovar Typhi (27).

In the past few years, the complete nucleotide sequences have been published for *E. coli* K12 (6), *E. coli* O157:H7 (*E. coli* O157:H7 strain EDL933 and *E. coli* O157:H7 strain Sakai-VT2) (17, 34), *S. enterica* serovar Typhimurium LT2 (30), and *S. enterica* serovar Typhi CT18 (33). Pulsed-field gel electrophoresis showed that serovar Typhi Ty2 differs from *S. enterica* serovar Typhimurium LT2 by an inversion over the TER region (27). We have made sequence comparisons which show that the same inversion in serovar Typhi strain CT18 is due to homologous recombination between two of the 25 IS*200* elements in serovar Typhi CT18. PCR analysis of representative strains revealed that all *S. enterica* serovar Typhi strains tested, but no other *Salmonella* strains, have an inversion at that point.

MATERIALS AND METHODS

Bacterial strains and cultivation conditions. The strains, which are maintained in 15% glycerol at −70°C in the collection of the *Salmonella* Genetic Stock Center (www.ucalgary.ca/~kesander), are shown together with their sources in Table 1. Single colony isolates were used in all experiments. All strains were grown at 37°C in Luria-Bertani medium; 1.5% agar was added for solid media.

* Corresponding author. Mailing address: Department of Biological Sciences, University of Calgary, 2500 University Dr. N.W., Calgary, Alberta T2N 1N4, Canada. Phone: (403) 220-6792. Fax: (403) 289-9311. E-mail: kesander@ucalgary.ca.

JOURNAL OF BACTERIOLOGY, Apr. 2003, p. 2131–2142 Vol. 185, No. 7
0021-9193/03/$08.00+0 DOI: 10.1128/JB.185.7.2131–2142.2003
Copyright © 2003, American Society for Microbiology. All Rights Reserved.

Genomic Diversification among Archival Strains of *Salmonella enterica* Serovar Typhimurium LT7

Gui-Rong Liu,[1,2] Kelly Edwards,[3] Abraham Eisenstark,[3] Ying-Mei Fu,[4] Wei-Qiao Liu,[5] Kenneth E. Sanderson,[5] Randal N. Johnston,[6] and Shu-Lin Liu[1,2]*

Departments of Microbiology and Infectious Diseases,[1] Biological Sciences,[5] and Biochemistry and Molecular Biology,[6] University of Calgary, Calgary, T2N 4N1 Alberta, Canada; Cancer Research Center and University of Missouri, Columbia, Missouri 65201[3]; Department of Microbiology, Harbin Medical University, Harbin 150086,[4] and Department of Microbiology, Peking University School of Basic Medical Sciences, Beijing 100083,[2] China

Received 6 May 2002/Accepted 7 January 2003

To document genomic changes during long periods of storage, we analyzed *Salmonella enterica* serovar Typhimurium LT7, a mutator strain that was previously reported to have higher rates of mutations compared to other serovar Typhimurium strains such as LT2. Upon plating directly from sealed agar stabs that had been stocked at room temperature for up to four decades, many auxotrophic mutants derived from LT7 gave rise to colonies of different sizes. Restreaking from single colonies consistently yielded colonies of diverse sizes even when we repeated single-colony isolation nine times. Colonies from the first plating had diverse genomic changes among and even within individual vials, including translocations, inversions, duplications, and point mutations, which were detected by rare-cutting endonuclease analysis with pulsed-field gel electrophoresis. Interestingly, even though the colony size kept diversifying, all descendents of the same single colonies from the first plating had the same sets of detected genomic changes. We did not detect any colony size or genome structure diversification in serovar Typhimurium LT7 stocked at −70°C or in serovar Typhimurium LT2 stocked either at −70°C or at room temperature. These results suggest that, although colony size diversification occurred during rapid growth, all detected genomic changes took place during the storage at room temperature and were carried over to their descendents without further changes during rapid growth in rich medium. We constructed a genomic cleavage map on the LT7 strain that had been stocked at −70°C and located all of the detected genomic changes on the map. We speculated on the significance of mutators for survival and evolution under environmentally stressed conditions.

Comparative studies of bacteria have demonstrated the high level of conservation of the basic genome structure, i.e., the physical arrangement of DNA segments on the genome, in evolution. The earliest known example comes from the comparison of *Salmonella enterica* serovar Typhimurium and *Escherichia coli*, bacteria of two genera that have diverged for over 100 million years (6, 8, 39) but still have very similar genome structures (19). Specifically, they have similar genome sizes, similar sets of genes, and similar gene orders on the genome. Bacteria with closer phylogenetic relationships have even greater similarity. For instance, wild-type strains of serovar Typhimurium isolated from different sources have an indistinguishable genome structure as measured by I-*Ceu*I cleavage patterns (25).

Genomic diversification does occur among cells of the same clone in culture and presumably also in nature, including duplication and inversion of genomic segments, at frequencies as high as 10^{-5} to 10^{-3} (3, 13). However, most of these types of genomic changes are selected against in nature and therefore cannot be easily detected. In order to capture such genomic changes for the elucidation of the basic rules in genomic diversification during evolution, we examined serovar Typhimurium cultures that had been stocked for several decades in sealed agar stabs at room temperature, a condition allowing slow growth for some time until the nutrients become exhausted. This archival system of serovar Typhimurium cultures provides a unique chance to detect genetic and genomic changes. Assuming that the originally uniform medium would become distinct in different parts of the stab with the growth of the bacteria and their competition with one another, we would expect to see survivors with unique sets of spontaneous genomic changes selected in different parts of the stab in adaptation to the local specific ecological conditions. We aim at detecting the hypothesized genomic changes and documenting the genomic diversification in this system. We have a collection of spontaneous mutants of serovar Typhimurium (43), including those derived from strain LT2 (16) and those from strain LT7 (15, 16, 35). When a program of developing a chromosomal map of serovar Typhimurium was initiated a half century ago, it was recognized that auxotrophic mutants selected from the LT2 strain had low rates of reversion to prototrophy. However, auxotrophs selected from LT7 had high reversion rates, making it difficult to distinguish recombinants from revertants upon transduction with phage P22. Therefore, the resulting chromosomal map was constructed with LT2, not LT7.

The LT7 strain was initially designated a phenotypic mutator and later shown to be due to a *mut* defect (15, 35). This genotype would indicate a possibility that populations within the LT7 culture might have greater diversity than those within the LT2 culture. In a preliminary parallel study with LT2 and LT7 mutants, we found great uniformity with LT2 mutants;

* Corresponding author. Mailing address: Department of Microbiology and Infectious Diseases, University of Calgary, 3330 Hospital Dr., NW, Calgary, Alberta T2N 4N1, Canada. Phone: (403) 220-3799. Fax: (403) 270-0834. E-mail: slliu@ucalgary.ca.

BMC Genomics

BioMed Central

Research article

Open Access

Wavelet to predict bacterial *ori* and *ter*: a tendency towards a physical balance

Jiuzhou Song[1], Antony Ware[2] and Shu-Lin Liu*[1,3]

Address: [1]Departments of Microbiology and Infectious Diseases, University of Calgary, Calgary, Canada, [2]Mathematics and Statistics, University of Calgary, Calgary, Canada and [3]Department of Microbiology, Peking University School of Basic Medical Sciences, Beijing, China

Email: Jiuzhou Song - songj@ucalgary.ca; Antony Ware - ware@math.ucalgary.ca; Shu-Lin Liu* - slliu@ucalgary.ca

* Corresponding author

Published: 5 May 2003

BMC Genomics 2003, 4:17

Received: 6 January 2003

Accepted: 5 May 2003

This article is available from: http://www.biomedcentral.com/1471-2164/4/17

© 2003 Song et al; licensee BioMed Central Ltd. This is an Open Access article: verbatim copying and redistribution of this article are permitted in all media for any purpose, provided this notice is preserved along with the article's original URL.

Abstract

Background: Chromosomal DNA replication in bacteria starts at the origin (*ori*) and the two replicores propagate in opposite directions up to the terminus (*ter*) region. We hypothesize that the two replicores need to reach *ter* at the same time to maintain a physical balance; DNA insertion would disrupt such a balance, requiring chromosomal rearrangements to restore the balance. To test this hypothesis, we needed to demonstrate that *ori* and *ter* are in a physical balance in bacterial chromosomes. Using wavelet analysis, we documented GC skew, AT skew, purine excess and keto excess on the published bacterial genomic sequences to locate the turning (minimum and maximum) points on the curves. Previously, the minimum point had been supposed to correlate with *ori* and the maximum to correlate with *ter*.

Results: We observed a strong tendency of the bacterial chromosomes towards a physical balance, with the minima and maxima corresponding to the known or putative *ori* and *ter* and being about half chromosome separated in most of the bacteria studied. A nonparametric method based on wavelet transformation was employed to perform significance tests for the predicted loci.

Conclusions: The wavelet approach can reliably predict the *ori* and *ter* regions and the bacterial chromosomes have a strong tendency towards a physical balance between *ori* and *ter*.

Background

Replication of the bacterial chromosomal DNA starts at the origin (*ori*) and the two replication forks (or replicores) propagate in opposite directions up to the terminus (*ter*) region, as demonstrated in *Escherichia coli* [1-7]. Obviously, the two replication forks need to reach the *ter* region at the same time to optimize the replication process. It is therefore reasonable to assume that *ori* and *ter* should have a physical balance between them, i.e., opposite to each other, on the chromosome to guarantee a synchronous completion of the bi-directional chromosomal replication. Based on this assumption, we hypothesize that lateral transfer of large blocks of DNA into a bacterial chromosome would disrupt such a balance, making necessary the rearrangements of the chromosome to restore the balance. We have observed and reported the large insertions and the striking chromosomal rearrangements in *Salmonella typhi* [8-10]. The 180° physical balance between *ori* and *ter* has been seen in the complete sequence of *Escherichia coli* K12 [11] and a number of other bacteria sequenced subsequently. To address the importance of such a physical balance of the bacterial chromosomes in evolution, we proposed a model of bacterial speciation, i.e., the Adopt-Adapt Model [12,13]. However, some sequenced chromosomes, such as that of *Bacillus subtilis* [14], show significant deviation of *ori* and *ter* from the

JOURNAL OF BACTERIOLOGY, May 2004, p. 3214–3223 Vol. 186, No. 10
0021-9193/04/$08.00+0 DOI: 10.1128/JB.186.10.3214–3223.2004
Copyright © 2004, American Society for Microbiology. All Rights Reserved.

Salmonella enterica Serovar Typhi Strains from Which SPI7, a 134-Kilobase Island with Genes for Vi Exopolysaccharide and Other Functions, Has Been Deleted

Satheesh Nair,[1]* Suneetha Alokam,[1] Sushma Kothapalli,[1] Steffan Porwollik,[2] Emily Proctor,[2] Carmen Choy,[2] Michael McClelland,[2] Shu-Lin Liu,[3] and Kenneth E. Sanderson[1]

Department of Biological Sciences[1] and Department of Microbiology and Infectious Diseases,[3] University of Calgary, Calgary, Alberta, Canada T2N 1N4, and Sidney Kimmel Cancer Center, San Diego, California 92121[2]

Received 28 November 2003/Accepted 3 February 2004

***Salmonella enterica* serovar Typhi has a 134-kb island of DNA identified as salmonella pathogenicity island 7 (SPI7), inserted between *pheU* and *'pheU* (truncated), two genes for tRNA^{Phe}. SPI7 has genes for Vi exopolysaccharide, for type IVB pili, for putative conjugal transfer, and for sopE bacteriophage. Pulsed-field gel electrophoresis following digestion with the endonuclease I-CeuI, using DNA from a set of 120 wild-type strains of serovar Typhi assembled from several sources, identified eight strains in which the I-CeuI G fragment, which contains SPI7, had a large deletion. In addition, agglutination tests with Vi antiserum and phage typing with Vi phages show that all eight strains are Vi negative. We therefore tested these strains for deletion of SPI7 by multiplex PCR, by microarray analysis, and by sequencing of PCR amplicons. Data show that seven of the eight strains are precise deletions of SPI7: a primer pair flanking SPI7 results in a PCR amplicon containing a single *pheU* gene; microarrays show that all SPI7 genes are deleted. Two of the strains produce amplicons which have A derived from *pheU* at bp 27, while five have C derived from *'pheU* at this position; thus, the position of the crossover which results in the deletion can be inferred. The deletion in the eighth strain, TYT1669, removes 175 kb with junction points in genes STY4465 and STY4664; the left junction of SPI7 and adjacent genes, as well as part of SPI7 including the *viaB* operon for Vi exopolysaccharide, was removed, while the right junction of SPI7 was retained. We propose that these deletions occurred during storage following isolation.**

Of the more than 2,300 closely related *Salmonella* serovars recognized, *Salmonella enterica* serovar Typhi (referred to hereafter as serovar Typhi) is the only one which grows exclusively in humans and causes typhoid enteric fever. The closely related serovar *S. enterica* serovar Typhimurium is a host-generalist able to grow on a wide range of animals, and is causal agent of gastroenteritis rather than enteric fevers. In most enteric bacteria there is a strong conservation of chromosomal gene order, but serovar Typhi is an exception, because its chromosome shows major rearrangements in gene order in wild-type strains due to homologous recombination between the *rrn* operons (23). These rearrangements were detected by pulsed-field gel electrophoresis (PFGE) analysis involving complete and partial digestion of genomic DNA with intron-encoded endonuclease I-CeuI which cuts only in the *rrn* genes (20). PFGE analysis also revealed the presence of insertions in serovar Typhi, one predicted to be about 120 kb, carrying the *viaB* locus for Vi exopolysaccharide synthesis which is missing from most other *Salmonella* species (21, 23). Further analysis showed that this island contains genes for the type IV pili (37, 38).

This island is now shown in strain CT18 to be a 134-kb pathogenicity island, identified as SPI7, which is inserted between two genes which code for tRNA^{Phe}, *pheU* and *'pheU* (truncated) (29, 31) (Fig. 1A). Distribution of the island seems to be limited in *S. enterica*, with only serovar Typhi, serovar Dublin, and serovar Paratyphi C harboring it at the same *pheU* site; in *Citrobacter freundii* it can be inserted in the *glyU* gene for tRNA (31). The island is a mosaic structure and has been characterized into six distinct regions: the *'pheU* to *ssb* region with genes for conjugal DNA transfer; *pil* genes for type IVB pili; genes which might determine DNA conjugational transfer; sopE bacteriophage genes; *viaB* operon for Vi exopolysaccharide; and integrases and *pheU* gene (31). The presence of genes for type IVB pili and for DNA transfer, suggests that SPI7 might have been obtained by *Salmonella* by horizontal transfer, perhaps as a conjugative transposon (31).

The *viaB* locus in serovar Typhi in SPI7 consists of 10 genes: *tviBCDE* for Vi polysaccharide biosynthesis and *vexABCDE* for export, as well as *tviA*, which is activated by unlinked regulators *rcsB-rcsC* (2, 17) and *ompR-envZ*, which are themselves controlled by pH and osmolarity levels (30). Recently microarray work by Boyd et al. (4) and PCR analysis by Pickard et al. (31) have revealed that the 134-kb island is deleted from a serovar Typhi strain, SARB 64, one of the strains in the SARB set of strains constructed by Boyd et al. (3). The stability of SPI7 is of great interest as the Vi exopolysaccharide is currently used as a component for typhoid vaccines.

Previous analysis carried out by our research group on a set of 120 wild-type strains of serovar Typhi by endonuclease I-CeuI digestion followed by PFGE revealed that some of these strains had reductions in the size of fragment I-CeuI G which contains the *viaB* operon; some of these strains were also

* Corresponding author. Mailing address: Department of Biological Sciences, University of Calgary, 2500 University Dr., Calgary, Alberta T2N 1N4, Canada. Phone: (403) 220-3572. Fax: (403) 289-9311. E-mail: nair@ucalgary.ca.

JOURNAL OF BACTERIOLOGY, Apr. 2005, p. 2638–2650 Vol. 187, No. 8
0021-9193/05/$08.00+0 doi:10.1128/JB.187.8.2638–2650.2005
Copyright © 2005, American Society for Microbiology. All Rights Reserved.

Diversity of Genome Structure in *Salmonella enterica* Serovar Typhi Populations†

Sushma Kothapalli,[1] Satheesh Nair,[1] Suneetha Alokam,[1] Tikki Pang,[2] Rasik Khakhria,[3]‡ David Woodward,[3] Wendy Johnson,[4] Bruce A. D. Stocker,[5]§ Kenneth E. Sanderson,[1]* and Shu-Lin Liu[1,6,7]

Department of Biological Sciences[1] and Department of Microbiology and Infectious Diseases,[6] University of Calgary, Calgary, and Bacteriology and Enteric Diseases Program, National Microbiology Laboratory, Health Canada,[3] and Cangene Corporation,[4] Winnipeg, Manitoba, Canada; Research Policy and Cooperation, World Health Organization, Geneva, Switzerland[2]; Department of Medical Microbiology, Stanford University, Stanford, California[5]; and Department of Microbiology Peking University School of Basic Medical Sciences, Beijing, China[7]

Received 24 September 2004/Accepted 6 January 2005

The genomes of most strains of *Salmonella* and *Escherichia coli* are highly conserved. In contrast, all 136 wild-type strains of *Salmonella enterica* serovar Typhi analyzed by partial digestion with I-CeuI (an endonuclease which cuts within the *rrn* operons) and pulsed-field gel electrophoresis and by PCR have rearrangements due to homologous recombination between the *rrn* operons leading to inversions and translocations. Recombination between *rrn* operons in culture is known to be equally frequent in *S. enterica* serovar Typhi and *S. enterica* serovar Typhimurium; thus, the recombinants in *S. enterica* serovar Typhi, but not those in *S. enterica* serovar Typhimurium, are able to survive in nature. However, even in *S. enterica* serovar Typhi the need for genome balance and the need for gene dosage impose limits on rearrangements. Of 100 strains of genome types 1 to 6, 72 were only 25.5 kb off genome balance (the relative lengths of the replichores during bidirectional replication from *oriC* to the termination of replication [Ter]), while 28 strains were less balanced (41 kb off balance), indicating that the survival of the best-balanced strains was greater. In addition, the need for appropriate gene dosage apparently selected against rearrangements which moved genes from their accustomed distance from *oriC*. Although rearrangements involving the seven *rrn* operons are very common in *S. enterica* serovar Typhi, other duplicated regions, such as the 25 IS*200* elements, are very rarely involved in rearrangements. Large deletions and insertions in the genome are uncommon, except for deletions of *Salmonella* pathogenicity island 7 (usually 134 kb) from fragment I-CeuI-G and 40-kb insertions, possibly a prophage, in fragment I-CeuI-E. The phage types were determined, and the origins of the phage types appeared to be independent of the origins of the genome types.

Salmonella enterica serovar Typhi is host restricted, for it grows only in humans, where it causes typhoid enteric fever (13, 51). The annual global incidence of typhoid fever is estimated to be 21.6 million cases, with more than 220,000 deaths (10). The emergence of antibiotic-resistant strains (8) and the increased incidence of typhoid fever in human immunodeficiency virus type 1-infected persons are causes for concern. The genus *Salmonella* is separated into two species and more than 2,500 serovars (52) on the basis of the somatic and flagellar antigens. Many of the serovars, such as *S. enterica* serovar Typhimurium, are host generalists, growing in many different animal species and humans and causing gastroenteritis.

S. enterica serovar Typhi is more homogeneous than most serovars of *Salmonella*. Using multilocus enzyme electrophoresis, Reeves et al. (54) and Selander et al. (58) showed that *S. enterica* serovar Typhi strains constitute only one or two clones that are widely separated from the other serovars in subspecies I. Membrane protein profiles (15, 17) and plasmids (42) show homogeneity. Multilocus sequence typing of housekeeping genes has suggested that *S. enterica* serovar Typhi evolved only about 50,000 years ago from other *Salmonella* serovars (30).

The orders of orthologous genes in *Escherichia coli* K-12 and *S. enterica* serovar Typhimurium LT2 are almost identical, although the genera diverged about 100 to 160 million years ago (38, 48, 59, 62). Within the genus *Salmonella*, the gene order of *S. enterica* serovar Paratyphi B (33) and the gene order of *S. enterica* serovar Enteritidis (36) are very similar to the gene order of *S. enterica* serovar Typhimurium LT2, and chromosomes are also conserved in 17 independent strains of *S. enterica* serovar Typhimurium (39). During growth in laboratory culture, duplications of segments of the chromosome occur at high frequencies (10^{-2} to 10^{-5}) (4, 23), and some inversions, especially those with endpoints in the *rrn* operons, are common (22). Such remarkable conservation of the chromosome during evolution, in spite of the high frequency of

* Corresponding author. Mailing address for Kenneth E. Sanderson: Department of Biological Sciences, University of Calgary, Calgary T2N 1N4, Canada. Phone: (403) 220-6792. Fax: (403) 289-9311. E-mail: kesander@ucalgary.ca. Mailing address for Shu-Lin Liu: Department of Microbiology and Infectious Diseases, University of Calgary, Calgary T2N 1N4, Canada. Phone: (403) 220-3799. Fax: (403) 270-2772. E-mail: slliu@ucalgary.ca.

† Supplemental material for this article may be found at http://jb.asm.org/.

‡ Present address: 32 Amberwood Crescent, Nepean, Ontario, Canada.

§ Deceased.

JOURNAL OF BACTERIOLOGY, July 2005, p. 4720–4727 Vol. 187, No. 14
0021-9193/05/$08.00+0 doi:10.1128/JB.187.14.4720–4727.2005
Copyright © 2005, American Society for Microbiology. All Rights Reserved.

The Genome of *Salmonella enterica* Serovar Gallinarum: Distinct Insertions/Deletions and Rare Rearrangements

Kai-Yu Wu,[1] Gui-Rong Liu,[1,2] Wei-Qiao Liu,[3] Austin Q. Wang,[1] Sen Zhan,[1] Kenneth E. Sanderson,[3] Randal N. Johnston,[4] and Shu-Lin Liu[1,2]*

Departments of Microbiology and Infectious Diseases,[1] Biological Sciences,[3] and Biochemistry and Molecular Biology,[4] University of Calgary, Calgary, Alberta, Canada, and Department of Microbiology, Peking University Health Science Center, Beijing, China[2]

Received 4 October 2004/Accepted 19 April 2005

***Salmonella enterica* serovar Gallinarum is a fowl-adapted pathogen, causing typhoid fever in chickens. It has the same antigenic formula (1,9,12:—:—) as *S. enterica* serovar Pullorum, which is also adapted to fowl but causes pullorum disease (diarrhea). The close relatedness but distinct pathogeneses make this pair of fowl pathogens good models for studies of bacterial genomic evolution and the way these organisms acquired pathogenicity. To locate and characterize the genomic differences between serovar Gallinarum and other salmonellae, we constructed a physical map of serovar Gallinarum strain SARB21 by using I-CeuI, XbaI, and AvrII with pulsed-field gel electrophoresis techniques. In the 4,740-kb genome, we located two insertions and six deletions relative to the genome of *S. enterica* serovar Typhimurium LT2, which we used as a reference *Salmonella* genome. Four of the genomic regions with reduced lengths corresponded to the four prophages in the genome of serovar Typhimurium LT2, and the others contained several smaller deletions relative to serovar Typhimurium LT2, including regions containing *srfJ*, *std*, and *stj* and gene clusters encoding a type I restriction system in serovar Typhimurium LT2. The map also revealed some rare rearrangements, including two inversions and several translocations. Further characterization of these insertions, deletions, and rearrangements will provide new insights into the molecular basis for the specific host-pathogen interactions and mechanisms of genomic evolution to create a new pathogen.**

Salmonella species are important bacterial pathogens. To date, more than 2,500 *Salmonella* serovars have been identified (39). Genetic evidence shows that all *Salmonella* serovars are closely related (3, 16). For example, comparisons of housekeeping genes indicate 96 to 99% sequence identity among the *Salmonella* serovars (5). According to microarray data, 2,244 potential genes are present in all 24 examined strains of 12 *S. enterica* serovars and 2 strains of *S. bongori* (2); similar observations have also been made by Porwollik and his colleagues (40). Such genes are termed core genes and are assumed to play key roles in many typical cellular functions, e.g., metabolism, biosynthesis, and DNA replication. On the other hand, although the *Salmonella* serovars are closely related by phylogeny, they differ significantly in biology, including factors such as host range and disease spectrum. For instance, serovar Typhimurium infects a broad range of hosts, causing enteritis in humans and typhoid fever in mice, whereas serovar Typhi infects only humans and causes only typhoid fever. It is thus of great interest to ask what genetic differences in the *Salmonella* genomes have caused such phenotypic diversity among these close relatives.

Genomic comparisons between different *Salmonella* serovars have revealed that there are numerous serovar-specific insertions, deletions, inversions, translocations, and pseudogenes in the genomes (4, 20, 22–26, 30, 34, 35, 38). The insertions usually have G+C contents that differ from the average for the whole genome, an indication of exogenous origin. Some insertions have been designated *Salmonella* pathogenicity islands (SPIs) because they contain virulence genes contributing to bacterial pathogenicity. SPI-7, one of the recently identified SPIs, for instance, encodes Vi antigen in serovar Typhi (36, 38). Genomic sequence analysis has revealed many pseudogenes in the genome of serovar Typhi, which may account at least in part for its host specificity.

Serovars Gallinarum and Pullorum are fowl-adapted pathogens and the only known nonflagellate (and thus nonmotile) *Salmonella* lineages. They have the same antigenic formula (1,9,12:—:—) and are indeed very closely related. However, they cause very different diseases, with serovar Gallinarum causing fowl typhoid fever and serovar Pullorum causing pullorum disease. Fowl typhoid fever is a chronic disease of adult chickens, but pullorum disease is an acute diarrheal illness in chicks. Fowl typhoid fever is usually spread by the ingestion of contaminated food or water, whereas pullorum disease can be transferred vertically through eggs in carrier hens (17, 43). The close relatedness, common host specificity, and different pathogeneses of serovars Gallinarum and Pullorum make them good models in comparative genomics for exploration of the evolutionary events converting nonpathogenic bacteria into different pathogens. It is reasonable to suppose that some genomic features shared only by the two *Salmonella* lineages may be responsible for their common phenotypes, such as host range, and other genomic features unique to each of them may account for their distinct pathogeneses. In this study, we aim at finding such respective common and distinct genomic features of serovars Gallinarum and Pullorum.

* Corresponding author. Mailing address: Department of Microbiology and Infectious Diseases, University of Calgary, 3330 Hospital Dr. NW, Calgary, Alberta T2N 4N1, Canada. Phone: (403) 220-3799. Fax: (403) 270-0834. E-mail: slliu@ucalgary.ca.

Genome Plasticity and *ori-ter* Rebalancing in *Salmonella typhi*

Gui-Rong Liu,†‡ Wei-Qiao Liu,§ Randal N. Johnston,‖ Kenneth E. Sanderson,§ Shao-Xian Li,‡[1] and Shu-Lin Liu*†‡*

*Department of Microbiology, Peking University Health Science Center, Beijing, China; †Department of Microbiology and Infectious Diseases, University of Calgary, Calgary, Alberta, Canada; ‡Department of Microbiology, Harbin Medical University, Harbin, China; §Department of Biological Sciences, University of Calgary, Calgary, Alberta, Canada; and ‖Department of Biochemistry and Molecular Biology, University of Calgary, Calgary, Alberta, Canada

Genome plasticity resulting from frequent rearrangement of the bacterial genome is a fascinating but poorly understood phenomenon. First reported in *Salmonella typhi*, it has been observed only in a small number of *Salmonella* serovars, although the over 2,500 known *Salmonella* serovars are all very closely related. To gain insights into this phenomenon and elucidate its roles in bacterial evolution, especially those involved in the formation of particular pathogens, we systematically analyzed the genomes of 127 wild-type *S. typhi* strains isolated from many places of the world and compared them with the two sequenced strains, Ty2 and CT18, attempting to find possible associations between genome rearrangement and other significant genomic features. Like other host-adapted *Salmonella* serovars, *S. typhi* contained large genome insertions, including the 134 kb *Salmonella* pathogenicity island, SPI7. Our analyses showed that SPI7 disrupted the physical balance of the bacterial genome between the replication origin (*ori*) and terminus (*ter*) when this DNA segment was inserted into the genome, and rearrangement in individual strains further changed the genome balance status, with a general tendency toward a better balanced genome structure. In a given *S. typhi* strain, genome diversification occurred and resulted in different structures among cells in the culture. Under a stressed condition, bacterial cells with better balanced genome structures were selected to greatly increase in proportion; in such cases, bacteria with better balanced genomes formed larger colonies and grew with shorter generation times. Our results support the hypothesis that genome plasticity as a result of frequent rearrangement provides the opportunity for the bacterial genome to adopt a better balanced structure and thus eventually stabilizes the genome during evolution.

Introduction

Physical structure of the bacterial genome has been known to be highly conservative during evolution in many cases such as in *Escherichia coli* and *Salmonella*, in which genomic comparisons were possible by linkage analysis (Taylor and Thoman 1964; Sanderson and Demerec 1965), physical mapping (Kohara, Akiyama, and Isono 1987; Smith et al. 1987; Liu and Sanderson 1992; Wong and McClelland 1992), and sequencing (McClelland et al. 2001, 2004; Parkhill et al. 2001; Deng et al. 2003). *Escherichia coli* and *Salmonella* have diverged for over 100 MYR (Ochman and Wilson 1987; Doolittle et al. 1996; Feng, Cho, and Doolittle 1997) but their genome structures remain highly similar (Krawiec and Riley 1990; Liu, Hessel, and Sanderson 1993). Within *Salmonella*, the conservation is even higher: strains across all eight major *Salmonella* subgroups usually have a common genome structure (Liu et al. 1999). However, a small number of *Salmonella* serovars are puzzling exceptions in that they have remarkably diverse genome structures, with the DNA segments being rearranged in many different ways, as observed in *Salmonella typhi* (Liu and Sanderson 1996; Kothapalli et al. 2005) and some other host-adapted *Salmonella* pathogens (Liu and Sanderson 1998; Liu et al. 2003). We speculated that rearrangements leading to genome plasticity in these bacteria might reflect or contribute to some special evolutionary processes in the creation of new pathogens.

[1] This paper is dedicated to the memory of Professor Sho-Xian Li, who deceased on November 21, 2004.

Key words: *Salmonella typhi*, genome plasticity, *ori-ter* rebalancing, I-CeuI, genome rearrangements, typhoid.

E-mail: slliu@bjmu.edu.cn.

Mol. Biol. Evol. 23(2):365–371. 2006
doi:10.1093/molbev/msj042
Advance Access publication October 19, 2005

© The Author 2005. Published by Oxford University Press on behalf of the Society for Molecular Biology and Evolution. All rights reserved. For permissions, please e-mail: journals.permissions@oxfordjournals.org

Previously, in an attempt to correlate genome rearrangement with any other genomic features for clues that might give insights into the phenomenon, we compared the genome maps between *S. typhi* and other *Salmonella* serovars that have stable genomes. Most outstanding of the few extraordinary genomic features that we found in *S. typhi* was a large insertion (Liu and Sanderson 1995*b*), later identified as *Salmonella* pathogenicity island SPI7 with a size of 134 kb (Parkhill et al. 2001; Nair et al. 2004). We postulated that this insertion, while presumably conferring phenotypic benefits to the bacteria, would nevertheless disrupt the physical balance of the circular genome between origin (*ori*) and terminus (*ter*) of DNA replication, delaying the completion of DNA replication cycles and slowing the bacterial growth (Liu and Sanderson 1995*b*, 1995*d*). Based on this postulation, we hypothesized that a physical balance between *ori* and *ter* would normally exist on the bacterial genome for simultaneous completion of DNA replication in the two directions, and rearrangement of genomic DNA segments would help reestablish the balance once it is disrupted (Liu and Sanderson 1995*d*). The first half of this hypothesis has gained substantial support from genomic sequence analyses in numerous bacteria, such as *Haemophilus influenzae* Rd (Fleischmann et al. 1995), *E. coli* K12 (Blattner et al. 1997), *Salmonella typhimurium* LT2 (McClelland et al. 2001), and *Salmonella paratyphi* A (McClelland et al. 2004), which all have the circular genome divided into equal halves by *ori* and *ter*. Consistent with the hypothesis, bacteria with a balanced genome do not exhibit rearrangement, as demonstrated by a uniform genome structure among populations of *S. typhimurium* (Liu and Sanderson 1995*c*) and of *S. paratyphi* A (Liu and Sanderson 1995*a*). Wavelet analysis also reveals a general tendency of the bacterial genomes toward a physical balance between *ori* and *ter* (Song, Ware, and Liu

Author's personal copy

ELSEVIER

Available online at www.sciencedirect.com

ScienceDirect

Genomics 90 (2007) 542–549

GENOMICS

www.elsevier.com/locate/ygeno

Spontaneous conversion between *mutL* and 6 bpΔ*mutL* in *Salmonella typhimurium* LT7: Association with genome diversification and possible roles in bacterial adaptation

Jun Gong [a], Wei-Qiao Liu [b], Gui-Rong Liu [a,b], Fang Chen [a], Jun-Qian Li [a], Guo-Min Xu [a], Ling Wang [a], Randal N. Johnston [c], Abraham Eisenstark [d], Shu-Lin Liu [a,b,*]

[a] *Department of Microbiology, Peking University Health Science Center, Beijing 100083, China*
[b] *Department of Microbiology and Infectious Diseases, University of Calgary, Calgary, Canada AB T2N 4N1*
[c] *Department of Biochemistry and Molecular Biology, University of Calgary, Calgary, Canada AB T2N 4N1*
[d] *Cancer Research Center, University of Missouri at Columbia, Columbia, MO 65211, USA*

Received 14 March 2007; accepted 26 June 2007
Available online 3 August 2007

Abstract

Previously, we reported the phenomenon of genome diversification in *Salmonella typhimurium* LT7, i.e., individual strains derived from LT7 kept changing the genome structure by inversions, translocations, duplications, and mutations. To elucidate the genetic basis, we sequenced selected genes of the mismatch repair (MMR) system for correlations between MMR defects and genome diversification. We chose *S. typhimurium* LT7 mutants 8111F2 and 9052D1 for *mut* gene sequence analyses and found that both mutants had a deletion of one of three tandem 6-bp repeats, GCTGGC GCTGGC GCTGGC, within *mutL*, which was designated 6 bpΔ*mutL*. *mutS* and *mutH* genes were unchanged in the mutants analyzed. Some sublines of 8111F2 and 9052D1 spontaneously stopped the genome diversification process at certain stages during single-colony restreaking passages, and in these strains the 6 bpΔ*mutL* genotype also became wild-type *mutL*. We conclude that conversion between *mutL* and 6 bpΔ*mutL* occurs spontaneously and that transient defects of *mutL* facilitate genome diversification without leading to the accumulation of multiple detrimental genetic changes. Spontaneous conversion between *mutL* and 6 bpΔ*mutL* may be an important mechanism used by bacteria to regulate genetic stability in adaptation to changing environments.
© 2007 Elsevier Inc. All rights reserved.

Keywords: *mutL*; *Salmonella*; Genome diversification; Bacterial adaptation; Mutator

Bacteria of the family *Enterobacteriaceae*, such as those in the genera *Salmonella* and *Escherichia*, usually have stable genome structures as revealed by physical mapping [1,2] and sequencing [3–9]. However, in a previous study, we found that archival strains of *Salmonella typhimurium* LT7, stocked at room temperature in agar stabs for about 4 decades, had diversifying genomes, i.e., individual strains had kept changing the genome structure, leading to mixtures of cells with differently organized genomes [10]. However, the genetic basis of this phenomenon remained unknown.

S. typhimurium LT7 was reported to have a defect in a gene, responsible for an increase in mutation frequency for many loci [11]. The defective gene, or mutator locus, was initially mapped to a genomic region near and upstream of *thr* [12] and was later characterized as part of the mismatch repair (MMR) system, which plays a key role in maintaining genetic stability by correcting DNA biosynthetic errors [13–16]. The basic components in MMR are conserved from bacteria to humans. Three proteins in the MMR system, MutS, MutL, and MutH, are important for initiating the mismatch repair process. MutS is an ATPase that recognizes and binds to mismatched regions of DNA. MutL is also an ATPase and acts as a coordinator between MutS and MutH. MutH is a sequence-specific and methyl-dependent endonuclease that cleaves the newly synthesized and

* Corresponding author. Fax: +86 10 8280 2961.
E-mail address: slliu@ucalgary.ca (S.-L. Liu).

0888-7543/$ - see front matter © 2007 Elsevier Inc. All rights reserved.
doi:10.1016/j.ygeno.2007.06.009

BMC Genomics

BioMed Central

Research article

Open Access

Diverse genome structures of *Salmonella paratyphi* C

Wei-Qiao Liu†[1,2], Gui-Rong Liu†[1,2,3], Jun-Qian Li†[1], Guo-Min Xu[1], Danni Qi[3], Xiao-Yan He[1], Juan Deng[1], Feng-Min Zhang[3], Randal N Johnston[4] and Shu-Lin Liu*[1,2,3]

Address: [1]Microbiology, Peking University Health Science Center, Beijing, China, [2]Microbiology and Infectious Diseases, University of Calgary, Calgary, Canada, [3]Microbiology, Harbin Medical University, Harbin, China and [4]Biochemistry and Molecular Biology, University of Calgary, Calgary, Canada

Email: Wei-Qiao Liu - wqliu@ucalgary.ca; Gui-Rong Liu - grliu@ucalgary.ca; Jun-Qian Li - lijunqian@263.net.cn; Guo-Min Xu - XGM410@163.com; Danni Qi - danni_qi@yahoo.com.cn; Xiao-Yan He - hexiaoyan1970@163.com; Juan Deng - dj5718@sina.com; Feng-Min Zhang - fengminzhang@hotmail.com; Randal N Johnston - rnjohnst@ucalgary.ca; Shu-Lin Liu* - slliu@ucalgary.ca

* Corresponding author † Equal contributors

Published: 27 August 2007

BMC Genomics 2007, **8**:290 doi:10.1186/1471-2164-8-290

Received: 26 March 2007
Accepted: 27 August 2007

This article is available from: http://www.biomedcentral.com/1471-2164/8/290

© 2007 Liu et al; licensee BioMed Central Ltd.
This is an Open Access article distributed under the terms of the Creative Commons Attribution License (http://creativecommons.org/licenses/by/2.0), which permits unrestricted use, distribution, and reproduction in any medium, provided the original work is properly cited.

Abstract

Background: *Salmonella paratyphi* C, like *S. typhi*, is adapted to humans and causes typhoid fever. Previously we reported different genome structures between two strains of *S. paratyphi* C, which suggests that *S. paratyphi* C might have a plastic genome (large DNA segments being organized in different orders or orientations on the genome). As many but not all host-adapted *Salmonella* pathogens have large genomic insertions as well as the supposedly resultant genomic rearrangements, bacterial genome plasticity presents an extraordinary evolutionary phenomenon. Events contributing to genomic plasticity, especially large insertions, may be associated with the formation of particular *Salmonella* pathogens.

Results: We constructed a high resolution genome map in *S. paratyphi* C strain RKS4594 and located four insertions totaling 176 kb (including the 90 kb SPI7) and seven deletions totaling 165 kb relative to *S. typhimurium* LT2. Two rearrangements were revealed, including an inversion of 1602 kb covering the *ter* region and the translocation of the 43 kb I-CeuI F fragment. The 23 wild type strains analyzed in this study exhibited diverse genome structures, mostly as a result of recombination between *rrn* genes. In at least two cases, the rearrangements involved recombination between genomic sites other than the *rrn* genes, possibly homologous genes in prophages. Two strains had a 20 kb deletion between *rrlA* and *rrlB*, which is a highly conservative region and no deletion has been reported in this region in any other *Salmonella* lineages.

Conclusion: *S. paratyphi* C has diverse genome structures among different isolates, possibly as a result of large genomic insertions, e.g., SPI7. Although the *Salmonella* typhoid agents may not be more closely related among them than each of them to other *Salmonella* lineages, they may have evolved in similar ways, i.e., acquiring typhoid-associated genes followed by genome structure rearrangements. Comparison of multiple *Salmonella* typhoid agents at both single sequenced genome and population levels will facilitate the studies on the evolutionary process of typhoid pathogenesis, especially the identification of typhoid-associated genes.

OPEN ACCESS Freely available online PLoS one

Salmonella paratyphi C: Genetic Divergence from *Salmonella choleraesuis* and Pathogenic Convergence with *Salmonella typhi*

Wei-Qiao Liu[1,2¶], Ye Feng[3,4¶], Yan Wang[2¶¤a], Qing-Hua Zou[5], Fang Chen[5], Ji-Tao Guo[5], Yi-Hong Peng[5], Yan Jin[2¤b], Yong-Guo Li[6], Song-Nian Hu[3,4], Randal N. Johnston[7], Gui-Rong Liu[1,2,5*], Shu-Lin Liu[1,2,5,6*]

1 Genomics Research Center, Harbin Medical University, Harbin, China, **2** Microbiology and Infectious Diseases, University of Calgary, Calgary, Alberta, Canada, **3** JD Watson Institute of Genome Sciences, Zhejiang University, Hangzhou, China, **4** Beijing Institute of Genomics, Chinese Academy of Sciences, Beijing, China, **5** Department of Microbiology, Peking University Health Science Center, Beijing, China, **6** Depatment of Infectious Diseases, First Hospital, Harbin Medical University, Harbin, China, **7** Departments of Biochemistry and Molecular Biology, University of Calgary, Calgary, Alberta, Canada

Abstract

Background: Although over 1400 *Salmonella* serovars cause usually self-limited gastroenteritis in humans, a few, e.g., *Salmonella typhi* and *S. paratyphi* C, cause typhoid, a potentially fatal systemic infection. It is not known whether the typhoid agents have evolved from a common ancestor (by divergent processes) or acquired similar pathogenic traits independently (by convergent processes). Comparison of different typhoid agents with non-typhoidal *Salmonella* lineages will provide excellent models for studies on how similar pathogens might have evolved.

Methodologies/Principal Findings: We sequenced a strain of *S. paratyphi* C, RKS4594, and compared it with previously sequenced *Salmonella* strains. RKS4594 contains a chromosome of 4,833,080 bp and a plasmid of 55,414 bp. We predicted 4,640 intact coding sequences (4,578 in the chromosome and 62 in the plasmid) and 152 pseudogenes (149 in the chromosome and 3 in the plasmid). RKS4594 shares as many as 4346 of the 4,640 genes with a strain of *S. choleraesuis*, which is primarily a swine pathogen, but only 4008 genes with another human-adapted typhoid agent, *S. typhi*. Comparison of 3691 genes shared by all six sequenced *Salmonella* strains placed *S. paratyphi* C and *S. choleraesuis* together at one end, and *S. typhi* at the opposite end, of the phylogenetic tree, demonstrating separate ancestries of the human-adapted typhoid agents. *S. paratyphi* C seemed to have suffered enormous selection pressures during its adaptation to man as suggested by the differential nucleotide substitutions and different sets of pseudogenes, between *S. paratyphi* C and *S. choleraesuis*.

Conclusions: *S. paratyphi* C does not share a common ancestor with other human-adapted typhoid agents, supporting the convergent evolution model of the typhoid agents. *S. paratyphi* C has diverged from a common ancestor with *S. choleraesuis* by accumulating genomic novelty during adaptation to man.

Citation: Liu W-Q, Feng Y, Wang Y, Zou Q-H, Chen F, et al. (2009) *Salmonella paratyphi* C: Genetic Divergence from *Salmonella choleraesuis* and Pathogenic Convergence with *Salmonella typhi*. PLoS ONE 4(2): e4510. doi:10.1371/journal.pone.0004510

Editor: Malcolm James Horsburgh, University of Liverpool, United Kingdom

Received October 25, 2008; **Accepted** December 15, 2008; **Published** February 20, 2009

Copyright: © 2009 Liu et al. This is an open-access article distributed under the terms of the Creative Commons Attribution License, which permits unrestricted use, distribution, and reproduction in any medium, provided the original author and source are credited.

Funding: This work was supported by a Canadian Institutes of Health Research grant to RNJ; and a grant of Harbin Medical University, National Natural Science Foundation of China grants (NSFC30370774, NSFC30870098), a 985 Project grant of Peking University Health Science Center, a Specialized Research Fund for the Doctoral Program of Higher Education (No. 20030001029), and a Discovery Grant from Natural Sciences and Engineering Research Council of Canada to SLL. The funders had no role in study design, data collection and analysis, decision to publish, or preparation of the manuscript.

Competing Interests: The authors have declared that no competing interests exist.

* E-mail: grliu@ucalgary.ca (G-RL); slliu@ucalgary.ca (S-LL)

¤a Current address: Department of Microbiology, Harbin Medical University, Harbin, China
¤b Current address: Laboratory of Medical Genetics, Harbin Medical University, Harbin, China

¶ These authors contributed equally to this work.

Introduction

Salmonella are important human and animal pathogens [1,2], and over 1400 serovars have the potential to cause human gastroenteritis, which is essentially a self-limited disease. However, a few *Salmonella* serovars, such as *S. typhi* and *S. paratyphi* A, B and C, elicit typhoid, which is a serious systemic infection with high mortality rates [3,4]. *S. paratyphi* C as a typhoid agent [5–7] is not reported as frequently as *S. typhi* or *S. paratyphi* A or B, partly because this pathogen shares the antigenic formula 6,7:c:1,5 with *S. choleraesuis* and *S. typhisuis* and clinical identification of *Salmonella* isolates usually does not go beyond serotyping, although molecular methods are available to reliably distinguish *S. paratyphi* C from other Group C members [8]. As the gastroenteritis-causing and typhoidal *Salmonella* serovars are all closely related, sharing up to about 90% of their genetic contents [9–14], it is natural to ask how typhoid pathogenicity has developed in just a few of the thousands of *Salmonella* serovars. Specifically, are these similar pathogens the products of divergent (recent common ancestry) or convergent (common pathogenic

RESEARCH LETTER

A genome map of *Salmonella enterica* serovar Agona: numerous insertions and deletions reflecting the evolutionary history of a human pathogen

Fang Chen[1], Cornelis Poppe[2], Gui-Rong Liu[1,3,4], Yong-Guo Li[5], Yi-Hong Peng[1], Kenneth E. Sanderson[4], Randal N. Johnston[6] & Shu-Lin Liu[1,3,4,5]

[1]Department of Microbiology, Peking University Health Science Center, Beijing, China; [2]Laboratory for Foodborne Zoonoses, Public Health Agency of Canada, Guelph, ON, Canada; [3]Genomics Research Center (one of The State-Province Key Laboratories of Biomedicine-Pharmaceutics of China), Harbin Medical University, Harbin, China; [4]Department of Microbiology and Infectious Diseases, University of Calgary, Calgary, AB, Canada; [5]Department of Infectious Diseases, First Hospital, Harbin Medical University, Harbin, China; and [6]Department of Biochemistry and Molecular Biology, University of Calgary, Calgary, AB, Canada

Correspondence: Shu-Lin Liu, Genomics Research Center (one of The State-Province Key Laboratories of Biomedicine-Pharmaceutics of China), First Hospital, Harbin Medical University, 194 Xuefu Road, Harbin 150081, China. Tel.: +86 451 866 691 50; fax: +86 451 875 063 80; e-mail: slliu@ucalgary.ca

Received 12 November 2008; accepted 21 January 2009.
First published online March 2009.

DOI:10.1111/j.1574-6968.2009.01539.x

Editor: Ross Fitzgerald

Keywords
Salmonella Agona; genomic evolution; physical map.

Abstract

Salmonella enterica serovar Agona is an important zoonotic pathogen, causing serious human illness worldwide, but knowledge about its genetics and evolution, especially regarding the genomic events that might have contributed to the formation of *S.* Agona as an important pathogen, is lacking. As a first step toward understanding this pathogen and characterizing its genomic differences with other salmonellae, we constructed a physical map of *S.* Agona in strain SARB1 using I-CeuI, XbaI, AvrII and Tn*10* insertions with pulsed-field gel electrophoresis techniques. On the 4815-kb genomic map, we located 82 genes, revealed one inversion of about 1000 kb and resolved seven deletions and seven insertions ranging from 10 to 67 kb relative to the genome of *Salmonella typhimurium* LT2. These genomic features clearly distinguish *S.* Agona from other previously analyzed salmonellae and provide clues to the molecular basis for its genomic divergence. Additionally, these kinds of physical maps, combined with emerging high-speed sequencing technologies, such as the Solexa or SOLiD techniques, which require a pre-existing high-resolution physical map such as the *S.* Agona map reported here, will play important roles in genomic comparative studies of bacteria involving large numbers of strains.

Introduction

Of the > 2500 closely related *Salmonella* lineages recognized to date, *Salmonella enterica* serovar Agona (antigenic formula, 1,4,12:f,g,s:- -) is an important pathogen, causing serious human illness worldwide (Threlfall *et al.*, 1996; Taylor *et al.*, 1998), and has been implicated in various food-borne outbreaks leading to deaths (Killalea *et al.*, 1996; Shohat *et al.*, 1996; CDC, 1998; Brouard *et al.*, 2007). This *Salmonella* lineage was first identified from cattle in Ghana (Guinee *et al.*, 1961), and then it emerged as a public health concern on a global level. The *Salmonella* Surveillance Annual Summary of the Centers for Disease Control and Prevention (CDC) reported *S.* Agona as one of the top 20 *Salmonella* serovars isolated from human sources, the most frequently reported *Salmonella* serovars from clinical nonhuman sources and the most frequently reported *Salmonella* serovars from nonclinical nonhuman sources during the years 1997–2002 (http://www.cdc.gov/ncidod/dbmd/phlisdata/Salmonella.htm). Many animals, including cattle, swine, chicken and turkey, have frequently been found to be infected with *S.* Agona, and milk, snacks and vegetarian foods have also been identified as sources of infection. Transmission of *S.* Agona to humans commonly occurs by ingestion of such contaminated foods.

During the past few years, increasing numbers of *S.* Agona isolates from humans and animals have been reported and, frequently, the *S.* Agona isolates harbor a huge variety of gene complexes that confer resistance to antimicrobial agents (Angulo *et al.*, 2000; Doublet *et al.*, 2004;

© 2009 Federation of European Microbiological Societies
Published by Blackwell Publishing Ltd. All rights reserved

Wang et al. BMC Microbiology 2010, 10:115
http://www.biomedcentral.com/1471-2180/10/115

BMC Microbiology

RESEARCH ARTICLE Open Access

Production of enterodiol from defatted flaxseeds through biotransformation by human intestinal bacteria

Cheng-Zhi Wang[1†], Xiao-Qing Ma[2†], Dong-Hui Yang[2*], Zhi-Rong Guo[1], Gui-Rong Liu[3,5], Ge-Xin Zhao[1], Jie Tang[1], Ya-Nan Zhang[1], Miao Ma[2], Shao-Qing Cai[2], Bao-Shan Ku[4], Shu-Lin Liu[1,3,5*]

Abstract

Background: The effects of enterolignans, e.g., enterodiol (END) and particularly its oxidation product, enterolactone (ENL), on prevention of hormone-dependent diseases, such as osteoporosis, cardiovascular diseases, hyperlipemia, breast cancer, colon cancer, prostate cancer and menopausal syndrome, have attracted much attention. To date, the main way to obtain END and ENL is chemical synthesis, which is expensive and inevitably leads to environmental pollution. To explore a more economic and eco-friendly production method, we explored biotransformation of enterolignans from precursors contained in defatted flaxseeds by human intestinal bacteria.

Results: We cultured fecal specimens from healthy young adults in media containing defatted flaxseeds and detected END from the culture supernatant. Following selection through successive subcultures of the fecal microbiota with defatted flaxseeds as the only carbon source, we obtained a bacterial consortium, designated as END-49, which contained the smallest number of bacterial types still capable of metabolizing defatted flaxseeds to produce END. Based on analysis with pulsed field gel electrophoresis, END-49 was found to consist of five genomically distinct bacterial lineages, designated Group I-V, with Group I strains dominating the culture. None of the individual Group I-V strains produced END, demonstrating that the biotransformation of substrates in defatted flaxseeds into END is a joint work by different members of the END-49 bacterial consortium. Interestingly, Group I strains produced secoisolariciresinol, an important intermediate of END production; 16S rRNA analysis of one Group I strain established its close relatedness with *Klebsiella*. Genomic analysis is under way to identify all members in END-49 involved in the biotransformation and the actual pathway leading to END-production.

Conclusion: Biotransformation is a very economic, efficient and environmentally friendly way of mass-producing enterodiol from defatted flaxseeds.

Background

Early in the 1980s, enterodiol (END) and enterolactone (ENL) were first detected in the serum, urine and bile of humans and several animals [1,2]. They were classified as phytoestrogens due to their origins from plants and their estrogenic as well as antiestrogenic activities in humans. Epidemiologic and pharmacologic studies have shown that END and particularly its oxidation product ENL have preventive effects on osteoporosis, cardiovascular diseases, hyperlipemia, breast cancer, colon cancer, prostate cancer and menopausal syndrome [3-7]. Unlike other plant-derived lignans, they are also known as mammalian lignan or enterolignan, because they are mainly found in mammals. Numerous studies have indicated that END and ENL can be produced from several plants, such as flaxseed, by bacteria in the intestinal tract of humans and animals. Thompson et al. tested 68 common plant foods and found that flaxseed flour and its defatted meal produced the highest yield of END and ENL *in vitro*, up to 800 times higher than that from others [8].

* Correspondence: ydhui@bjmu.edu.cn; slliu@ucalgary.ca
† Contributed equally
[1]Department of Microbiology, Peking University Health Science Center, Beijing 100191, China
[2]Department of Natural Medicines, School of Pharmaceutical Sciences, Peking University Health Science Center, Beijing 100191, China

BioMed Central

© 2010 Wang et al; licensee BioMed Central Ltd. This is an Open Access article distributed under the terms of the Creative Commons Attribution License (http://creativecommons.org/licenses/by/2.0), which permits unrestricted use, distribution, and reproduction in any medium, provided the original work is properly cited.

and bronchial hyperresponsiveness: Interactions with passive smoke exposure. *J Allergy Clin Immunol* 2005;115:1169–1175.

7. Colilla S, Nicolae D, Pluzhnikov A, Blumenthal MN, Beaty TH, Bleecker ER, Lange EM, Rich SS, Meyers DA, Ober C, Cox NJ. Evidence for gene-environment interactions in a linkage study of asthma and smoking exposure. *J Allergy Clin Immunol* 2003;111:840–846.
8. Bhalla DK, Hirata F, Rishi AK, Gairola CG. Cigarette smoke, inflammation, and lung injury: a mechanistic perspective. *J Toxicol Environ Health* 2009;12:45–64.
9. Cozen W, Diaz-Sanchez D, Gauderman JW, Zadnic J, Cockburn MG, Gill PS, Masood R, Hamilton AS, Jyrala M, Mack TM. Th1 and Th2 cytokines and IgE levels in identical twins with varying levels of cigarette consumption. *J Clin Immunol* 2004;6:617–622.
10. Nouri-Shirazi M, Tinajero R, Guinet E. Nicotine alters the biological activities of developing mouse bone marrow-derived dendritic cells (DCs). *Immunol Lett* 2007;109:155–164.
11. Nureki S, Miyazaki E, Ando M, Kumamoto T, Tsuda T. CC chemokine receptor 4 ligand production by bronchoalveolar lavage fluid Wells in cigarette-smoke-associated acute eosinophilic pneumonia. *Clin Immunol* 2005;116:83–93.
12. Vassallo R, Tamada K, Lau JS, Kroening PR, Chen L. Cigarette smoke extract suppresses human dendritic cell function leading to preferential induction of Th-2 priming. *J Immunol* 2005;175:2684–2691.
13. Larsson L, Szponar B, Pehrson C. Tobacco smoking increases dramatically air concentrations of endotoxin. *Indoor Air* 2004;14: 421–424.

Compromised T-Cell Immunity and Virus-like Structure in a Patient with Pulmonary Hypertension

To the Editor:

HIV infection is widely recognized as one of the causes for the pathogenesis of pulmonary arterial hypertension (PAH) (1, 2). In a previous study of HIV-related pulmonary hypertension, the authors pointed out that the pathogenesis of HIV-PAH is believed to be associated with viral proteins such as Nef, Tat, and gp120 (3). HIV-1 Nef protein, perhaps in conjunction with persistent immune dysregulation, contributes to the development of pulmonary vasculature remodeling by inducing secretion of inflammatory cytokines (4). However, whether other types of viruses, especially those that cannot be routinely identified in clinical practice, can also play an important role in the pathogenesis of PAH has not been investigated until now. At the same time, there has been little direct evidence of the pathogens' action during the pathogenic process of PAH. Therefore, we report a case of a previously healthy 11-year-old girl in whom PAH was diagnosed 3 months after an upper respiratory tract infection caused by an undetermined virus. Thirteen months after diagnosis of PAH, the girl died of right heart failure. Blood tests revealed the increase of D-dimer, which indicated the possibility of embolism in this patient. Immunophenotyping showed that function of T-cell immunity was compromised with the decreased cell count of CD3 (50.7% decrease, normal value 60–85%) and CD8 (17.8% decrease, normal value 18.5–42.1%) but with a normal cell count of CD4 (29.0%, normal value 24.5–48.8%). In addition, we found the same phenomenon in the other 6 of 8 (75%) patients with chronic thromboembolic pulmonary hypertension when performing T-cell immunity testing in 30 patients with pulmonary embolism with or without PAH. Meanwhile, enveloped mulberry-like structures were detected in the cytoplasm of T lymphocytes, accompanied by budding and proliferation under electron microscopy observation. The size of these structures is similar to virus. The dynamic process of adhering to and departing from T lymphocytes for these structures was in line with the process of virus pullulation and release to and from T cells (Figure 1). Thus, we supposed that the compromised T cell–mediated immunity function is associated with the infection of these viruslike structures with the exclusion of other causes clinically in this patient.

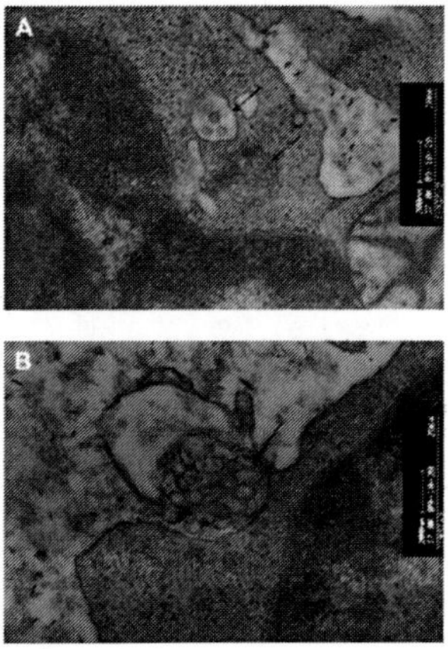

Figure 1. (*A*) Round structures with intact capsules and different densities of granules in the cytoplasm of T cells (*arrow*). (*B*) Mulberry-like pathogenic microorganisms tpenetrated through the T-cell membrane and pullulated (*arrow*).

We previously showed that T-cell immunity function–associated genes were down-regulated in patients with pulmonary embolism by means of gene profiling analyses (5). Therefore, we hypothesize that not only HIV infection but also other types of viral infections might lead to pulmonary hypertension through deteriorating host T-cell immunity function and ensuing events. This special case offers a clinical clue for studies of the etiology of pulmonary hypertension and needs to be further verified.

Author Disclosure: None of the authors has a financial relationship with a commercial entity that has an interest in the subject of this manuscript.

Lemin Wang
Zhu Gong
Aibin Liang
Yuan Xie
Tongji Hospital, School of Medicine, Tongji University, Shanghai, China

Shu-Lin Liu
Harbin Medical University, Harbin, China

Zhang Yu
Shanghai Medical College, Fudan University, Shanghai, China

Ling Wang
Medical College, Peking University, Beijing
and
Yenan Wang
Tongji Hospital, School of Medicine, Tongji University, Shanghai, China

References

1. Aarons EJ, Nye FJ. Primary pulmonary hypertension and HIV infection. *AIDS* 1991;5:1276–1277.

RESEARCH LETTER

mutL as a genetic switch of bacterial mutability: turned on or off through repeat copy number changes

Fang Chen[1,2], Wei-Qiao Liu[1,3], Zhen-Hong Liu[1,4], Qing-Hua Zou[2], Ye Wang[2], Yong-Guo Li[5], Jin Zhou[5], Abraham Eisenstark[6], Randal N. Johnston[7], Gui-Rong Liu[1], Bao-Feng Yang[4] & Shu-Lin Liu[1,2,3,5]

[1]Genomics Research Center (one of the State-Province Key Laboratories of Biomedicine-Pharmaceutics of China), Harbin Medical University, Harbin, China; [2]Department of Microbiology, Peking University Health Science Center, Beijing, China; [3]Departments of Microbiology and Infectious Diseases, University of Calgary, Calgary, Canada; [4]Department of Pharmacology, Harbin Medical University, Harbin, China; [5]Genetic Detection Laboratory of First Hospital, Harbin Medical University, Harbin, China; [6]Cancer Research Center, University of Missouri, Columbia, MO, USA; and [7]Departments of Biochemistry and Molecular Biology, University of Calgary, Calgary, Canada

Correspondence: Shu-Lin Liu, Genomics Research Center, Harbin Medical University, 194 Xuefu Road, Harbin 150081, China. Tel.: +864 518 666 9150; fax: +864 518 750 6380; e-mail: slliu@ucalgary.ca

Received 17 April 2010; revised 14 August 2010; accepted 24 August 2010.
Final version published online 27 September 2010.

DOI:10.1111/j.1574-6968.2010.02107.x

Editor: Jeff Cole

Keywords
mutL; mutability; *Salmonella*; evolution; genetic switch.

Abstract

Bacterial adaptation to changing environments can be achieved through the acquisition of genetic novelty by accumulation of mutations and recombination of laterally transferred genes into the genome, but the mismatch repair (MMR) system strongly inhibits both these types of genetic changes. As mutation and recombination do occur in bacteria, it is of interest to understand how genetic novelty may be achieved in the presence of MMR. Previously, we observed associations of a defective MMR genotype, 6bpΔ*mutL*, with greatly elevated bacterial mutability in *Salmonella typhimurium*. To validate these observations, we experimentally converted the *mutL* gene between the wild-type and 6bpΔ*mutL* in *S. typhimurium* and inspected the bacterial mutability status. When 6bpΔ*mutL* was converted to *mutL*, the originally highly mutable *Salmonella* strains regained genetic stability; when *mutL* was converted to 6bpΔ*mutL*, the mutability was elevated 100-fold. Interestingly, *mutL* cells were found to grow out of 6bpΔ*mutL* cells; the new *mutL* cells eventually replaced the original 6bpΔ*mutL* population. As conversion between *mutL* and 6bpΔ*mutL* may occur readily during DNA replication, it may represent a previously unrecognized mechanism to modulate bacterial mutability at the population level, allowing bacteria to respond rapidly to changing environments while minimizing the risks associated with persistent hypermutability.

Introduction

Previously, we observed the peculiar phenomenon of genome diversification, i.e. mutants of *Salmonella typhimurium* LT7 stored at room temperature kept changing the physical structure of the genome (Liu *et al.*, 2003). We have since concentrated on identifying the genetic basis responsible for this phenomenon, with a focus on mismatch repair (MMR) genes including *mutL*, *mutS* and *mutH*. Our initial work showed that all screened *S. typhimurium* LT7 mutants had intact *mutS* and *mutH* genes, but a deletion was found in *mutL*; this genotype was designated 6bpΔ*mutL* (Gong *et al.*, 2007).

MutL has been suggested to function as a master coordinator or molecular matchmaker in the MMR system. It has a weak ATPase function, binds to DNA, interacts directly with MutS, MutH and UvrD, and is required for initiation as well as subsequent steps in MMR processes (Ban & Yang, 1998; Hall *et al.*, 1998; Ban *et al.*, 1999; Spampinato & Modrich, 2000). The deleted sequence that we identified in *mutL* is one of three tandem 6-bp repeats, GCTGGC GCTGGC GCTGGC. Similar repeats were reported in *Escherichia coli*, although they were presented as G CTGGCG CTGGCG CTGGCG (Shaver & Sniegowski, 2003). The sequence (G)CTGGC GCTGGC GCTGGC C in *Salmonella* and (G) CTGGCG CTGGCG CTGGCG in *E. coli* both code for the amino acid sequence LALALA, which lies in a region of MutL that forms the lid of the ATP-binding pocket (Ban & Yang, 1998; Ban *et al.*, 1999; Yang, 2000; Yang *et al.*, 2000). In our case, the deletion of one of the 6-bp repeats will lead to

FEMS MICROBIOLOGY LETTERS

© 2010 Federation of European Microbiological Societies
Published by Blackwell Publishing Ltd. All rights reserved

Chen *et al. BMC Evolutionary Biology* 2010, **10**:277
http://www.biomedcentral.com/1471-2148/10/277

BMC Evolutionary Biology

RESEARCH ARTICLE Open Access

Multiple genetic switches spontaneously modulating bacterial mutability

Fang Chen[1,2], Wei-Qiao Liu[1,3], Abraham Eisenstark[4], Randal N Johnston[5], Gui-Rong Liu[1*], Shu-Lin Liu[1,2,3*]

Abstract

Background: All life forms need both high genetic stability to survive as species and a degree of mutability to evolve for adaptation, but little is known about how the organisms balance the two seemingly conflicting aspects of life: genetic stability and mutability. The DNA mismatch repair (MMR) system is essential for maintaining genetic stability and defects in MMR lead to high mutability. Evolution is driven by genetic novelty, such as point mutation and lateral gene transfer, both of which require genetic mutability. However, normally a functional MMR system would strongly inhibit such genomic changes. Our previous work indicated that MMR gene allele conversion between functional and non-functional states through copy number changes of small tandem repeats could occur spontaneously *via* slipped-strand mis-pairing during DNA replication and therefore may play a role of genetic switches to modulate the bacterial mutability at the population level. The open question was: when the conversion from functional to defective MMR is prohibited, will bacteria still be able to evolve by accepting laterally transferred DNA or accumulating mutations?

Results: To prohibit allele conversion, we "locked" the MMR genes through nucleotide replacements. We then scored changes in bacterial mutability and found that *Salmonella* strains with MMR locked at the functional state had significantly decreased mutability. To determine the generalizability of this kind of mutability 'switching' among a wider range of bacteria, we examined the distribution of tandem repeats within MMR genes in over 100 bacterial species and found that multiple genetic switches might exist in these bacteria and may spontaneously modulate bacterial mutability during evolution.

Conclusions: MMR allele conversion through repeats-mediated slipped-strand mis-pairing may function as a spontaneous mechanism to switch between high genetic stability and mutability during bacterial evolution.

Background

A balance between genetic stability and mutability is essential for bacteria to both retain species identities over long evolutionary times and enable adaptability to changing environments, but little is known about the mechanisms for establishing, maintaining and modulating such a balance. It is richly documented that, under usual growth conditions, genetic stability is largely assured by the functional DNA replication and repair systems. Conversely, when the environment becomes stressful, genetic modifications through mutation or acquisition of exogenous DNA may provide novel traits for greater adaptability of organisms.

Among the known systems for maintaining genetic stability, the DNA mismatch repair (MMR) machinery is the most powerful contributor to the inhibition of mutation and recombination events [1-6]. Bacteria that have elevated mutation rates due to defects in MMR genes, e.g., *mutS, mutL* or *mutH*, are termed mutators or hypermutators and have been isolated from various human pathogens or commensals [7-11]. The mutator genotype may confer a temporary selective advantage for the bacteria under stressful conditions, as it allows for the creation of genetic novelties, including stochastic mutations and incorporation of a great diversity of exogenous DNAs [12,13]. However, as most mutations or intruding DNAs are likely to be harmful, the continuous existence of defective MMR alleles would eventually lead to loss of

* Correspondence: grliunatsumi@gmail.com; slliu@ucalgary.ca
[1]Genomics Research Center (one of The State-Province Key Laboratories of Biomedicine-Pharmaceutics of China), Harbin Medical University, Harbin, China
Full list of author information is available at the end of the article

BioMed Central © 2010 Chen et al; licensee BioMed Central Ltd. This is an Open Access article distributed under the terms of the Creative Commons Attribution License (http://creativecommons.org/licenses/by/2.0), which permits unrestricted use, distribution, and reproduction in any medium, provided the original work is properly cited.

Zou *et al. BMC Genomics* 2010, **11**:729
http://www.biomedcentral.com/1471-2164/11/729

BMC Genomics

RESEARCH ARTICLE Open Access

SPC-P1: a pathogenicity-associated prophage of *Salmonella paratyphi* C

Qing-Hua Zou[1†], Qing-Hai Li[2,6†], Hong-Yun Zhu[1], Ye Feng[2,6], Yong-Guo Li[3], Randal N Johnston[4], Gui-Rong Liu[2,6*], Shu-Lin Liu[1,2,3,5,6*]

Abstract

Background: *Salmonella paratyphi* C is one of the few human-adapted pathogens along with *S. typhi*, *S. paratyphi* A and *S. paratyphi* B that cause typhoid, but it is not clear whether these bacteria cause the disease by the same or different pathogenic mechanisms. Notably, these typhoid agents have distinct sets of large genomic insertions, which may encode different pathogenicity factors. Previously we identified a novel prophage, SPC-P1, in *S. paratyphi* C RKS4594 and wondered whether it might be involved in pathogenicity of the bacteria.

Results: We analyzed the sequence of SPC-P1 and found that it is an inducible phage with an overall G+C content of 47.24%, similar to that of most *Salmonella* phages such as P22 and ST64T but significantly lower than the 52.16% average of the RKS4594 chromosome. Electron microscopy showed short-tailed phage particles very similar to the lambdoid phage CUS-3. To evaluate its roles in pathogenicity, we lysogenized *S. paratyphi* C strain CN13/87, which did not have this prophage, and infected mice with the lysogenized CN13/87. Compared to the phage-free wild type CN13/87, the lysogenized CN13/87 exhibited significantly increased virulence and caused multi-organ damages in mice at considerably lower infection doses.

Conclusions: SPC-P1 contributes pathogenicity to *S. paratyphi* C in animal infection models, so it is possible that this prophage is involved in typhoid pathogenesis in humans. Genetic and functional analyses of SPC-P1 may facilitate the study of pathogenic evolution of the extant typhoid agents, providing particular help in elucidating the pathogenic determinants of the typhoid agents.

Background

The bacterial genus *Salmonella* contains more than 2600 very closely related serovars, classified by the Kauffmann-White Scheme according to their differences in the somatic (O) and flagellar (H) antigens [1,2]. Although essentially all *Salmonella* bacteria are pathogens, they may have different host ranges or cause different diseases.

Over 1400 *Salmonella* serovars may infect humans, with most of them causing self-limiting gastroenteritis. On the other hand, a few *Salmonella* serovars, such as *Salmonella typhi*, *S. paratyphi* A, *S. paratyphi* B and *S. paratyphi* C, are adapted to humans and cause typhoid fever, a serious and potentially fatal systemic infection [3]. It is not clear whether these *Salmonella* typhoid agents use the same, similar or totally different pathogenic traits to infect the same host and cause the disease. Genomic comparisons between *S. typhi* and *S. paratyphi* A did not reveal a common genetic basis possibly responsible for human adaptation or typhoid pathogenesis [4,5]. Notably, various *Salmonella* pathogenicity islands (SPIs) or prophages have been identified in the *Salmonella* typhoid agents, e.g., SPI-7 in *S. typhi* [6,7] and *S. paratyphi* C [8], and SPA-1, SPA-2 and SPA-3 in *S. paratyphi* A [4], but their specific roles in typhoid pathogenesis have not been well established.

In a previous study, we located several insertions in the genome of *S. paratyphi* C strain RKS4594 by comparing it with other *Salmonella* genomes [9], including one, SPC-P1, which was a prophage present only in *S. paratyphi* C among all sequenced *Salmonella* strains [8]. In this study,

* Correspondence: grliu.natsumi@gmail.com; slliu@ucalgary.ca
† Contributed equally
[1]Department of Microbiology, Peking University Health Science Center, Beijing, PR China
[2]Genomics Research Center (one of The State-Province Key Laboratories of Biomedicine-Pharmaceutics of China), Harbin Medical University, Harbin, PR China
Full list of author information is available at the end of the article

BioMed Central

© 2010 Zou et al; licensee BioMed Central Ltd. This is an Open Access article distributed under the terms of the Creative Commons Attribution License (http://creativecommons.org/licenses/by/2.0), which permits unrestricted use, distribution, and reproduction in any medium, provided the original work is properly cited.

Microbial Pathogenesis 51 (2011) 121–132

Contents lists available at ScienceDirect

Microbial Pathogenesis

journal homepage: www.elsevier.com/locate/micpath

Tn5AraOut mutagenesis for the identification of *Yersinia pestis* genes involved in resistance towards cationic antimicrobial peptides

Jitao Guo [b,1], Manoj K.M. Nair [a], Estela M. Galván [a,2], Shu-Lin Liu [b,3], Dieter M. Schifferli [a,*]

[a] *Department of Pathobiology, University of Pennsylvania, School of Veterinary Medicine, Philadelphia, PA 19104, USA*
[b] *Department of Microbiology, Peking University Health Science Center, Beijing 100191, China*

ARTICLE INFO

Article history:
Received 23 March 2010
Received in revised form
21 April 2011
Accepted 29 April 2011
Available online 7 May 2011

Keywords:
Yersinia pestis
Minitransposon
Polymyxin B
Protamine
LL-37

ABSTRACT

Bacterial pathogens display a variety of protection mechanisms against the inhibitory and lethal effects of host cationic antimicrobial peptides (CAMPs). To identify *Yersinia pestis* genes involved in CAMP resistance, libraries of DSY101 (KIM6 *caf1 pla psa*) minitransposon Tn5AraOut mutants were selected at 37 °C for resistance to the model CAMPs polymyxin B or protamine. This approach targeted genes that needed to be repressed (null mutations) or induced (upstream P_{BAD} insertions) for the detection of CAMP resistance, and predictably for improved pathogen fitness in mammalian hosts. Ten mutants demonstrated increased resistance to polymyxin B or protamine, with the mapped mutations pointing towards genes suspected to participate in modifying membrane components, genes encoding transport proteins or enzymes, or the regulator of a ferrous iron uptake system (*feoC*). Not all the mutants were resistant to both CAMPs used for selection. None of the polymyxin B- and only some protamine-resistant mutants, including the *feoC* mutant, showed increased resistance to rat bronchoalveolar lavage fluid (rBALF) known to contain cathelicidin and β-defensin 1. Thus, findings on bacterial resistance to polymyxin B or protamine don't always apply to CAMPs of the mammalian innate immune system, such as the ones in rBALF.

© 2011 Elsevier Ltd. All rights reserved.

1. Introduction

Yersinia pestis is best known as the causative agent of bubonic plague, a disease transmitted by the bite of infected fleas. However, if inhaled, this pathogen also produces a severe primary pneumonia known as pneumonic plague, which is contagious and most often lethal. This bacterial agent uses an arsenal of virulence factors that render its entrance into the host as surreptitious as possible. These tools are thought to be most important during the first few hours following infection to avoid alarming the innate immune system and to avoid phagocytosis. We and others have previously shown that in addition to being antiphagocytic, the surface proteins F1 and Psa inhibit bacterial uptake by respiratory tract epithelial cells or macrophages [1–3]. The antiphagocytic mechanism of Psa was suggested to be due to Psa binding to host receptors that don't direct internalization [4]. *Y. pestis* injects several antiphagocytic proteins directly into host cells through its type III secretion system (T3SS) [5,6], some of which have strong anti-inflammatory properties [6–11]. In addition, *Y. pestis* also makes a non-inflammatory LPS at mammalian body temperature, thereby escaping the typical LPS-induced stimulation of TLR4 [12,13]. Although the anti-inflammatory activities of *Y. pestis* also affect DCs and their migratory properties [14,15], *Y. pestis* delivered through a fleabite still spreads to the local lymph node, causing lymphadenitis (bubo). Further spreading steps leading to bacteremia or septicemia are not infrequent, particularly when bubonic plague remains untreated. Plague lethality is generally assumed to be due to sepsis. Dissemination is facilitated by core LPS, the Psa fimbriae, the outer membrane adhesin Ail and the plasminogen activator outer membrane protein Pla [16–20]. Pla acts as a protease that cleaves plasminogen to plasmin and mediates bacterial binding to extracellular matrix proteins [21,22]. It is essential for bubonic plague, (but not for septicemic plague) after flea-mediated transmission [18,19,23,24]. Pla is also essential for the development of (but not for the dissemination from) primary pneumonic plague [25].

Y. pestis has not only evolved to survive but also to thrive in a hostile host environment that includes the antimicrobial peptides

* Corresponding author. Tel.: +1 215 898 1685; fax: +1 215 898 7887.
E-mail addresses: jitaoguo@bjmu.edu.cn (J. Guo), egalvan@leloir.org.ar (E.M. Galván), slliu@ucalgary.ca (S.-L. Liu), dmschiff@vet.upenn (D.M. Schifferli).
[1] Tel.: +86 10 8280 2963; fax: +86 10 8280 5465.
[2] Present address: Fundación Instituto Leloir, University of Buenos Aires and CONICET, C1405BWE Buenos Aires, Argentina.
[3] Present address: Genomics Research Center, Harbin Medical University, 157 Baojian Road, Harbin 150081, China.

0882-4010/$ – see front matter © 2011 Elsevier Ltd. All rights reserved.
doi:10.1016/j.micpath.2011.04.010

OPEN ACCESS Freely available online PLoS one

Gene Decay in *Shigella* as an Incipient Stage of Host-Adaptation

Ye Feng[1], **Zhe Chen**[2], **Shu-Lin Liu**[1,3,4]*

1 Genomics Research Center, Harbin Medical University, Harbin, China, 2 National Clinical Research Base,Zhejiang Hospital of Traditional Chinese Medicine, Hangzhou, China, 3 Department of Microbiology, Peking University Health Science Center, Beijing, China, 4 Department of Microbiology and Infectious Diseases, University of Calgary, Calgary, Canada

Abstract

Background: Many facultative bacterial pathogens have undergone extensive gene decay processes, possibly due to lack of selection pressure during evolutionary conversion from free-living to intracellular lifestyle. *Shigella*, the causative agents of human shigellosis, have arisen from different *E. coli*-like ancestors independently by convergent paths. As these bacteria all have lost large numbers of genes by mutation or deletion, they can be used as ideal models for systematically studying the process of gene function loss in different bacteria living under similar selection pressures.

Methodologies/Principal Findings: We compared the sequenced *Shigella* genomes and re-defined decayed genes (pseudogenes plus deleted genes) in these bacteria. Altogether, 85 genes are commonly decayed in the five analyzed *Shigella* strains and 1456 genes are decayed in at least one *Shigella* strain. Genes coding for carbon utilization, cell motility, transporter or membrane proteins are prone to be inactivated. Decayed genes tend to concentrate in certain operons rather than distribute averagely across the whole genome. Genes in the decayed operon accumulated more non-synonymous mutations than the rest genes and meanwhile have lower expression levels.

Conclusions: Different *Shigella* lineages underwent convergent gene decay processes, and inactivation of one gene would lead to a lesser selection pressure for the other genes in the same operon. The pool of superfluous genes for *Shigella* may contain at least two thousand genes and the gene decay processes may still continue in *Shigella* until a minimum genome harboring only essential genes is reached.

Citation: Feng Y, Chen Z, Liu S-L (2011) Gene Decay in *Shigella* as an Incipient Stage of Host-Adaptation. PLoS ONE 6(11): e27754. doi:10.1371/journal.pone.0027754

Editor: David Liberles, University of Wyoming, United States of America

Received February 12, 2011; **Accepted** October 24, 2011; **Published** November 16, 2011

Copyright: © 2011 Feng et al. This is an open-access article distributed under the terms of the Creative Commons Attribution License, which permits unrestricted use, distribution, and reproduction in any medium, provided the original author and source are credited.

Funding: This work was supported by a grant from Harbin Medical University, grants of National Natural Science Foundation of China (NSFC30870098, 30970119, 81030029) and Specialized Research Fund for the Doctoral Program of Higher Education (SRFDP, 20092307110001) to SLL. The funders had no role in study design, data collection and analysis, decision to publish, or preparation of the manuscript.

Competing Interests: The authors have declared that no competing interests exist.

* E-mail: slliu@ucalgary.ca

Introduction

Bacterial genomes are usually tightly packed with protein-coding genes and other functional elements. From the evolutionary point of view, a bacterial genome stays at a general balance in terms of genetic material gains and losses. On the one hand, it receives exogenous DNA in order to acquire extra fitness traits for better adapting to the external environment, and on the other hand the genome itself is undergoing a shrinking process, mainly in the forms of pseudogenization and deletion. Supporting evidence includes the finding that the majority of pseudogenes are newly-born genes and the derived young pseudogenes may be expelled out of genome soon [1,2]. Direct deletion can also occur to throw out DNA fragments of various sizes [3].

When bacteria evolve from free-living to an intracellular lifestyle, a balance between DNA flowing in and out to maintain a certain genomic size may vanish. In this process, some bacterial pathogens may accumulate a large number of pseudogenes, such as *Mycobacterium leprae* [4], which has half of its genes inactivated, and some others may even get rid of all non-essential genes to keep a minimum genome, such as *Mycoplasma genitalium* [5]. Perhaps the most important cause leading to genome shrinking is natural selection: genes that no longer make significant contributions to bacterial fitness may subject to decay (including pseudogene formation and complete deletion). Genetic drift is another important factor [6,7,8]. Especially for some highly pathogenic bacteria, which typically require only small inocula to elicit infection in their host, the effective population size is dramatically reduced. Such extreme population bottleneck greatly diminishes the efficacy of selection, under which even beneficial genes are prone to be eliminated. In addition, loss of certain genes will sometimes contribute to fitness, so the bacteria would tend not to express these genes. Such "adaptive loss" has been reported in *Shigella*. For example, expression of *cadA* in *Shigella* would inhibit the enterotoxin activity, therefore reducing the virulence. So this gene is usually inactivated in *Shigella* [9].

Shigella are human-restricted pathogens that are highly contagious. According to the traditional taxonomy, the *Shigella* genus consists of four species: *S. dysenteriae*, *S. flexneri*, *S. boydii* and *S. sonnei* [10]. However, modern genotyping methods, especially comparative genomic studies, have revealed that the four *Shigella* species are phylogenetically interwoven with the *E. coli* lineages, suggesting

JB
Journals.ASM.org

GENOME ANNOUNCEMENT

Complete Genome Sequence of *Salmonella enterica* Serovar Pullorum RKS5078

Ye Feng,[a] Hua-Feng Xu,[a] Qing-Hai Li,[a] Si-Yao Zhang,[a] Chun-Xiao Wang,[a] Da-Ling Zhu,[b] Feng-Lin Cao,[c] Yong-Guo Li,[c] Randal N. Johnston,[d] Jin Zhou,[c] Gui-Rong Liu,[a,c] and Shu-Lin Liu[a,c,e,f]

Genomics Research Center,[a] Institute of Biopharmaceutical Sciences, College of Pharmacy,[b] and Genetic Detection Center, First Hospital,[c] Harbin Medical University, Harbin, China; Departments of Biochemistry and Molecular Biology[d] and Microbiology and Infectious Diseases,[e] University of Calgary, Calgary, Alberta, Canada; and Department of Microbiology, Peking University Health Science Center, Beijing, China[f]

***Salmonella enterica* serovar Pullorum is a chicken-adapted pathogen, causing pullorum disease. Its strict host adaptation has been suspected to result in gene decay. To validate this hypothesis and identify the decayed genes, we sequenced the complete genome of *S.* Pullorum RKS5078. We found 263 pseudogenes in this strain and conducted functional analyses of the decayed genes.**

Downloaded from http://jb.asm.org/ on April 23, 2012 by guest

Salmonellae are important pathogenic bacteria infecting humans or animals. *Salmonella enterica* serovar Pullorum, a strictly chicken-adapted pullorum agent, is one of the more than 2,500 documented *Salmonella* lineages (4). It is very closely related to another chicken pathogen, *Salmonella enterica* serovar Gallinarum, and, to a lesser degree, to a host generalist, *Salmonella enterica* serovar Enteritidis. Therefore, *S.* Pullorum has the special genetic and pathogenic features suitable for studies to elucidate the genetic basis and evolution of host adaptation and acquisition of novel pathogenicity in *Salmonella*. To this end, we sequenced the genome of *S.* Pullorum RKS5078 and carried out systematic analyses.

The sequenced *S.* Pullorum strain RKS5078 was obtained from R. K. Selander. The genomic DNA was sheared into 3-kb fragments by the Hydroshear instrument and then was sequenced on a SOLiD sequencer by the mate-pair strategy (2 × 50 bp), as detailed in the manual for the instrument (Applied Biosystems). The final coverage depth reached 325-fold for an estimated genome size of 4.6 Mb. The derived color space reads were assembled by SOLiD *de novo* accessory tools V2.0. The relationships between contigs were determined following the physical map published earlier (3), and the gaps between contigs were closed by PCR amplification of the genomic DNA and sequencing. To avoid potential misassembly caused by the short-reads sequencing platform, we compared the finished genome with that of *S.* Gallinarum 287/91 (accession no. AM933173.1): all nucleotide differences longer than 50 bp (e.g., insertions and deletions) were further validated by PCR.

The chromosome of *S.* Pullorum RKS5078 was 4,637,962 bp, and its average G+C content was 52.2%. The sequence was submitted to the web service RAST for automatic annotation (1) followed by manual checking. For identification of pseudogenes, *S.* Enteritidis P125109 (accession no. AM933172.1) was used as a reference for comparison by the Psi-Fi Perl script (2). Genes that contain frameshifts, nonsense mutations, truncations, or insertion/deletions (indels) that altered >20% of the amino acid sequence in comparison with the reference sequence were treated as pseudogenes.

On the chromosome of *S.* Pullorum RKS5078, we annotated 4,325 protein-coding genes and 263 pseudogenes. The genome was highly syntenic with those of *S.* Enteritidis P125109 and *S.* Gallinarum 287/91, with average nucleotide identities of 99.7% to the former and 99.8% to the latter. More detailed comparative analyses with additional *Salmonella* strains will provide further insights into the evolution of the genetically related but pathogenically distinct *Salmonella* lineages.

Nucleotide sequence accession number. The genome sequence of *S.* Pullorum RKS5078 has been deposited in GenBank under accession no. CP003047.

ACKNOWLEDGMENTS

We thank R. K. Selander for the kind gift of the bacterial strains used in this study.

This work was supported by a Canadian Institutes of Health Research grant to R.N.J., a grant from the National Natural Science Foundation of China (NSFC30970078) and a grant from the Natural Science Foundation of Heilongjiang Province of China to G.R.L.; a grant from Harbin Medical University, grants from the National Natural Science Foundation of China (NSFC30870098, -30970119, and -81030029), a 985 Project grant from the Beijing University Health Science Center, and a Specialized Research Fund for the Doctoral Program of Higher Education (no. 20092307110001) to S.L.L.; and a grant from the Harbin Medical University Innovation Program in Graduate Education (HCXB2009016) to H.-F.X.

REFERENCES

1. **Aziz RK, et al.** 2008. The RAST Server: rapid annotations using subsystems technology. BMC Genomics 9:75.
2. **Lerat E, Ochman H.** 2004. Psi-Phi: exploring the outer limits of bacterial pseudogenes. Genome Res. 14:2273–2278.
3. **Liu GR, et al.** 2002. The evolving genome of *Salmonella enterica* serovar Pullorum. J. Bacteriol. 184:2626–2633.
4. **Shivaprasad HL.** 2000. Fowl typhoid and pullorum disease. Rev. Sci. Tech. 19:405–424.

Received 10 November 2011 **Accepted** 18 November 2011
Address correspondence to Jin Zhou, jinzhouh65@163.com, or Shu-Lin Liu, slliu@ucalgary.ca.
Y. Feng and H.-F. Xu contributed equally to this work.
Copyright © 2012, American Society for Microbiology. All Rights Reserved.
doi:10.1128/JB.06507-11

Author's personal copy

Infection, Genetics and Evolution 12 (2012) 1058–1063

Contents lists available at SciVerse ScienceDirect

Infection, Genetics and Evolution

journal homepage: www.elsevier.com/locate/meegid

Inheritance of the *Salmonella* virulence plasmids: Mostly vertical and rarely horizontal

Ye Feng [a,1], Ji Liu [a,1], Yong-Guo Li [b], Feng-Lin Cao [b], Randal N. Johnston [c], Jin Zhou [b,*], Gui-Rong Liu [a,*], Shu-Lin Liu [a,b,d,e,*]

[a] Genomics Research Center, The State-Province Key Laboratories of Biomedicine-Pharmaceutics, Harbin Medical University, Harbin, China
[b] Genetic Detection Center, First Hospital, Harbin Medical University, Harbin, China
[c] Department of Biochemistry and Molecular Biology, University of Calgary, Calgary, Canada
[d] Department of Microbiology and Infectious Diseases, University of Calgary, Calgary, Canada
[e] Department of Microbiology, Peking University Health Science Center, Beijing, China

ARTICLE INFO

Article history:
Received 11 November 2011
Received in revised form 3 March 2012
Accepted 6 March 2012
Available online 23 March 2012

Keywords:
Salmonella
Virulence plasmid
Horizontal transfer

ABSTRACT

Salmonella virulence plasmids (VPs) contribute to pathogenesis during the systemic phase of infection. Only eight serovars have been found to contain VP, and the size of VP is unique to the host serovar, suggesting VPs are mainly transmitted vertically. According to this hypothesis, VPs should have the same phylogenetic relationships as the chromosomes among the bacteria that carry the VPs. To test this hypothesis, we sequenced VPs from the serovar Enteritidis and Pullorum, named pSENV and pSPUV, respectively, and compared them with VPs from other *Salmonella* serovars. The overall results supported our hypothesis with the exception of pSENV, which was more similar to VPs from the more distantly related serovars Typhimuirum, Choleraesuis and Paratyphi C than to those from the very closely related serovars Dublin and Gallinarum/Pullorum with regard to either gene content or nucleotide similarity. These findings demonstrate that Enteritidis acquired pSENV by horizontal transfer.

© 2012 Elsevier B.V. All rights reserved.

1. Introduction

Salmonella enterica are animal and zoonotic pathogens of worldwide importance. Over 2600 serovars have been classified according to the somatic and flagellar antigens. Different *Salmonella* serovars may have distinct host ranges and can cause a variety of human diseases, ranging from self-limiting gastroenteritis to life-threatening typhoid and bacteremia, all of which are collectively called salmonellosis. Virulence plasmids (VPs) have been shown to express virulence during the systemic phase of infection by the bacteria in their specific hosts, i.e., *Salmonella enterica* serovar Choleraesuis in swine (Danbara et al., 1992), serovar Dublin in cattle (Libby et al., 1997), serovar Gallinarum/Pullorum in poultry (Barrow and Lovell, 1988; Barrow et al., 1987), and serovar Typhimurium and Enteritidis in mice (Gulig and Curtiss, 1987; Nakamura et al., 1985). All these VPs invariably carry the *spv* operon (Gulig et al., 1993), indicative of *spv* being a virulent determinant. The importance of *spv* genes has also been shown by *in vivo* expression technology, in which *spv* genes are induced during infection (Heithoff et al., 1997). Additionally, signature-tagged mutagenesis has also identified them as essential virulence genes (Hensel et al., 1995).

To date, eight *Salmonella* serovars, i.e. Abortusovis, Choleraesuis, Paratyphi C, Dublin, Enteritidis, Gallinarum/Pullorum, Sendai, and Typhimurium, are known to harbor VPs (Akiba et al., 1999; Barrow and Lovell, 1988; Barrow et al., 1987; Danbara et al., 1992; Gulig and Curtiss, 1987; Libby et al., 1997; Liu et al., 2009; Nakamura et al., 1985; Ou et al., 1990). Despite many common properties among them (Montenegro et al., 1991), each VP seems to be specific to its host as suggested by the fact that the plasmid size is unique to the host, ranging from the largest VP (from Sendai, 285 kb) to the smallest (from Choleraesuis, 50 kb). This phenomenon actually suggests that VPs can hardly transfer between different serovars, or else more than one type of VP would be detected in the same serovar. All VPs have different degrees of degradation in the *tra* operon except in pSTMV (from Typhimurium). While the deletion of the *tra* operon leads to the different VP sizes, it also explains why most VPs are non-conjugative. It has been reported that pSCSV (from Choleraesuis) and pSDUV (from Dublin) could not be transferred by conjugation, and pSGAV (from Gallinarum) could merely be mobilized with assistance from F or F-like plasmids (Ou et al., 1994). Only pSTMV is somehow self-transmissible, although the conjugation frequency is quite low (Ahmer et al.,

* Corresponding authors. Address: Genomics Research Center, Harbin Medical University, 157 Baojian Road, Harbin 150081, China. Tel.: +86 451866614075; fax: +86 45187502720.

E-mail addresses: jinzhouh85@163.com (J. Zhou), grliu.natsumi@gmail.com (G.-R. Liu), slliu@ucalgary.ca (S.-L. Liu).

[1] These authors contributed equally to this work.

1567-1348/$ - see front matter © 2012 Elsevier B.V. All rights reserved.
http://dx.doi.org/10.1016/j.meegid.2012.03.004

Antonie van Leeuwenhoek (2012) 101:67–72
DOI 10.1007/s10482-011-9680-0

PERSPECTIVE

The 3Cs provide a novel concept of bacterial species: messages from the genome as illustrated by *Salmonella*

Le Tang · Shu-Lin Liu

Received: 7 September 2011 / Accepted: 13 November 2011 / Published online: 24 November 2011
© Springer Science+Business Media B.V. 2011

Abstract A key issue troubling bacterial taxonomy and systematics is the lack of a biological species definition. Criteria to be used for defining bacterial species on genetic and biological bases should be able to reveal clear-cut boundaries among clusters of bacteria. To date, DNA–DNA re-association assays and ribosomal RNA sequence comparison have been useful in determining relative evolutionary distances among bacteria but the data are continuous and thus cannot define bacterial clusters as taxonomic units to be called species. Using *Salmonella* as models, we have looked for definite genetic and biologic uniqueness of clusters of bacteria. Based on our findings that each *Salmonella* lineage has a unique genome structure shared by strains of the same lineage but not overlapping with strains of other *Salmonella* lineages, we conclude that this is a result of genetic isolation following divergence of the bacteria. We propose that there should be genetic boundaries between different species of bacteria at the genomic level, which awaits further genomic information for validation.

Keywords Bacterial species · Bacterial systematics · Bacterial taxonomy · Bacterial nomenclature · *Salmonella* genome

L. Tang · S.-L. Liu (✉)
Genomics Research Center (One of the State-Province Key Laboratories of Biomedicine-Pharmaceutics of China), Harbin Medical University, 157 Baojian Road, Harbin 150081, China
e-mail: slliu@ucalgary.ca

L. Tang · S.-L. Liu
Genetic Detection Center of First Affiliated Hospital, Harbin Medical University, Harbin, China

S.-L. Liu
Department of Microbiology and Infectious Diseases, University of Calgary, Calgary, Canada

S.-L. Liu
Department of Microbiology, Peking University Health Science Center, Beijing, China

A brief historical review of bacterial species concepts

In 1684, Antonie van Leeuwenhoek, a Dutch amateur microscope builder, for the first time saw the long suspected "wee animalcules", later called bacteria, using his extremely simple but at that time the finest microscope. Bacteria are now known to be ubiquitous, living in various environments and consisting of the largest biomass with greatest biological diversity in the biosphere. Over the past three centuries, more than ten thousand distinct kinds of bacteria have been documented, the majority having no known significant activities and a very small number of them causing diseases in humans, animals or plants. However, it has been a long unanswered question: how "distinct" a group of like bacteria from others should be in order to

Journal of Applied Microbiology

Journal of Applied Microbiology ISSN 1364-5072

ORIGINAL ARTICLE

Production of secoisolariciresinol from defatted flaxseed by bacterial biotransformation

M.-X. Li[1], H.-Y. Zhu[2], D.-H. Yang[1], X.-Q. Ma[1], C.-Z. Wang[2], S.-Q. Cai[1], G.-R. Liu[3], B.-S. Ku[2] and S.-L. Liu[2,3,4]

1 State Key Laboratory of Natural and Biomimetic Drugs, School of Pharmaceutical Sciences, Peking University, Beijing, China
2 School of Basic Medical Sciences, Peking University, Beijing, China
3 Genomics Research Center, Harbin Medical University, Harbin, China
4 Department of Microbiology and Infectious Diseases, University of Calgary, Calgary, AB Canada

Keywords
Bacteroides uniformis, biotransformation, flaxseed, intestinal bacteria, secoisolariciresinol, secoisolariciresinol diglucoside.

Correspondence
Dong-Hui Yang, State Key Laboratory of Natural and Biomimetic Drugs, School of Pharmaceutical Sciences, Peking University, 38 Xueyuan Road, Beijing 100191, China. E-mail: ydhui@bjmu.edu.cn
Shu-Lin Liu, Genomics Research Center, Harbin Medical University, 157 Baojian Road, Harbin 150081, China. E-mail: slliu@ucalgary.ca

M.X.L. and H.Y.Z. contributed equally to this work.

2012/0978: received 30 May 2012, revised 3 August 2012 and accepted 17 August 2012

doi:10.1111/j.1365-2672.2012.05436.x

Abstract

Aims: Secoisolariciresinol (SECO) is increasingly recognized for potential clinical application because of its preventive effects against breast and colon cancers, atherosclerosis and diabetes, and its production through biotransformation has been attempted. However, previously reported bacteria all required stringent anaerobic culture conditions, precluding large-scale production. Here, we report the isolation and characterization of bacteria that produce SECO under less stringent anaerobic culture conditions.
Methods and Results: Using defatted flaxseed as raw material, we isolated a facultative anaerobic bacterium from human faeces that hydrolysed secoisolariciresinol diglucoside-3-hydroxy-3-methyl glutaric acid (SDG-HMGA) oligomers in flaxseed to produce SECO. Both conventional assays and 16S rRNA gene sequence analysis demonstrated its close relatedness with *Bacteroides uniformis*. The transformation efficiency of SDG in defatted flaxseed to SECO was more than 80% by this bacterial strain. We investigated factors that might influence fermentation, such as redox potential and pH, for large-scale fermentation of defatted flaxseed to produce SECO.
Conclusions: The method to produce SECO through biotransformation of defatted flaxseed with this bacterial strain is highly efficient and economic.
Significance and Impact of the Study: This bacterial strain can transform SDG to SECO under less stringent anaerobic culture conditions, which will greatly facilitate industry-scale production of SECO.

Introduction

Lignans have phyto-oestrogenic activities and are effective in the prevention of breast and colon cancers, atherosclerosis and diabetes (Thompson 1998; Prasad 1999, 2001; Prasad *et al.* 2000). Flaxseed is a rich source of lignans, containing 75–800 times more secoisolariciresinol diglucoside (SDG) than other food materials (Thompson *et al.* 1991; Mazura *et al.* 1996). However, SDG in flaxseed is present as part of an oligomeric structure composed of five SDG residues interconnected by four 3-hydroxy-3-methyl glutaric acid (HMGA) residues (Kamal-Eldin *et al.* 2001) (Fig. 1). Extraction of the lignans in flaxseed involves multiple steps with organic solvent, including dissolving the SDG oligomer and liberating SDG monomers by base hydrolysis and the release of secoisolariciresinol (SECO) by acid or β-glucuronidase treatment (Obermeyer *et al.* 1995; Mazur and Adlercreutz 1998; Setchell *et al.* 1999; Johnsson *et al.* 2000; Eliasson *et al.* 2003), which, however, may not completely hydrolyse the lignans. More importantly, the stability of the products from acid hydrolysis has recently been questioned, because SECO may be partially converted to its anhydrous form anhydrosecoisolariciresinol

Journal of Basic Microbiology
Environment · Health · Techniques

600 Ji Liu *et al.*

Research Paper

The type VI secretion system gene cluster of *Salmonella typhimurium*: Required for full virulence in mice

Ji Liu[1,2*], Ji-Tao Guo[3], Yong-Guo Li[4], Randal N. Johnston[5], Gui-Rong Liu[1] and Shu-Lin Liu[1,2,3,4,6]

[1] Genomics Research Center, Harbin, China
[2] Faculty of Pharmacy, Department of Biopharmaceutics, Harbin Medical University, Harbin, China
[3] Department of Microbiology, Peking University Health Science Center, Beijing, China
[4] Genetic Diagnosis Center of First Affiliated Hospital, Harbin Medical University, Harbin, China
[5] Department of Biochemistry and Molecular Biology, University of Calgary, Calgary, Canada
[6] Department of Microbiology and Infectious Diseases, University of Calgary, Calgary, Canada

Type VI secretion system (T6SS) has increasingly been believed to participate in the infection process for many bacterial pathogens, but its role in the virulence of *Salmonella typhimurium* remains unclear. To look into this, we deleted the T6SS cluster from the genome of *S. typhimurium* 14028s and analyzed the phenotype of the resulting T6SS knockout mutant (T6SSKO mutant) *in vitro* and *in vivo*. We found that the T6SSKO mutant exhibited reduced capability in colonizing the spleen and liver in an *in vivo* colonization competition model in BALB/c mice infected by the oral route. Additionally, infection via intraperitoneal administration also showed that the T6SSKO mutant was less capable of colonizing the mouse spleen and liver than the wild-type strain. We did not detect significant differences between the T6SSKO and wild-type strains in epithelial cell invasion tests. However, in the macrophage RAW264.7 cell line, the T6SSKO mutant survived and proliferated significantly more poorly than the wild-type strain. These findings indicate that T6SS gene cluster is required for full virulence of *S. typhimurium* 14028s in BALB/c mice, possibly due to its roles in bacterial survival and proliferation in macrophages.

Keywords: Bacterial secretion systems / Mouse model / *Salmonella typhimurium* / T6SS / Virulence

Received: January 25, 2012; accepted: June 6, 2012

DOI 10.1002/jobm.201200047

Introduction

Salmonella are important human and animal pathogens, with individual serovars causing local or systemic infections, e.g., gastroenteritis, typhoid, or septicemia in the host. To date, a number of virulence factors have been characterized in *Salmonella* but a full picture of pathogenic traits contributing to salmonellosis is still yet to be elucidated. *Salmonella typhimurium* is a leading etiological agent in *Salmonella* food-poisoning outbreaks, causing heavy economic losses globally [1]. Additionally, due to the relatively rich genetic information available on this pathogen since the 1960s [2–6], *S. typhimurium* has been a well-used model for investigating the pathogenesis of *Salmonella* infections.

S. typhimurium causes typhoid in mice but gastroenteritis in humans and calves, demonstrating that it uses different subsets of virulence factors in infecting different hosts, which makes *S. typhimurium* especially suitable for revealing the full spectrum of virulence factors in a *Salmonella* pathogen [7, 8]. In orally infected mice, *S. typhimurium* colonizes the intestinal tract, penetrates the intestinal epithelium and disseminates to deeper tissues, such as the liver and spleen. As a facultative intracellular pathogen, *S. typhimurium* is able to survive and grow within macrophages [9, 10]. Using both animals and cultured cell lines, researchers have identified a variety of virulence factors in *Salmonella*, including the two type III secretion systems (T3SS), which are encoded on *Salmonella*

*Current address: Clinical Laboratory of the Affiliated Hospital of Medical College Qingdao University, 266003 Qingdao, Shandong, China.
Correspondence: Gui-Rong Liu and Shu-Lin Liu, Genomics Research Center, Harbin Medical University, 157 Baojian Road, Harbin 150081, China
E-mail: grliu.natsumi@gmail.com (G.-R. L.); slliu@ucalgary.ca (S.-L. L.)
Phone: +86 451866614075
Fax: +86 45187502720

© 2013 WILEY-VCH Verlag GmbH & Co. KGaA, Weinheim

Molecular Biomarkers & Diagnosis

Li et al., J Mol Biomark Diagn 2013, 4:2
http://dx.doi.org/10.4172/2155-9929.1000144

Research Article Open Access

Identification of a Location at Chromosome 19p in a Big Chinese Family with Charcot-Marie-Tooth Disease

Fei-Feng Li[1], Xu-dong Wang[2], Min-wei Zhu[3], Hui-wen Xiao[1], Quan Yang[1] Xin Shao[4], Hong-lin Feng[2*], Zhi-Guo Lin[3*] and Shu-Lin Liu[1,5,6*]

[1]Genomics Research Center, Harbin Medical University, China
[2]Department of Neurology, The First Affiliated Hospital, Harbin Medical University, China
[3]Department of Neurosurgery, The First Affiliated Hospital, Harbin Medical University, China
[4]Department of Colorectal Surgery, the Second Affiliated Hospital of Harbin Medical University, China
[5]Genetic Detection Center of the First Clinical College, Harbin Medical University, China
[6]Department of Microbiology and Infectious Diseases, University of Calgary, Calgary, Canada

Abstract

Background: Autosomal dominant Charcot Marie Tooth disease (CMT) diseases is an inherited peripheral neuropathies disease, the prevalence is 17-40 per 100,000 individuals 17-40 per 100,000 individuals. The complex genetic mode and large number of CMT causing genes and loci made it is very hard for clinicians and researchers when trying to determine the underlying genetic diagnosis. In this work, we want to identify the cause for a Chinese family with Charcot-Marie-Tooth disease.

Methods: Family history data were recorded. Clinical and Electromyography examinations were performed on the ten affected and ten unaffected family members. All the members were genotyped with microsatellite markers at loci considered to be associated with CMT. Two-point LOD scores were calculated using the Linkage software after genotyping. Some highly suspect genes were excluded by direct sequencing.

Results and Conclusions: The clinical and pathological features were relatively gently, but which became gradually worse, with the increased genetic generation, and the onset age of the affected members. Linkage analysis was obtained at markers D19S433 (LOD score [Z]=2.03, recombination fraction [θ]=0.0) and D19S916 (Z=1.6, θ=0.0). Sequencing the dynamin 2 gene (*DNM2*) didn't found any variation in the translated region. There may be some other gene or loci associated with this disease.

Keywords: CMT; Linkage analysis; Gene mutation; DNM2; MNCV

Introduction

Charcot-Marie-Tooth (CMT) disease is a genetically and clinically heterogeneous inherited disease, affecting peripheral neuropathies [1,2]. The prevalence of the disease is 17-40 per 100,000 people [3]. So far, more than 40 genes and 900 loci have been identified for their association with the disease (http://www.molgen.ua.ac.be/CMTMutations/Mutations/MutByGene.cfm). The hereditary modes of CMT include Autosomal Dominant (AD) demyelinating (CMT1), AD axonal (CMT2), autosomal recessive and X-linked (CMTX) forms. The highly complex genetic modes and extraordinary large number of loci to cause CMT make it difficult for clinicians and researchers to determine the actual underlying genetic etiology. CMT is also known as hereditary motor and sensory neuropathy (HMSN), because it also affects the motor and sensory nerves. Variable ages of onset and progressive distal muscle weakness and atrophy are the main clinical characteristics, usually starting from the lower limbs and subsequently affecting the upper extremities [4]. The most typical features of the disease are gradual atrophy of distal muscles of the feet and legs, and the thin legs have been likened to an "inverted champagne bottle".

Point mutations and sequence deletions in the *dynamin 2* (*DNM2*) genes have been associated with the CMT disease. In 2005, the DNM2 gene was first reported to be associated with CMT [5]. Since then, three point mutations and two sequence deletions in the *DNM2* gene have been described in *DNM2* related CMT disease [5,6]. But the full spectrum of genetic changes leading to this disease is yet unknown. Here, we report a 4-generational Han Chinese family with CMT; we located the responsible locus at chromosome 19p13.2-19q12, which is flanked by markers D19S433 and D19S916.

Materials and Methods

Affected and unaffected individuals in the family

We ascertained a 4-generational Chinese Han family with non-syndromic CMT (Figure 1) at the First Affiliated Hospital of Harbin Medical University, Harbin, China. Informed consent was obtained from each participant, consistent with the Declaration of Helsinki. We recorded their medical history in detail. Physical and electromyography examination was carried out on each of the family members. Genomic DNA was extracted from peripheral blood leukocytes using standard protocols.

Genotyping

Polymerase Chain Reactions (PCRs) were carried out with microsatellite markers close to candidate loci associated with autosomal

***Corresponding authors:** Hong-ling Feng, Department of Neurology, The First Affiliated Hospital, Harbin Medical University, China, E-mail: fenghonglin5678@sina.com

Zhi-Guo Lin, Department of Neurosurgery, The First Affiliated Hospital, Harbin Medical University, China, E-mail: linzhiguo@sohu.com

Shu-Lin Liu, Genomics Research Center, Harbin Medical University, China, E-mail: slliu@ucalgary.ca

Received June 12, 2013; **Accepted** July 25, 2013; **Published** July 27, 2013

Citation: Li FF, Wang X, Zhu M, Xiao H, Yang Q, et al. (2013) Identification of a Location at Chromosome 19p in a Big Chinese Family with Charcot-Marie-Tooth Disease. J Mol Biomark Diagn 4: 144. doi:10.4172/2155-9929.1000144

Copyright: © 2013 Li FF, et al. This is an open-access article distributed under the terms of the Creative Commons Attribution License, which permits unrestricted use, distribution, and reproduction in any medium, provided the original author and source are credited

OPEN ACCESS Freely available online

PLOS ONE

Genomic Comparison between *Salmonella* Gallinarum and Pullorum: Differential Pseudogene Formation under Common Host Restriction

Ye Feng[1], Randal N. Johnston[2], Gui-Rong Liu[1], Shu-Lin Liu[1,3]*

1 Genomics Research Center (one of The State-Province Key Laboratories of Biomedicine-Pharmaceutics of China), Harbin Medical University, Harbin, China, 2 Department of Biochemistry and Molecular Biology, University of Calgary, Calgary, Canada, 3 Department of Microbiology and Infectious Diseases, University of Calgary, Calgary, Canada

Abstract

Background: *Salmonella* serovars Enteritidis and Gallinarum are closely related, but their host ranges are very different: the former is host-promiscuous and the latter can infect poultry only. Comparison of their genomic sequences reveals that Gallinarum has undergone much more extensive degradation than Enteritidis. This phenomenon has also been observed in other host restricted *Salmonella* serovars, such as Typhi and Paratyphi A. The serovar Gallinarum can be further split into two biovars: Gallinarum and Pullorum, which take poultry as their common host but cause distinct diseases, with the former eliciting typhoid and the latter being a dysentery agent. Genomic comparison of the two pathogens, with a focus on pseudogenes, would provide insights into the evolutionary processes that might have facilitated the formation of host-restricted *Salmonella* pathogens.

Methodologies/Principal Findings: We sequenced the complete genome of Pullorum strains and made comparison with Gallinarum and other *Salmonella* lineages. The gene contents of Gallinarum and Pullorum were highly similar, but their pseudogene compositions differed considerably. About one fourth of pseudogenes had the same inactivation mutations in Gallinarum and Pullorum but these genes remained intact in Enteritidis, suggesting that the ancestral Gallinarum may have already been restricted to poultry. On the other hand, the remaining pseudogenes were either in the same genes but with different inactivation sites or unique to Gallinarum or Pullorum, reflecting unnecessary functions in infecting poultry.

Conclusions: Our results support the hypothesis that the divergence between Gallinarum and Pullorum was initiated and facilitated by host restriction. Formation of pseudogenes instead of gene deletion is the major form of genomic degradation. Given the short divergence history of Gallinarum and Pullorum, the effect of host restriction on genomic degradation is huge and rapid, and such effect seems to be continuing to work. The pseudogenes may reflect the unnecessary functions for *Salmonella* within the poultry host.

Citation: Feng Y, Johnston RN, Liu G-R, Liu S-L (2013) Genomic Comparison between *Salmonella* Gallinarum and Pullorum: Differential Pseudogene Formation under Common Host Restriction. PLoS ONE 8(3): e59427. doi:10.1371/journal.pone.0059427

Editor: Dipshikha Chakravortty, Indian Institute of Science, India

Received December 6, 2012; **Accepted** February 14, 2013; **Published** March 15, 2013

Copyright: © 2013 Feng et al. This is an open-access article distributed under the terms of the Creative Commons Attribution License, which permits unrestricted use, distribution, and reproduction in any medium, provided the original author and source are credited.

Funding: This work was supported by a grant from the National Science Foundation of China (NSFC81201248) to YF; a grant of National Natural Science Foundation of China (NSFC30970078) and a grant of Natural Science Foundation of Heilongjiang Province of China to GRL; and a start-up grant from Harbin Medical University, grants of the National Natural Science Foundation of China (NSFC30970119, 81030029, 81271786), a grant of the National Natural Science Foundation of China and National Institutes of Health of United States of America (NSFC-NIH 81161120416), and a Specialized Research Fund for the Doctoral Program of Higher Education (SRFDP, 20092307110001) to SLL. The funders had no role in study design, data collection and analysis, decision to publish, or preparation of the manuscript.

Competing Interests: The authors have declared that no competing interests exist.

* E-mail: slliu@ucalgary.ca

Introduction

Salmonella are important pathogenic bacteria infecting humans or animals. Different *Salmonella* serovars may either infect a variety of animals or be restricted to a single host. Take serovars from serogroup D for example, Enteritidis can infect multiple hosts whereas Gallinarum can only infect chickens, though they are very similar to each other genetically. Two contrary scenarios in terms of comparative genomics may explain their differences in host range. One is that the Last Common Ancestor (LCA) of Enteritidis and Gallinarum infected chickens only; during evolution, Enteritidis acquired certain mobile genetic elements and thereby became capable of infecting other hosts. The other is that their LCA was a host-generalist; after divergence, Gallinarum evolved to infect birds only, whereas Enteritidis remained the same. Recently, comparative genome analyses have revealed that Gallinarum contained a much greater number of pseudogenes than Enteritidis [1], providing support to the latter scenario.

The serovar Gallinarum can be further divided into two biovars: bv. Gallinarum (abbr. bvGa) and bv. Pullorum (abbr. bvPu). The two biovars are both non-motile and have nearly identical biochemical characteristics except that bvPu can produce rapid decarboxylation of ornithine. Clinically, they both infect chickens only, with bvGa causing typhoid but bvPu causing pullorum disease. We have genotyped a large number of bvGa and bvPu strains by pulsed field gel electrophoresis and found that the

Mol Genet Genomics
DOI 10.1007/s00438-013-0762-8

ORIGINAL PAPER

Genomic comparison of *Salmonella typhimurium* DT104 with non-DT104 strains

Er-Ying Zhao · Hong-Xia Bao · Le Tang · Qing-Hua Zou · Wei-Qiao Liu · Da-Ling Zhu · Jessica Chin · Ying-Ying Dong · Yong-Guo Li · Feng-Lin Cao · Cornelis Poppe · Kenneth E. Sanderson · Randal N. Johnston · Daoguo Zhou · Gui-Rong Liu · Shu-Lin Liu

Received: 13 April 2013 / Accepted: 15 June 2013
© Springer-Verlag Berlin Heidelberg 2013

Abstract DT104 emerged as a new branch of *Salmonella typhimurium* with resistance to multiple antimicrobials. To reveal some general genomic features of DT104 for clues of evolutionary events possibly associated with the emergence of this relatively new type of this pathogen, we mapped 11 independent DT104 strains and compared them with non-DT104 *S. typhimurium* strains. We found that all 11 DT104 strains contained three insertions absent in non-DT104 strains, i.e., the previously reported ST104, ST104B and ST64B. However, SGI-1, a genomic island known to be responsible for DT104 multidrug resistance, was not present in all DT104 strains examined in this study: one DT104 strain did not contain SGI-1 but carried a 144 kb plasmid, suggesting possible evolutionary relationships between the two DNA elements in the development of antimicrobial resistance.

Communicated by D. Ussery.

E.-Y. Zhao, H.-X. Bao, and L. Tang contributed equally to this work.

E.-Y. Zhao · H.-X. Bao · L. Tang · Q.-H. Zou (✉) ·
G.-R. Liu (✉) · S.-L. Liu (✉)
Genomics Research Center (one of The State-Province Key Laboratories of Biomedicine-Pharmaceutics of China), Harbin Medical University, 157 Baojian Road, 150081 Harbin, China
e-mail: zouqinghua2002@yahoo.com.cn

G.-R. Liu
e-mail: grliu.natsumi@gmail.com

S.-L. Liu
e-mail: slliu@ucalgary.ca

H.-X. Bao · L. Tang · S.-L. Liu
HMU-UCFM Centre for Infection and Genomics, Harbin Medical University, Harbin, China

Q.-H. Zou · S.-L. Liu
Department of Microbiology, Peking University Health Science Center, Beijing, China

Keywords *Salmonella typhimurium* · DT104 · Antimicrobial resistance · SGI-1

Introduction

Salmonellae are important pathogens for humans and animals. Since their divergence from *Escherichia coli* more than 100 million years ago (Ochman and Wilson 1987; Feng et al. 1997), *Salmonella* have developed into more than 2,500 serotypes classified according to the Kauffmann–White Scheme (Kauffmann and Edwards 1957; Popoff 2001). The *Salmonella* serotypes are traditionally treated as individual species with typical Latinized scientific names, although, due to *Salmonella* nomenclature changes in 1980s, most *Salmonella* species were reclassified as mere serovars of a newly named species *Salmonella enterica*, with *Salmonella bongori* remaining as a separate

W.-Q. Liu · J. Chin · Y.-Y. Dong · K. E. Sanderson · S.-L. Liu
Departments of Microbiology and Infectious Diseases, University of Calgary, Calgary, Canada

Present Address:
W.-Q. Liu
Department of Neurology, Vancouver General Hospital, Vancouver, Canada

D.-L. Zhu · S.-L. Liu
Department of Biopharmaceuticals, Faculty of Pharmacy, Harbin Medical University, Harbin, China

Y.-G. Li · F.-L. Cao · S.-L. Liu
Genetic Diagnosis Laboratory of First Hospital, Harbin Medical University, Harbin, China

Published online: 11 August 2013

Tang *et al. BMC Genomics* 2013, **14**:489
http://www.biomedcentral.com/1471-2164/14/489

BMC Genomics

RESEARCH ARTICLE **Open Access**

Defining natural species of bacteria: clear-cut genomic boundaries revealed by a turning point in nucleotide sequence divergence

Le Tang[1,2,3], Yang Li[1], Xia Deng[1], Randal N Johnston[4], Gui-Rong Liu[1,2,3*] and Shu-Lin Liu[1,2,3,5*]

Abstract

Background: Bacteria are currently classified into arbitrary species, but whether they actually exist as discrete natural species was unclear. To reveal genomic features that may unambiguously group bacteria into discrete genetic clusters, we carried out systematic genomic comparisons among representative bacteria.

Results: We found that bacteria of *Salmonella* formed tight phylogenetic clusters separated by various genetic distances: whereas over 90% of the approximately four thousand shared genes had completely identical sequences among strains of the same lineage, the percentages dropped sharply to below 50% across the lineages, demonstrating the existence of clear-cut genetic boundaries by a steep turning point in nucleotide sequence divergence. Recombination assays supported the genetic boundary hypothesis, suggesting that genetic barriers had been formed between bacteria of even very closely related lineages. We found similar situations in bacteria of *Yersinia* and *Staphylococcus*.

Conclusions: Bacteria are genetically isolated into discrete clusters equivalent to natural species.

Keywords: Natural species, *Salmonella*, Genetic boundary

Background

Bacteria are classified into species, which are organized into higher taxonomic ranks such as genera, families, orders, etc., based on levels of similarity among them. However, the definition of the fundamental taxonomic unit, the species, is still an unsolved issue. Over the past three centuries since their discovery, bacteria have been classified in numerous ways based on morphological, serological, biochemical or genetic properties, with the species being defined differently according to the method used for the classification. As a result, a bacterial pathogen may at one time be defined as an independent species or at another time as a variant of a species along with many other bacteria that share phenotypic or genetic similarities. For example, the human typhoid agent was originally treated as a species with a Latinized scientific name *Salmonella typhi* but later was re-classified as merely a serovar of another species, *Salmonella enterica*, together with over 2000 other "serovars" [1-3]; these 2000 plus serovars are mostly mild or non-pathogenic to humans and were, like *S. typhi*, initially also classified as separate species. Inclusion of the deadly human pathogen *S. typhi* in a species together with thousands of pathogenically very different bacteria has in fact caused enormous confusions in the clinical as well as basic research settings. In addition to medicine, the recognition of natural bacterial species is also important for research and applications in industrial and agricultural areas. Essentially, all such confusions have resulted from the lack of theory-based species concept and of objective criteria-supported species definition.

Currently an expedient way is to categorize bacteria into taxonomic species by arbitrary cut-off values at 70% DNA-DNA association and 97% 16S rRNA sequence identity [4,5]. However, since both kinds of data are continuous, the 70% and 97% criteria can hardly assign bacteria into discrete genetic groupings. More seriously, the wide ranges of genomic variation set by the 70% and 97% criteria would unavoidably classify a great diversity of phylogenetically different bacteria into the same

* Correspondence: grliu.natsumi@gmail.com; slliu@ucalgary.ca
[1]Genomics Research Center (one of The State-Province Key Laboratories of Biomedicine-Pharmaceutics of China), Harbin, China
[2]HMU-UCFM Centre for Infection and Genomics, Harbin, China
Full list of author information is available at the end of the article

BioMed Central

© 2013 Tang et al.; licensee BioMed Central Ltd. This is an Open Access article distributed under the terms of the Creative Commons Attribution License (http://creativecommons.org/licenses/by/2.0), which permits unrestricted use, distribution, and reproduction in any medium, provided the original work is properly cited.

Genomics 102 (2013) 331–337

Contents lists available at ScienceDirect

Genomics

journal homepage: www.elsevier.com/locate/ygeno

Genetic boundaries to delineate the typhoid agent and other *Salmonella* serotypes into distinct natural lineages

Le Tang [a], Chun-Xiao Wang [a], Song-Ling Zhu [a], Yang Li [a], Xia Deng [a], Randal N. Johnston [b], Gui-Rong Liu [a,*], Shu-Lin Liu [a,c,d,e,*]

[a] *Genomics Research Center (one of The State-Province Key Laboratories of Biomedicine-Pharmaceutics of China), Harbin Medical University, Harbin, China*
[b] *Department of Biochemistry and Molecular Biology, University of Calgary, Calgary, Canada*
[c] *HMU-UCFM Center for Infection and Genomics, Harbin Medical University, Harbin, China*
[d] *Department of Biopharmaceutics, Harbin Medical University, Harbin, China*
[e] *Department of Microbiology and Infectious Diseases, University of Calgary, Calgary, Canada*

ARTICLE INFO

Article history:
Received 8 June 2013
Accepted 24 July 2013
Available online 6 August 2013

Keywords:
Bacterial species
Genetic boundary
Genomic divergence

ABSTRACT

The deadly human typhoid agent was initially classified as a species called *Salmonella typhi* but later reclassified as a serovar of *Salmonella enterica* together with other pathogenically diverse serovars. The dynamic changes of *Salmonella* taxonomy reflect the need to clarify the phylogenetic status of the *Salmonella* serovars: are they discrete lineages or variants of a genetic lineage? To answer this question, we compared *S. typhi* and other *Salmonella* serotypes. We found that the *S. typhi* and *Salmonella typhimurium* strains had over 90% and ca. 80%, respectively, of their genes identical; however, between *S. typhi* and *S. typhimurium*, this percentage dropped to 6%, suggesting the existence of genetic boundaries between them. We conclude that *S. typhi* and the other compared *Salmonella* serovars have developed into distinct lineages circumscribed by the genetic boundary. This concept and methods may be used to delineate other *Salmonella* serotypes, many of which are polyphyletic, needing differentiation.

© 2013 Elsevier Inc. All rights reserved.

1. Introduction

Typhoid is a serious infectious disease with high morbidity and mortality [39]. The causative agent was first isolated in 1881 and was classified as a bacterial species [4,11,12], initially with multiple names and subsequently with the Latinized scientific name *Salmonella typhi*. In the 1980s, *S. typhi* was reclassified as a serological variant (called serovar) of a new species, *Salmonella enterica* [17–19,40], together with other "serological variants" that, though genetically similar, are pathogenically diverse. While the new name of the typhoid agent, *S. enterica* subspecies *enterica* serovar Typhi, has been widely adopted, many authors continue using the previous nomenclature [44], due largely to several uncertainties of the new *Salmonella* taxonomy such as cutoffs for delineating bacteria into phylogenetic groupings. Regarding the typhoid agent, we ask a fundamental question: does this pathogen exist as a natural cluster of bacteria phylogenetically separated from other (and closely related) bacteria? Answering this question requires the identification of some kind of genetic boundary that may circumscribe the typhoid agent unambiguously from its close relatives.

Bacteria, like animals and plants, are categorized into species, based initially on phenotypic similarities and later also, and mainly, on genetic relatedness. However, unlike most animals and plants, which are classified into species based largely on objective criteria such as sexual reproduction potential [33,34], bacteria are essentially asexual organisms, which makes the adopted classification system problematic. The use of DNA–DNA association and 16S rDNA sequence comparison to define bacterial species has revolutionized bacterial classification [8,46,50]. However, evidence is needed to demonstrate that bacteria do exist in discrete natural clusters with unambiguous genetic boundaries separating each of them from others. As it is now increasingly recognized that bacterial species delineated by the modern taxonomy system are essentially complexes with great intra-"species" diversity [47], the current bacterial species definition may categorize multiple natural bacterial clusters into the same "species", hence inevitably causing confusions in many theoretical as well as applied areas. In addition, new advances of bacterial systematics tend to change the taxonomy and nomenclature of bacteria radically, moving some taxa back and forth from one species to another. As a result, a so-named species may contain both mild or non-pathogens and deadly pathogens, as exemplified by the *Salmonella* taxonomy [14,19]. Currently, over 2000 serological types of bacteria are documented under *S. enterica*, most of which are mild or virtually non-pathogenic to humans. Inclusion of the deadly human pathogen *S. typhi* together with them in the same species needs to be re-justified.

All these confusions have stepped from the lack of an answer to a long-asked question: do bacteria exist as discrete phylogenetic clusters? Many lines of evidence, including those from surveys of wild microbial populations, very convincingly indicate the existence of

* Corresponding authors at: Genomics Research Center, Harbin Medical University, 157 Baojian Road, Harbin 150081, China. Fax: +86 451866614075.
E-mail addresses: grliu.natsumi@gmail.com (G.-R. Liu), slliu@ucalgary.ca (S.-L. Liu).

0888-7543/$ – see front matter © 2013 Elsevier Inc. All rights reserved.
http://dx.doi.org/10.1016/j.ygeno.2013.07.014

OPEN ACCESS Freely available online PLOS ONE

Identification of Genes to Differentiate Closely Related *Salmonella* Lineages

Qing-Hua Zou[1], Ren-Qing Li[2], Ye-Jun Wang[3], Shu-Lin Liu[1,3,4]*

1 Department of Microbiology, School of Basic Medical Sciences, Peking University Health Science Center, Beijing, China, 2 Institute of Immunology, Beijing Center for Disease Control and Prevention, Beijing, China, 3 Genomics Research Center (one of The State-Province Key Laboratories of Biomedicine-Pharmaceutics of China), Harbin Medical University, Harbin, China, 4 Department of Microbiology and Infectious Diseases, University of Calgary, Calgary, Alberta, Canada

Abstract

Background: *Salmonella* are important human and animal pathogens. Though highly related, the *Salmonella* lineages may be strictly adapted to different hosts or cause different diseases, from mild local illness like gastroenteritis to fatal systemic infections like typhoid. Therefore, rapid and accurate identification of *Salmonella* is essential for timely and correct diagnosis of *Salmonella* infections. The current identification methods such as 16S rRNA sequencing and multilocus sequence typing are expensive and time consuming. Additionally, these methods often do not have sufficient distinguishing resolution among the *Salmonella* lineages.

Methodologies/Principal Findings: We compared 27 completely sequenced *Salmonella* genomes to identify possible genomic features that could be used for differentiation of individual lineages. We concatenated 2372 core genes in each of the 27 genomes and constructed a neighbor-joining tree. On the tree, strains of each serotype were clustered tightly together and different serotypes were unambiguously separated with clear genetic distances, demonstrating systematic genomic divergence among the *Salmonella* lineages. We made detailed comparisons among the 27 genomes and identified distinct sets of genomic differences, including nucleotide variations and genomic islands (GIs), among the *Salmonella* lineages. Two core genes STM4261 and *entF* together could unambiguously distinguish all *Salmonella* lineages compared in this study. Additionally, strains of a lineage have a common set of GIs and closely related lineages have similar sets of GIs.

Conclusions: *Salmonella* lineages have accumulated distinct sets of mutations and laterally acquired DNA (e.g., GIs) in evolution. Two genes *entF* and STM4261 have diverged sufficiently among the *Salmonella* lineages to be used for their differentiation. Further investigation of the distinct sets of mutations and GIs will lead to novel insights into genomic evolution of *Salmonella* and greatly facilitate the elucidation of pathogeneses of *Salmonella* infections.

Citation: Zou Q-H, Li R-Q, Wang Y-J, Liu S-L (2013) Identification of Genes to Differentiate Closely Related *Salmonella* Lineages. PLoS ONE 8(2): e55988. doi:10.1371/journal.pone.0055988

Editor: Michael Hensel, University of Osnabrueck, Germany

Received July 5, 2012; **Accepted** January 7, 2013; **Published** February 18, 2013

Copyright: © 2013 Zou et al. This is an open-access article distributed under the terms of the Creative Commons Attribution License, which permits unrestricted use, distribution, and reproduction in any medium, provided the original author and source are credited.

Funding: This work was supported by a project of National Natural Science Foundation of China (31100134). The funders had no role in study design, data collection and analysis, decision to publish, or preparation of the manuscript.

Competing Interests: The authors have declared that no competing interest exist.

* E-mail: slliu@ucalgary.ca

Introduction

The bacterial genus *Salmonella* encompasses a large number of lineages that cause a variety of diseases in humans or animals. In the United States, for example, *Salmonella* infections result in 15,000 hospitalizations and more than 400 deaths annually [1]. To date, more than 2500 lineages (Each *Salmonella* lineage was treated as individual species up to the 1930s, as both species and serotypes by the 1980s, and as serovars of one or two *Salmonella* species since late 1980s; currently a large number of journals still treat *Salmonella* lineages as species. See details in [2]) have been documented in the *Salmonella* genus [3]. All *Salmonella* bacteria are closely related but the individual lineages may differ greatly in pathogenic features, such as in host range or in the nature of diseases caused. For example, *Salmonella enterica* subspecies *enterica* serovar Typhi (*S.* Typhi) and *S.* Paratyphi A are strictly adapted to humans and cause typhoid, a serious systemic infection with a high mortality rate [4], whereas *S.* Typhimurium is a broad host-range pathogen, causing systemic infection in mice but only gastroenteritis in humans [5]. Similarly, the fowl-specific lineage *S.* Gallinarum causes typhoid-like disease and its close relative *S.* Pullorum, also fowl-specific, causes dysentery [6]. Although identification methods, such as the Kauffman-White scheme for serotyping [7] and DNA analysis for multilocus sequence typing [8], have been developed to differentiate the highly related but pathogenically distinct *Salmonella* lineages, these methods are either not available to most clinical laboratories or tedious and expensive. Therefore, in-depth comparative analyses of the *Salmonella* genomes are necessary to reveal unique features on them for possible use in convenient and accurate identification of these bacteria.

Genomic comparisons among representative *Salmonella* pathogens, based on physical mapping [9,10], provided the first evidence indicating that genomes of individual *Salmonella* lineages differ mainly in their specific sets of insertions [11,12,13,14,15,16,17,18]. Rearrangements of the genomes have been characterized in host-adapted *Salmonella* pathogens such as *S.* Typhi [19,20,21] and *S.* Paratyphi C [22], but they are likely the consequence rather than the cause of genomic divergence, thus

Author's personal copy

DNA Repair 12 (2013) 864–869

Contents lists available at ScienceDirect

DNA Repair

journal homepage: www.elsevier.com/locate/dnarepair

Brief communication

Characterization of the defects in the ATP lid of *E. coli* MutL that cause transient hypermutability

Monica C. Pillon[a], Michelle Dubinsky[a], Randal N. Johnston[b], Shu-Lin Liu[c,d], Alba Guarné[a,*]

[a] Department of Biochemistry and Biomedical Sciences, McMaster University, Hamilton, ON, Canada
[b] Department of Biochemistry and Molecular Biology, University of Calgary, Calgary, AB, Canada
[c] Department of Microbiology and Infectious Diseases, University of Calgary, Calgary, AB, Canada
[d] Genomics Research Center, Harbin Medical University, Harbin, China

ARTICLE INFO

Article history:
Received 19 February 2013
Received in revised form 5 July 2013
Accepted 7 July 2013
Available online 2 August 2013

Keywords:
DNA mismatch repair
Mutagenesis
MutL
Genetic switch
K^+-Mg^{2+} tandem

ABSTRACT

Mutator strains spontaneously arise in bacterial populations under stress in an attempt to increase evolutionary adaptation. Inactivation of the ubiquitous DNA mismatch repair pathway, whose normal function is to correct replication errors and hence increase replication fidelity, is often the cause of the mutator phenotype. One of the essential genes in this pathway, *mutL*, includes a short tandem repeat that is prone to polymerase slippage during replication. While extensive work has established that this repetitive sequence is a genuine genetic switch, the mechanism of MutL inactivation remains unclear. This short tandem repeat is translated into a LALALA motif that resides near the ATPase active site of MutL. Therefore, changes in the length of this motif are presumed to alter the ATPase activity of MutL. We have engineered variants of *Escherichia coli* MutL with shorter/longer LALALA motifs and characterized their ATPase and DNA binding functions. We have found that the deletion or insertion of a single LA repeat did not compromise the structural integrity of the protein, nor did it affect MutS- or DNA-binding activity. However, it severely compromised ATP binding and, consequently, engagement of the N-terminal domains; both essential activities for proper DNA mismatch repair. These results are discussed in the context of the structure of MutL.

© 2013 Elsevier B.V. All rights reserved.

1. Introduction

Bacteria have evolved toward a low DNA mutation frequency in stable environments because mutations often have deleterious effects [1,2]. However, bacterial populations in a new environment are confronted with the need to adapt. Since asexual populations rely on mutagenesis to increase genetic variation, bacteria tend to have hotspots in antimutator genes, such as DNA repair genes [3]. To compensate for the inevitable deleterious impact of maintaining a high mutation rate, bacterial mutator phenotypes are often transient so the population can spontaneously revert back to a low mutation frequency [2].

Defects in the conserved post-replicative DNA mismatch repair (MMR) pathway are often the cause of reversible hypermutability in bacteria. MMR increases fidelity of DNA replication by repairing mismatched bases and small insertion/deletion loops introduced during DNA synthesis. Three key proteins initiate the repair response (reviewed in [4,5]). MutS recognizes and binds to a mismatch and recruits the molecular matchmaker MutL in an ATP-dependent manner [6]. The ATP-bound form of MutL can then activate the latent endonuclease MutH which, in turn, nicks the newly synthesized strand at the nearest hemimethylated GATC site [7,8]. The nick marks the nascent strand for repair by providing an entry point for the UvrD helicase and exonucleases to unwind and degrade the erroneous strand, thereby providing the replication machinery with a second chance to re-synthesize the strand correctly [5]. While MutS and MutL are evolutionary conserved, MutH is only present in a subset of gamma-proteobacteria including *Escherichia coli* (*E. coli*). In organisms lacking MutH, MutL harbors a latent endonuclease activity that uses the gap left by the removal of misincorporated ribonucleotides as the strand discrimination signal [9,10] and provides entry sites for downstream MMR factors [11–16].

Several independent studies have linked bacterial hypermutability to mutations in a conserved short tandem repeat at the beginning of the *mutL* gene [17–21]. Sequencing of the *E. coli mutL* gene from hypermutator strains revealed either a deletion or an insertion in a triple hexanucleotide tandem repeat

* Corresponding author at: Department of Biochemistry and Biomedical Sciences, HSC-4H32A, McMaster University, 1280 Main Street West, Hamilton, ON L8S 4K1, Canada. Tel.: +1 905 525 9140x26394; fax: +1 905 522 9033.
E-mail address: guarnea@mcmaster.ca (A. Guarné).

1568-7864/$ – see front matter © 2013 Elsevier B.V. All rights reserved.
http://dx.doi.org/10.1016/j.dnarep.2013.07.003

J Nat Med
DOI 10.1007/s11418-012-0655-x

NOTE

The antidepressant effect of secoisolariciresinol, a lignan-type phytoestrogen constituent of flaxseed, on ovariectomized mice

Ying-Feng Wang · Zhi-Kun Xu · Dong-Hui Yang · Hai-Yan Yao · Bao-Shan Ku · Xiao-Qing Ma · Cheng-Zhi Wang · Shu-Lin Liu · Shao-Qing Cai

Received: 3 November 2011 / Accepted: 28 February 2012
© The Japanese Society of Pharmacognosy and Springer 2012

Abstract Secoisolariciresinol (SECO) is a natural lignan-type phytoestrogen constituent mainly found in flaxseed. It can be metabolized in vivo to mammalian lignans of enterodiol and enterolactone, which have been proven to be effective in relieving menopausal syndrome. Depression is one of the most common symptoms of menopausal syndrome, and is currently treated with estrogen replacement and antidepressant therapy. However, due to the serious side-effects of such agents, there are urgent needs for safer and more tolerable treatments. In this paper, using two classical depression models, the forced swimming test and the tail suspension test, we report the antidepressant effect of SECO on ovariectomized (OVX) mice by intragastric administration for 14 consecutive days at doses of 5, 10 and 20 mg/kg. The results showed that SECO (10 mg/kg) treatment could significantly reduce the duration of immobility of OVX mice in these two models compared with the control group (OVX mice + vehicle), which was similar to the positive control imipramine. In addition, SECO treatment could substantially increase brain monoamine (norepinephrine and dopamine) levels in OVX mice. The present studies showed that SECO can reverse depressive-like behavior and exhibit monoamine-enhancing effects.

Keywords Secoisolariciresinol · Ovariectomized mice · Forced swimming · Tail suspension · Monoamine level

Y.-F. Wang · Z.-K. Xu
Department of Chemistry, Capital Normal University, 105 Xisanhuanbei Road, Beijing 100048, China

D.-H. Yang (✉) · X.-Q. Ma · S.-Q. Cai
State Key Laboratory of Natural and Biomimetic Drugs, School of Pharmaceutical Sciences, Peking University, 38 Xueyuan Road, Beijing 100191, China
e-mail: ydhui@bjmu.edu.cn

H.-Y. Yao · B.-S. Ku · C.-Z. Wang
School of Basic Medical Sciences, Peking University, 38 Xueyuan Road, Beijing 100191, China

S.-L. Liu
School of Pharmaceutical Sciences, Harbin Medical University, 194 Xuefu Road, Harbin 150081, China

Introduction

Menopause is a process of gradual decline of ovary function and estrogen level, as an inevitable stage every female must face, often leading to menopausal syndrome with manifestations such as hectic fever, night sweats and depression [1]. To date, hormone replacement therapy (HRT) by estrogen, often supplemented with antidepressant agents, has been the treatment of choice for depression syndrome in menopausal populations. However, long-term use of estrogen poses risks of endometrial and breast cancer [2]. Additionally, almost all the antidepressant agents, such as amitriptyline, fluoxetine and venlafaxine, have side-effects of drowsiness, dry mouth, blurred vision, constipation, rapid heartbeat, difficulty in urinating and so on. Moreover, overdose of antidepressant agents can cause acute poisoning and even death [3]. In recent years, natural products possessing phytoestrogen activities (two-way regulation of estrogen and anti-estrogen) have been the focus in treating menopausal depression symptoms [4].

Secoisolariciresinol (SECO) is a lignan-type phytoestrogen, which can be metabolized to enterodiol (END) and enterolactone (ENL) by the colon microflora of mammals in vivo [5]. END and ENL have been generally taken as phytoestrogens based on their weakly estrogenic and anti-

Published online: 03 April 2012

Appl Microbiol Biotechnol (2014) 98:2519–2531
DOI 10.1007/s00253-013-5111-7

BIOTECHNOLOGICALLY RELEVANT ENZYMES AND PROTEINS

Cloning, expression, and characterization of the β-glucosidase hydrolyzing secoisolariciresinol diglucoside to secoisolariciresinol from *Bacteroides uniformis* ZL1

Y.-L. Tao · D.-H. Yang · Y.-T. Zhang · Y. Zhang · Z.-Q. Wang · Y.-S. Wang · S.-Q. Cai · S.-L. Liu

Received: 16 May 2013 / Revised: 6 June 2013 / Accepted: 3 July 2013 / Published online: 15 August 2013
© Springer-Verlag Berlin Heidelberg 2013

Abstract Previously, from the human intestinal flora we isolated the bacterial strain *Bacteroides uniformis* ZL1, which could convert secoisolariciresinol diglucoside (SDG) to its aglycone secoisolariciresinol (SECO) in vivo. In this study, 24 putative β-glucosidase genes were screened from the genome of *B. uniformis* ATCC 8492, which were used as templates to design PCR primers for the target genes in *B. uniformis* ZL1. Fifteen genes (*bgl1–bgl15*) were amplified from strain ZL1, and among them we identified *bgl8* as the gene encoding the SDG-hydrolyzing β-glucosidase. We sequenced the *bgl8* gene, cloned it into the expression vector and then transformed *Escherichia coli* to construct the recombinant bacteria that could synthesize the target β-glucosidase (BuBGL8). We purified and characterized BuBGL8, which showed maximal activity and stability under the culture conditions of pH 6.0 and 30 °C. SDG (2.0 mg/ml) was converted to SECO by both the purified BuBGL8 (0.035 mg/ml) and crude enzyme extract (0.23 mg crude protein/ml) with the efficiency of more than 90 % after 90 min at the reaction conditions. This is, to our knowledge, the first report of using recombinant bacteria to synthesize the SDG-hydrolyzing β-glucosidase, which could be used to produce SECO from SDG conveniently and highly efficiently.

Keywords *Bacteroides uniformis* · β-glucosidase · Secoisolariciresinol diglucoside · Secoisolariciresinol · Recombinant bacteria

Y.-L. Tao · D.-H. Yang (✉) · Y.-T. Zhang · Y. Zhang · S.-Q. Cai
State Key Laboratory of Natural and Biomimetic Drugs, School of Pharmaceutical Sciences, Peking University, Beijing 100191, China
e-mail: ydhui@bjmu.edu.cn

Z.-Q. Wang · Y.-S. Wang
National Key Laboratory of Biochemical Engineering, Chinese Academy of Sciences, Institute of Process Engineering, Beijing 100190, China

S.-L. Liu (✉)
Genomics Research Center, Harbin Medical University, Harbin 150081, China
e-mail: slliu@ucalgary.ca

S.-L. Liu
Department of Microbiology and Infectious Diseases, University of Calgary, Calgary, AB T2N 4N1, Canada

Introduction

Enterodiol (END) and enterolactone (ENL), known as mammalian lignans, are phytoestrogens that may be used for the prevention of menopausal syndrome, cardiovascular diseases, and cancers of the colon, breast, and prostate (Kitts et al. 1999; Meagher and Beecher 2000; Wang 2002). The human intestines contain bacteria that are capable of converting plant lignans, such as secoisolariciresinol diglucoside (SDG), to END and ENL (Clavel et al. 2006; Wang et al. 2000; 2010).

Secoisolariciresinol (SECO) was found to be the first intermediate in the biotransformation pathways from SDG to END and ENL (Raffaelli et al. 2002). To date, several bacterial strains capable of converting SDG to SECO have been reported, including *Bacteroides distasonis* DSM 20701^T, *Bacteroides fragilis* DIfE-05, *Clostridium cocleatum* DSM 1551^T, *Clostridium ramosum* DSM 1402^T (Clavel et al. 2006), *Clostridium saccharogumia* (Clavel et al. 2007), and *Klebsiella* sp. (Wang et al. 2010). In our previous work, we isolated an active bacterial strain, *Bacteroides uniformis* ZL1, from human intestinal flora, which could effectively transform SDG in flaxseed to SECO, with a transformation efficiency of more than 80 % (Li et al. 2012). However, several factors limit the application of bacterial biotransformation in large scale, such as the low content of functional enzyme in the bacteria, which leads to the need of a huge system to meet the desired production. The anaerobic culture condition was also a serious

Process Biochemistry 49 (2014) 19–24

Contents lists available at ScienceDirect

Process Biochemistry

journal homepage: www.elsevier.com/locate/procbio

Biotransformation of the SDG in defatted flaxseed into END co-cultured by three single bacterial colonies

Hong-Yun Zhu[a,b,1], Miao-Xin Li[a,1], Dong-Hui Yang[a,*], Yi-Lun Tao[a], Ying Zhang[a], Shu-Lin Liu[b,c,d,**]

[a] State Key Laboratory of Natural and Biomimetic Drugs, School of Pharmaceutical Sciences, Peking University, Beijing 100191, China
[b] School of Basic Medical Sciences, Peking University, Beijing 100191, China
[c] Genomics Research Center, Harbin Medical University, Harbin 150081, China
[d] Department of Microbiology and Infectious Diseases, University of Calgary, Calgary, AB T2N 4N1, Canada

A R T I C L E I N F O

Article history:
Received 20 June 2013
Received in revised form 1 October 2013
Accepted 3 October 2013
Available online 17 October 2013

Keywords:
Enterodiol
Defatted flaxseed
Biotransformation
Bacteroides uniformis
Eubacterium limosum
Eggerthella lenta

A B S T R A C T

Enterodiol (END) possesses the estrogenic and antiestrogenic activities, which could prevent the development of breast cancer and prostate cancer, as well as menopausal syndrome.

Previous studies in our laboratory set up a bio-transformation method for largely yielding secoisolariciresinol (SECO) from the substrate of defatted flaxseeds by strain *Bacteroides uniformis* ZL-I. In this research, another two single colonies, designated as strain ZL-II and strain ZL-III, were isolated, which were closely related to *Eubacterium limosum* species (ZL-II), and *Eggerthella lenta* species (ZL-III) on the basis of 16S rRNA gene sequence data. Under the combining actions of strains ZL-(I + II + III), END could be produced from defatted flaxseed directly, ZL-II was proved to possess the activities of demethylation, while ZL-III had the activities of dehydroxylation. Secoisolariciresinol diglucoside (SDG) existed in the form of oligomeric with 3-hydroxy-3-methyl glutaric acid in flaxseed could be efficiently transformed into END under the co-culture of strains ZL-(I + II + III), with the conversion rate of more than 90%. The method for mass-producing END from defatted flaxseed reported here is meaningful not only for the medicinal values of END but also for the resource utilization of flaxseed materials.

© 2013 Published by Elsevier Ltd.

1. Introduction

Phytoestrogens are kinds of estrogen-like active compounds that usually presented in plants, such as the isoflavonoides in soy beans and lignans in flaxseed [1]. Enterodiol (END) is one of the lignan-type phytoestrogens, which had potent antiestrogenic effects on estrogen receptor-positive breast cancer, it can modulate the immune response by acting on nuclear factor-κB (NF-κB) signaling, which in turn resulted in decreased tumor necrosis factor-α (TNF-α) production [2,3]. In addition, END had antioxidant activity [4,5]. As known, END was mainly found from the biosamples of mammalians [6,7], it was proved that many lignanoid constituents in plant resources, such as secoisolariciresinol diglucoside (SDG), matairesinol [8], lariciresinol, isolariciresinol [9,10], 7-hydroxymatairesinol [11], pinoresinol, arctigenin, syringaresinol [12] and asarinin [13], could act as the precursors of END *in vivo*, and they could be transformed to END under the biological transformation of human intestinal bacteria. Flaxseed is the known richest resource of lignans, which contains approximately 6.1–11.3 mg g^{-1} SDG in dried mass [14]. However, the SDG in flaxseed was in the form of oligomeric structure composed of five SDG residues interconnected by four 3-hydroxy-3-methyl glutaric acid (HMGA) residues [15], which brought difficulties for the isolation of SDG from flaxseed by using the traditional chemical methods. Therefore, we tried to directly transform the SDG-HMGA residues in flaxseed into END by human intestinal bacteria *in vitro*, the method of microbial transformation has been proved workable [15,16]. As the single strain clones which were in charge of the whole catalytic reaction process among the microbiota were still unknown, in this study, three colonies with different morphology were isolated and identified from the active microbiota after repetitive subculturing and plate cultiviation, the END producing technology by taking defatted flaxseed as substrate which was co-cultured with the three colonies was also investigated.

* Corresponding author at: State Key Laboratory of Natural and Biomimetic Drugs, School of Pharmaceutical Sciences, Peking University, 38 Xueyuan Road, Beijing 100191, China. Tel.: +86 10 82801559.
** Corresponding author at: Genomics Research Center, Harbin Medical University, 157 Baojian Road, Harbin 150081, China. Tel.: +86 10 86614075.
E-mail addresses: ydhui@bjmu.edu.cn (D.-H. Yang), sliu@ucalgary.ca (S.-L. Liu).
[1] These authors contributed equally to this work.

1359-5113/$ – see front matter © 2013 Published by Elsevier Ltd.
http://dx.doi.org/10.1016/j.procbio.2013.10.003

Infection, Genetics and Evolution 26 (2014) 295–302

Contents lists available at ScienceDirect

Infection, Genetics and Evolution

journal homepage: www.elsevier.com/locate/meegid

Comparative genomic analysis between typhoidal and non-typhoidal *Salmonella* serovars reveals typhoid-specific protein families

Qing-Hua Zou [a], Ren-Qing Li [b], Gui-Rong Liu [c,*], Shu-Lin Liu [a,c,d,e,f,*]

[a] Department of Microbiology, School of Basic Medical Sciences, Peking University Health Science Center, Beijing, China
[b] Institute of Immunology, Beijing Center for Disease Control and Prevention, Beijing, China
[c] Genomics Research Center (one of The State-Province Key Laboratories of Biomedicine-Pharmaceutics of China), Harbin Medical University, Harbin, China
[d] HMU-UCFM Centre for Infection and Genomics, Harbin Medical University, Harbin, China
[e] Department of Biopharmaceutical Sciences, Faculty of Pharmacy, Harbin Medical University, Harbin, China
[f] Department of Microbiology and Infectious Diseases, University of Calgary, Calgary, Alberta, Canada

ARTICLE INFO

Article history:
Received 14 January 2014
Received in revised form 4 June 2014
Accepted 10 June 2014
Available online 18 June 2014

Keywords:
Salmonella
S. Typhi
S. Paratyphi A
S. Paratyphi B
S. Paratyphi C
Specific protein families

ABSTRACT

Background: The genus *Salmonella* contains more than 2600 serovars. While most cause a self-limiting gastroenteritis, four serovars, *S.* Typhi, *S.* Paratyphi A, B and C, elicit typhoid, a potentially fatal systemic infection. Because of the prevalence in certain regions, such as South Asia, and the disease severity of typhoidal *Salmonella* infections, comprehensive studies are needed to elucidate the pathogenesis of diseases caused by these typhoidal serovars.
Results: We performed comparative genomic analyses on eight human typhoidal strains and 27 non-human typhoidal *Salmonella* strains to elucidate their evolutionary relationships and identify the genes specific to the four typhoidal serovars. Our results indicate that *Salmonella* may have an open pan-genome. A core-genome based phylogeny demonstrated that divergence between *S.* Paratyphi A and *S.* Typhi took place not long ago and *S.* Paratyphi B shared a recent common ancestor with *S.* Paratyphi C. Of great interest, the divergence between *S.* Paratyphi B and *S.* Paratyphi C was shown to be more recent than that between *S.* Paratyphi A and *S.* Typhi. Alignment and comparisons of the genomes identified unique complements of protein families to each of the typhoidal serovars. Most of these protein families are phage related and some are candidate virulence factors. Importantly, we found 88 protein families specific to two to three of the four typhoidal serovars. All but two of the 88 genes are present in *S.* Typhi, with a few in the three paratyphoidal serovars but none in the non-human typhoidal serovars. Most of these genes are predicted to encode hypothetical proteins and some are known to code for virulence factors such as Vi polysaccharide related proteins.
Conclusions: By comprehensive genomic comparisons, we identified protein families specific to the human typhoidal serovars, which will greatly facilitate investigations on typhoid pathogenesis.
© 2014 Elsevier B.V. All rights reserved.

1. Introduction

Salmonella are important bacterial pathogens. Since their divergence from *Escherichia coli* over 100 million years ago (Doolittle et al., 1996), bacteria of the *Salmonella* genus have differentiated into more than 2600 antigenically distinct serovars (Beltran et al., 1988; Reeves et al., 1989). Many *Salmonella* serovars can cause gastroenteritis, which is essentially a self-limiting illness, a few *Salmonella* serovars, including *S.* Typhi, *S.* Paratyphi A, B and C, may elicit typhoid-like diseases, which are serious systemic infections (Parry et al., 2002). To date, numerous virulence factors important for the *Salmonella* serovars causing gastroenteritis have been identified using animal models and a variety of elegant genetic methods, including signature-tagged transposon mutagenesis (Bispham et al., 2001), in vivo expression technology and differential fluorescence induction (Stanley et al., 2000; Bumann 2001), etc. However, due to the lack of proper animal models for the human typhoidal serovars, the genetic traits or virulence factors associated with the typhoid pathogenesis remain largely unidentified.

Comparative genomics studies based upon full genome sequences have allowed the identification of *Salmonella*

* Corresponding authors. Address: Genomics Research Center, Harbin Medical University, 157 Baojian Road, Harbin 150081, China. Tel.: +86 45186669150; fax: +86 45187502720.
E-mail addresses: grliu.natsumi@gmail.com (G.-R. Liu), slliu@ucalgary.ca (S.-L. Liu).

http://dx.doi.org/10.1016/j.meegid.2014.06.008
1567-1348/© 2014 Elsevier B.V. All rights reserved.

Wang *et al. BMC Genomics* 2014, **15**:50
http://www.biomedcentral.com/1471-2164/15/50

BMC Genomics

RESEARCH ARTICLE Open Access

Prediction of bacterial type IV secreted effectors by C-terminal features

Yejun Wang[1*†], Xiaowei Wei[1†], Hongxia Bao[1] and Shu-Lin Liu[1,2*]

Abstract

Background: Many bacteria can deliver pathogenic proteins (effectors) through type IV secretion systems (T4SSs) to eukaryotic cytoplasm, causing host diseases. The inherent property, such as sequence diversity and global scattering throughout the whole genome, makes it a big challenge to effectively identify the full set of T4SS effectors. Therefore, an effective inter-species T4SS effector prediction tool is urgently needed to help discover new effectors in a variety of bacterial species, especially those with few known effectors, e.g., *Helicobacter pylori*.

Results: In this research, we first manually annotated a full list of validated T4SS effectors from different bacteria and then carefully compared their C-terminal sequential and position-specific amino acid compositions, possible motifs and structural features. Based on the observed features, we set up several models to automatically recognize T4SS effectors. Three of the models performed strikingly better than the others and T4SEpre_Joint had the best performance, which could distinguish the T4SS effectors from non-effectors with a 5-fold cross-validation sensitivity of 89% at a specificity of 97%, based on the training datasets. An inter-species cross prediction showed that T4SEpre_Joint could recall most known effectors from a variety of species. The inter-species prediction tool package, T4SEpre, was further used to predict new T4SS effectors from *H. pylori*, an important human pathogen associated with gastritis, ulcer and cancer. In total, 24 new highly possible *H. pylori* T4S effector genes were computationally identified.

Conclusions: We conclude that T4SEpre, as an effective inter-species T4SS effector prediction software package, will help find new pathogenic T4SS effectors efficiently in a variety of pathogenic bacteria.

Keywords: Type IV secretion system, Effector, Secretion signal prediction, Sequence analysis, Machine learning, *Helicobacter pylori*

Background

Type IV secretion system (T4SS) is a membrane-associated multi-component transporter complex, which plays important roles both in horizontal DNA transfer between different bacteria and in bacterial pathogenesis by translocating pathogenic substrates (DNA or protein) into host plant, animal or human cells [1,2]. A large number of T4SSs have been identified in a variety of bacterial species [1,2]. In many cases T4SSs have been implicated in protein delivery during the infection process, such as *Helicobacter* Cag-T4SS in human gastric ulcer and cancer, *Legionella* Dot/Icm-T4SS in Legionnaires' disease, and *Bartonella* VirB/VirD4 in cat scratch disease [3-8]. Recently, a large-scale screening study performed in over 1000 prokaryotic genomes disclosed a total of 949 T4SSs, among which 267 lacked relaxases and were considered as putative protein-exporting T4SSs, since the T4SSs involving horizontal DNA transfer require the activity of relaxases while known protein-exporting T4SSs do not need relaxes [9].

The proteins specifically secreted through T4SS conduit are called type IV secreted (T4S) effectors, which exert important functions in cytoplasm of infected eukaryotic cells [10,11]. A large number of T4S effectors have been characterized experimentally with assays involving genetic complementation, reporter protein fusion, secretion apparatus or chaperone interaction, etc. [12-16]. However, it is difficult and time-consuming to find new effectors purely based on experimental

* Correspondence: yejun.wang@gmail.com; slliu@ucalgary.ca
†Equal contributors
[1]Genomics Research Center, Harbin Medical University, Harbin, China
[2]Department of Microbiology and Infectious Diseases, University of Calgary, Calgary, Canada

BioMed Central

© 2014 Wang et al.; licensee BioMed Central Ltd. This is an open access article distributed under the terms of the Creative Commons Attribution License (http://creativecommons.org/licenses/by/2.0), which permits unrestricted use, distribution, and reproduction in any medium, provided the original work is properly cited.

Industrial Crops and Products 58 (2014) 31–35

Contents lists available at ScienceDirect

Industrial Crops and Products

journal homepage: www.elsevier.com/locate/indcrop

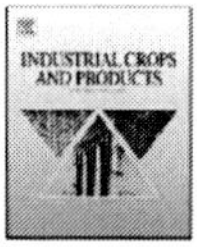

Functional groups and antioxidant activities of polysaccharides from five categories of tea

Zhan-Yi Zhao, Long-Tao Huangfu, Lu-Lu Dong*, Shu-Lin Liu*

College of Pharmacy, Harbin Medical University, Harbin 150081, China

ARTICLE INFO

Article history:
Received 11 November 2013
Received in revised form 14 March 2014
Accepted 6 April 2014

Keywords:
Tea polysaccharides
Functional group
Antioxidant
FT-IR

ABSTRACT

Ten polysaccharides were extracted from five categories of tea with hot water and further fractionated by stepwise ethanol precipitation. The polysaccharides were characterized by Fourier transform infrared spectroscopy (FT-IR) and the components including sulfuric radical, aminohexose and uronic acid were determined. All analyzed polysaccharides had antioxidant activities, with polysaccharides-II being stronger than polysaccharides-I and the antioxidant activity of the tea polysaccharides was closely related with the contents of functional groups in the polysaccharides. Our results suggest that the tea polysaccharides could be explored as a potential antioxidant agent for use in medicine or functional foods. On the other hand, the different antioxidant activities of samples provided an important reference for choosing the suitable kind of tea in application.

© 2014 Elsevier B.V. All rights reserved.

1. Introduction

As a daily beverage, tea is widely consumed in the world and is usually classified into unfermented (green tea – GT), slight-fermented (white tea – WT), semifermented (oolong tea – OT), fermented (black tea – BT), and post-fermented (dark green tea – DGT) forms (Tanaka et al., 2012; Zhu et al., 2002). Due to its validated as well as assumed beneficial effects on human health, it is planted as an important commercial crop in many areas in the world especially in China. In addition, tea has been used as a pharmaceutical to treat coma, to improve blood flow, and to eliminate toxins for many years (Balentine et al., 1997; Dufresne and Farnworth, 2000; Hara, 2011; Sewell, 1864). Recently, interest in tea is growing because of many other beneficial bioactivities, including its roles as an antioxidant (Wang et al., 2012c; Yang et al., 2012a), effects on angiogenesis (Maiti et al., 2003), and possible therapeutic values against cancers (Carvalho et al., 2010; Fan et al., 2011), mutagenesis (Geetha et al., 2004; Kuroda and Hara, 1999), hypertension (Antonello et al., 2007), and hyperglycemia (Han et al., 2011). These biological activities and health benefits are associated with the constituents of tea such as polysaccharides, polyphenols, caffeine, theanine and so on (Nie and Xie, 2011; Wang et al., 2012a).

In recent years, the association of bioactivities with structure of natural polysaccharides has caused great interest among researchers (Kishk and Al-Sayed, 2007; Klaus et al., 2011). Tea polysaccharides (TP) are among the most important components of tea. Although many of the bioactivities of tea mentioned above have been associated with TP, to date most of previous studies have been focused on green tea polysaccharides (Nie and Xie, 2011). Notably, the bioactivities and structures of the constituents from different categories of tea can be affected by the remaining enzymes originally contained in the leaves after different manufacturing processes (Tanaka et al., 2009, 2012). However, so far to our knowledge no comparative studies have been reported on the antioxidant activities and structures of TP from five categories of tea.

In this study, we analyzed the functional groups of ten TP samples from five types of tea by Fourier transform infrared (FT-IR) spectroscopy analysis, determined the contents of sulfuric radical, aminohexose and uronic acid, and investigated the antioxidant activities. Our work suggests that the tea polysaccharides, as potent antioxidant agents, have great potential for use in medicine or functional foods. Additionally, our results of different antioxidant activities of teas treated by different manufactural processes provide important guideline information for choosing the suitable kind of tea in different applications.

* Corresponding authors. Tel.: +86 45186699351; fax: +86 45186614073.
E-mail addresses: Zhanyi.Zhao@163.com (L.-L. Dong), slliu@ucalgary.ca (S.-L. Liu).

http://dx.doi.org/10.1016/j.indcrop.2014.04.004
0926-6690/© 2014 Elsevier B.V. All rights reserved.

Bao *et al. BMC Microbiology* 2014, **14**:157
http://www.biomedcentral.com/1471-2180/14/157

BMC Microbiology

RESEARCH ARTICLE **Open Access**

Differential efficiency in exogenous DNA acquisition among closely related *Salmonella* strains: implications in bacterial speciation

Hong-Xia Bao[1,2,3,8†], Le Tang[1,2,3,8†], Lu Yu[1,2,3], Xu-Yao Wang[1,2,3], Yang Li[1,2,3], Xia Deng[1,2,3], Yong-Guo Li[4], Ang Li[5], Da-Ling Zhu[2,6], Randal N Johnston[7], Gui-Rong Liu[1,2,3*], Ye Feng[1,2,3,9*] and Shu-Lin Liu[1,2,3,4,8*]

Abstract

Background: Acquisition of exogenous genetic material is a key event in bacterial speciation. It seems reasonable to assume that recombination of the incoming DNA into genome would be more efficient with higher levels of relatedness between the DNA donor and recipient. If so, bacterial speciation would be a smooth process, leading to a continuous spectrum of genomic divergence of bacteria, which, however, is not the case as shown by recent findings. The goal of this study was todetermine if DNA transfer efficiency is correlated with the levels of sequence identity.

Results: To compare the relative efficiency of exogenous DNA acquisition among closely related bacteria, we carried out phage-mediated transduction and plasmid-mediated transformation in representative *Salmonella* strains with different levels of relatedness. We found that the efficiency was remarkably variable even among genetically almost identical bacteria. Although there was a general tendency that more closely related DNA donor-recipient pairs had higher transduction efficiency, transformation efficiency exhibited over a thousand times difference among the closely related *Salmonella* strains.

Conclusion: DNA acquisition efficiency is greatly variable among bacteria that have as high as over 99% identical genetic background, suggesting that bacterial speciation involves highly complex processes affected not only by whether beneficial exogenous DNA may exist in the environment but also the "readiness" of the bacteria to accept it.

Keywords: Bacterial speciation, Homologous recombination, *Salmonella*, Transduction, Transformation

Background

Speciation of bacteria, i.e., their divergence from the ancestor and evolution into new species, is facilitated by incorporation of laterally acquired genetic material into the genome, as demonstrated by comparative studies of model bacteria, such as *Salmonella* and other enteric bacteria [1-3]. Bacteria of the *Salmonella* genus have been frequently used as ideal research models of bacterial genomic divergence and evolution owing to several advantages that fit such studies, including the close genetic relatedness and, conversely, distinct pathogenic properties of these bacteria. In addition, the extraordinarily large number of known genetic and pathogenic types of *Salmonella* makes the comparative studies informative and feasible.

Salmonella diverged from *Escherichia coli* more than 100 million years ago [4-6]; to date, more than 2500 serologically defined types, called serotypes or serovars, have been documented [7,8]. Genomic comparisons reveal that different *Salmonella* serotypes have highly similar overall genome structures, which are also similar to that of *E. coli* [9-12], validating the long speculated high level genomic conservation during long evolutionary times. When more detailed comparisons are made systematically

* Correspondence: grliu.natsumi@gmail.com; pandafengye@gmail.com; slliu@ucalgary.ca
† Equal contributors
[1] Genomics Research Center (one of The State-Province Key Laboratories of Biomedicine-Pharmaceutics of China), Harbin Medical University, 157 Baojian Road, Harbin 150081, China
[2] Department of Biopharmaceutical Sciences, Harbin Medical University, Harbin, China
[3] HMU-UCFM Centre for Infection and Genomics, Harbin Medical University, Harbin, China
Full list of author information is available at the end of the article

BioMed Central

© 2014 Bao et al.; licensee BioMed Central Ltd. This is an Open Access article distributed under the terms of the Creative Commons Attribution License (http://creativecommons.org/licenses/by/2.0), which permits unrestricted use, distribution, and reproduction in any medium, provided the original work is properly credited.

OPEN ACCESS Freely available online
PLOS ONE

CTAG-Containing Cleavage Site Profiling to Delineate *Salmonella* into Natural Clusters

Le Tang[1,2,3], Wei-Qiao Liu[4¤], Xin Fang[1,2,3], Qiang Sun[1,2,3], Song-Ling Zhu[1,2,3], Chun-Xiao Wang[1,2,3], Xiao-Yu Wang[1,2,3], Yong-Guo Li[3,5], Da-Ling Zhu[2,6], Kenneth E. Sanderson[4], Randal N. Johnston[7], Gui-Rong Liu[1,2,3]*, Shu-Lin Liu[1,2,3,4,5]*

1 Genomics Research Center (one of The State-Province Key Laboratories of Biomedicine-Pharmaceutics of China), Harbin Medical University, Harbin, China, **2** Department of Biopharmaceutical Sciences, Harbin Medical University, Harbin, China, **3** HMU-UCFM Centre for Infection and Genomics, Harbin Medical University, Harbin, China, **4** Department of Microbiology and Infectious Diseases, University of Calgary, Calgary, Canada, **5** Department of Infectious Diseases of First Affiliated Hospital, Harbin Medical University, Harbin, China, **6** College of Pharmacy, Daqing Campus, Harbin Medical University, Daqing, China, **7** Department of Biochemistry and Molecular Biology, University of Calgary, Calgary, Canada

Abstract

Background: The bacterial genus *Salmonella* contains thousands of serotypes that infect humans or other hosts, causing mild gastroenteritis to potentially fatal systemic infections in humans. Pathogenically distinct *Salmonella* serotypes have been classified as individual species or as serological variants of merely one or two species, causing considerable confusion in both research and clinical settings. This situation reflects a long unanswered question regarding whether the *Salmonella* serotypes exist as discrete genetic clusters (natural species) of organisms or as phenotypic (e.g. pathogenic) variants of a single (or two) natural species with a continuous spectrum of genetic divergence among them. Our recent work, based on genomic sequence divergence analysis, has demonstrated that genetic boundaries exist among *Salmonella* serotypes, circumscribing them into clear-cut genetic clusters of bacteria.

Methodologies/Principal Findings: To further test the genetic boundary concept for delineating *Salmonella* into clearly defined natural lineages (e.g., species), we sampled a small subset of conserved genomic DNA sequences, i.e., the endonuclease cleavage sites that contain the highly conserved CTAG sequence such as TCTAGA for XbaI. We found that the CTAG-containing cleavage sequence profiles could be used to resolve the genetic boundaries as reliably and efficiently as whole genome sequence comparisons but with enormously reduced requirements for time and resources.

Conclusions: Profiling of CTAG sequence subsets reflects genetic boundaries among *Salmonella* lineages and can delineate these bacteria into discrete natural clusters.

Citation: Tang L, Liu W-Q, Fang X, Sun Q, Zhu S-L, et al. (2014) CTAG-Containing Cleavage Site Profiling to Delineate *Salmonella* into Natural Clusters. PLoS ONE 9(8): e103388. doi:10.1371/journal.pone.0103388

Editor: Michiel Vos, University of Exeter Medical School, United Kingdom

Received February 12, 2014; **Accepted** June 30, 2014; **Published** August 19, 2014

Copyright: © 2014 Tang et al. This is an open-access article distributed under the terms of the Creative Commons Attribution License, which permits unrestricted use, distribution, and reproduction in any medium, provided the original author and source are credited.

Funding: This work was supported by a Heilongjiang Innovation Endowment Award for graduate studies (YJSCX2012-197HLJ) to LT; a National Natural Science Foundation of China (NSFC30970078) and a grant of Natural Science Foundation of Heilongjiang Province of China to GRL; a grant of Canadian Institutes of Health Research to RNJ; and grants of the National Natural Science Foundation of China (NSFC30970119, 81030029, 81271786, NSFC-NIH 81161120416) to SLL. The funders had no role in study design, data collection and analysis, decision to publish, or preparation of the manuscript.

Competing Interests: The authors have declared that no competing interests exist.

* Email: grliu.natsumi@gmailcom (GRL); slliu@ucalgary.ca (SLL)

¤ Current address: Department of Neurology, Vancouver General Hospital, Vancouver, Canada

Introduction

Since the first isolation of a *Salmonella* pathogen from a typhoid patient in 1881, more than 2500 different *Salmonella* types have been documented [1,2]. Based on their differences in the somatic (O) and flagellar (H) antigens, the *Salmonella* bacteria are classified into serotypes by the Kauffmann-White scheme [3]. Initially, the *Salmonella* serotypes were treated as individual species each having a Latinized scientific name such as *Salmonella typhi* and *Salmonella typhimurium*, but in the 1980s all *Salmonella* serotypes were combined into one species (*Salmonella enterica* [1]) or two species (*Salmonella enterica* and *Salmonella bongori* [5]) as serological variants (serovars [6]) due largely to the extraordinarily high genetic similarity among them, which has caused confusion in research and clinical settings. Indeed, all *Salmonella* serotypes have very similar genetic backgrounds as revealed by DNA-DNA re-association [7], comparison of genome structures [8,9] and genomic sequencing [10–12], but on the other hand they may differ radically in pathogenic properties. For example, whereas many *Salmonella* serotypes may cause self-limited gastroenteritis (such as *S. typhimurium*, *S. enteritidis*, etc.) or may be virtually non-pathogenic to humans, a few may elicit potentially fatal systemic infections, such as *S. typhi* that causes typhoid [13]. The dynamic and confusing *Salmonella* taxonomy reflects long lasting uncertainties about the phylogenetic status of *Salmonella*: do they dwell in nature as discrete genetic clusters of organisms or as phenotypic variants of a single (or two) natural species with a continuous spectrum of genetic divergence among them?

Liu et al. Journal of Ovarian Research 2014, 7:87
http://www.ovarianresearch.com/content/7/1/87

JOURNAL OF OVARIAN RESEARCH

RESEARCH Open Access

Reduced expression of SOX7 in ovarian cancer: a novel tumor suppressor through the Wnt/β-catenin signaling pathway

Huidi Liu[1,2,4], Zi-Qiao Yan[1], Bailiang Li[1], Si-Yuan Yin[1], Qiang Sun[1], Jun-Jie Kou[1], Dan Ye[1], Kelsey Ferns[1,5], Hong-Yu Liu[3] and Shu-Lin Liu[1,2,4*]

Abstract

Background: Products of the SOX gene family play important roles in the life process. One of the members, SOX7, is associated with the development of a variety of cancers as a tumor suppression factor, but its relevance with ovarian cancer was unclear. In this study, we investigated the involvement of SOX7 in the progression and prognosis of epithelial ovarian cancer (EOC) and the involved mechanisms.

Methods: Expression profiles in two independent microarray data sets were analyzed for SOX7 between malignant and normal tissues. The expression levels of SOX7 in EOC, borderline ovarian tumors and normal ovarian tissues were measured by immunohistochemistry. We also measured levels of COX2 and cyclin-D1 to examine their possible involvement in the same signal transduction pathway as SOX7.

Results: The expression of SOX7 was significantly reduced in ovarian cancer tissues compared with normal controls, strongly indicating that SOX7 might be a negative regulator in the Wnt/β-catenin pathway in ovarian cancer. By immunohistochemistry staining, the protein expression of SOX7 showed a consistent trend with that of the gene expression microarray analysis. By contrast, the protein expression level of COX2 and cyclin-D1 increased as the tumor malignancy progressed, suggesting that SOX7 may function through the Wnt/β-catenin signaling pathway as a tumor suppressor. In comparison between the protein expression levels of SOX7 with pathological features of the cancer, we found that SOX7 was down-regulated mainly in serous cystadenocarcinoma and advanced stages of the cancers.

Conclusions: The expression of SOX7 correlates with tumor progression as a tumor suppressor, possibly through the Wnt/β-catenin signaling pathway in ovarian cancers, suggesting that SOX7 may be a promising prognostic marker.

Keywords: SOX7, Tumor suppressor, Ovarian cancer, Wnt/β-catenin signaling pathway

Background

Ovarian cancer is one of the three most common cancers in female with high morbidity and mortality rates [1]. The disease is also among the most lethal cancers in females, primarily because of its aggressive metastasis within the peritoneal cavity. It is hardly detectable at the early stage, largely due to the lack of specific symptoms and reliable screening [2,3]. Among all types, epithelial ovarian cancer (EOC) is the most common, accounting for 85% to 90% of ovarian cancers [4], and this type is highly lethal. This situation calls for the investigation of pathogenesis of EOC and the identification of molecular markers for early diagnosis or for use as targets in treatment.

SOX7, a member of subfamily SOXF along with SOX17 and SOX18, has been identified as a developmental regulator in hematopoiesis and cardiogenesis [5-9]. The human SOX7 gene is located at the chromosomal region of 8p23.1 and is approximately 7.7 kbps in length [10]; a frequently methylated CpG island on the promoter region of

* Correspondence: slliu@ucalgary.ca
[1]Genomics Research Centre, Harbin Medical University, Harbin 150081, China
[2]HMU-UCFM Centre for Infection and Genomics, Harbin, China
Full list of author information is available at the end of the article

BioMed Central

© 2014 Liu et al.; licensee BioMed Central Ltd. This is an Open Access article distributed under the terms of the Creative Commons Attribution License (http://creativecommons.org/licenses/by/4.0), which permits unrestricted use, distribution, and reproduction in any medium, provided the original work is properly credited. The Creative Commons Public Domain Dedication waiver (http://creativecommons.org/publicdomain/zero/1.0/) applies to the data made available in this article, unless otherwise stated.

Bioinformatics Advance Access published August 26, 2014

Original Paper

Individual-level analysis of differential expression of genes and pathways for personalized medicine

Hongwei Wang[1], Qiang Sun[2], Wenyuan Zhao[1], Lishuang Qi[1], Yunyan Gu[1], Pengfei Li[1], Mengmeng Zhang[1], Yang Li[1], Shu-Lin Liu[2,3]* and Zheng Guo[1,4]*

[1]College of Bioinformatics Science and Technology, Harbin Medical University, Harbin, 150086, China
[2]Genomics Research Center, Harbin Medical University, Harbin, 150086, China
[3]Department of Microbiology and Infectious Diseases, University of Calgary, Calgary, AB, T2N 4N1, Canada
[4]Bioinformatics Department, Basic Medical College, Fujian Medical University, Fuzhou, 350004, China

Downloaded from http://bioinformatics.oxfordjournals.org/ at Purdue University Libraries ADMN on August 28, 2014

Associate Editor: Dr. Ziv Bar-Joseph

ABSTRACT

Motivation: The differential expression analysis focusing on inter-group comparison can only capture differentially expressed genes (DE genes) at the population level, which may mask the heterogeneity of differential expression in individuals. Thus, in order to provide patient-specific information for personalized medicine, it is necessary to conduct differential expression analysis at the individual level.

Results: We proposed a method to detect DE genes in individual disease samples by utilizing the disrupted ordering in individual disease samples. In both simulated data and real paired cancer-normal sample data, this method showed excellent performance. It was found to be insensitive to experimental batch effects and data normalization. The landscape of stable gene pairs in a particular type of normal tissue could be pre-determined using previously accumulated data, based on which dysregulated genes and pathways for any disease sample can be readily detected. The usefulness of the *RankComp* method in clinical settings was exemplified by the identification and application of prognostic markers for lung cancer.

Availability and Implementation: *RankComp* is implemented in R script that is freely available from Supplemental materials.

Contact: guoz@ems.hrbmu.edu.cn and slliu@ucalgary.ca

Supplementary Information: Supplementary data are available at Bioinformatics online.

1 INTRODUCTION

The differential expression analysis methods on inter-group comparison for identifying disease-related genes can classified into two broad categories: the intensity-based methods such as T-Test (JA, 1995), SAM (Tusher *et al.*, 2001) and Limma (Smyth, 2004), and the rank-based methods such as Wilcoxon signed rank test (Wilcoxon, 1945), Wilcoxon rank sum test (Hollander, 1973) and RP (Breitling *et al.*, 2004). Of the rank-based methods, there is a special type of method utilizing the fold-change ordering information, such as RP (Breitling *et al.*, 2004) RcoS (Navon *et al.*, 2009) and FCROS (Dembele and Kastner, 2014). In general, these methods first entail ranking fold-change values within each pairwise comparison between two types of samples, then calculate a fold-change rank ordering statistic for each gene. The significance of the observed statistic could be determined by using a permutation test (e.g., RP) or probability distribution function (e.g., FCROS). The rank-based methods usually have some advantages in comparison with the intensity-based methods, such as robustness against outlier values and favorable power efficiency in some cases (Lehmann, 1975). However, both the above-mentioned intensity-based and rank-based methods are designed to detect the population-level DE genes and cannot provide patient-specific differential expression information.

Taking the heterogeneous nature of disease into account, several outlier detection methods, including COPA(Tomlins *et al.*, 2005), OS (Tibshirani and Hastie, 2007), ORT (Wu, 2007), MOST (Lian, 2008) and others (Hu, 2008; Wang *et al.*, 2012; de Ronde *et al.*, 2013), are developed to detect genes that are dysregulated in subsets of disease samples. However, they are more sensitive to various technical artefacts, especially experimental batch effects caused by differences in laboratory conditions, reagent lots, and personnel (Leek *et al.*, 2010). In general, batch effects can introduce serious problems in translating experimental findings to clinical settings. For example, because of this problem, an optimized threshold value of the risk score summarizing the expression levels of signature genes determined from a set of training samples cannot be directly applied to other samples. Usually, in validation studies, data normalization is required for independently extracted samples in order to make all data having nearly the same scale as the training samples. However, current normalization methods that are used to adjust for systematic technical artefacts are usually not able to remove batch effects (Lazar *et al.*, 2012). They may even distort biological signals (Wang *et al.*, 2011). More fundamentally, large inter-individual variation in gene expression will exacerbate the problem of threshold setting for risk stratification. To tackle this difficult problem, researchers have proposed to make use of the relative ordering information of gene expression within each sample, considering that the relative ordering of gene expression within each sample would be rather robust against batch effects and insensitive to data normalization (Geman *et al.*, 2004; Tan *et al.*, 2005).

The relative ordering of gene expression is overall stable in a particular type of normal human tissue but widely disturbed in diseased tissue. Taking this into account, a method of detecting DE

*To whom correspondence should be addressed.

© The Author (2014). Published by Oxford University Press. All rights reserved. For Permissions, please email: journals.permissions@oup.com

Carbohydrate Polymers 119 (2015) 101–109

Contents lists available at ScienceDirect

Carbohydrate Polymers

journal homepage: www.elsevier.com/locate/carbpol

Optimization of ultrasound extraction of *Alisma orientalis* polysaccharides by response surface methodology and their antioxidant activities

Zhan-Yi Zhao[a], Qiang Zhang[b], Ya-Fang Li[a], Lu-Lu Dong[a,*], Shu-Lin Liu[a,c,*]

[a] College of Pharmacy, Harbin Medical University, Harbin 150081, China
[b] Harbin Medical University Library, Harbin 150081, China
[c] Genomics Research Center, Harbin Medical University, Harbin 150081, China

ARTICLE INFO

Article history:
Received 12 September 2014
Received in revised form 20 October 2014
Accepted 20 November 2014
Available online 3 December 2014

Keywords:
Rhizoma alismatis
Polysaccharides
Ultrasound extraction
Response surface methodology
Antioxidant activity

ABSTRACT

Rhizoma alismatis (the rhizome of *Alisma orientalis*) polysaccharides (RAP) have been reported to have a variety of important biological activities. However, effective extraction of RAP has been an unsolved issue. In this study, we used an ultrasound method for high yield extraction of RAP and optimized the conditions using the response surface methodology (RSM). Following multiple regression analyses of the experimental results, we applied the 3-D response surface and the contour plots to determine the optimal conditions, which were found to be ultrasound treatment at 76.1 °C for 75.2 min, and water to material ratio at 30.1 ml/g. Under such conditions, the yield was 6.90% which was much higher than traditional hot water extraction yield (3.41%). The fractionated RAPs following stepwise ethanol precipitation showed strong antioxidant activities. The results indicated that ultrasound extraction was a very effective method for the extraction of RAP and the polysaccharides could be explored as a potential antioxidant agent for use in medicine or functional food.

© 2014 Elsevier Ltd. All rights reserved.

1. Introduction

Rhizoma alismatis (RA) is the rhizome of *Alisma orientalis* (Sam.) Juzep, which belongs to the family *Alismataceae* and is mainly distributed in China, Japan, and India (Han et al., 2013; Wu, 2005). RA is recorded as a high-grade drug in Shennong Bencao Jing, the first drug monograph of ancient China (Gu, 2007). As a folk medicine, it has been prescribed for treatment of hypertension, hyperlipemia and diabetes (China, 2005; Li & Qu, 2012; Wu, 2005), and is included in the Pharmacopoeia of China as one of the traditional Chinese herbal medicines (China, 2005). Recently, interest in RA is growing, because many of its components, such as triterpene, alisol B, and especially polysaccharides, have been reported to have important bioactivities, including anti-hepatitis, anti-inflammatory, hypoglycemic and immunological effects (Han et al., 2013; Jiang et al., 2006; Lee et al., 2013; Li & Qu, 2012; Shimizu, Ohtsu, Tomoda, Gonda, & Ohara, 1994; Tomoda, Gonda, Shimizu, & Ohara, 1994).

The RA polysaccharides (RAP) have been documented for their effects of against lipid peroxidation (Li, Jin, & Zhang, 2008), which are potentially important for human health. However, there are few studies on effective extraction of RAP. Conventional methods, such as those by hot water, immersion or Soxhlet, are often time-consuming and expensive, with low yield of RAP or even loss of some of their pharmacological activities (Li, Ding, & Ding, 2007; Wang, Cheng, Mao, Fan, & Wu, 2009). Ultrasound extraction technology has several advantages, such as reasonably high extraction yield, moderate solvent requirement, relatively short extraction time, etc., and so has been used to extract high quality bioactive polysaccharides from plant materials (Hromadkova & Ebringerova, 2003; Hromadkova, Ebringerova, & Valachovic, 2002; Pan et al., 2010; Ying, Han, & Li, 2011). Hence, ultrasound extraction technique was used to improve the extraction yield of RAP with minimally impact on their bioactivity. To apply this method for RAP, we optimized the extraction conditions and procedure using the response surface methodology (RSM), which is an effective tool for optimizing the experimental process when many factors and interactions may affect extraction yield (Box & Wilson, 1951; Prakash Maran, Manikandan, Thirugnanasambandham, Vigna Nivetha, & Dinesh, 2013). The main advantage of RSM is the considerably reduced number of tests potentially needed for evaluating

* Corresponding authors at: Harbin Medical University, College of Pharmacy, Harbin 150081, China. Tel.: +86 45186699351; fax: +86 45186614073.
E-mail addresses: Zhaoyi.Zhao@163.com (L.-L. Dong), slliu@ucalgary.ca (S.-L. Liu).

http://dx.doi.org/10.1016/j.carbpol.2014.11.052
0144-8617/© 2014 Elsevier Ltd. All rights reserved.

Am J Cancer Res 2015;5(2):726-737
www.ajcr.us /ISSN:2156-6976/ajcr0003871

Original Article

Profile of differentially expressed intratumoral cytokines to predict the immune-polarizing side effects of tamoxifen in breast cancer treatment

Bailiang Li[1], Yang Li[2], Xiao-Yu Wang[1], Zi-Qiao Yan[1], Huidi Liu[1], Gui-Rong Liu[1], Shu-Lin Liu[1,3]

[1]*Genomics Research Center (One of The State-Province Key Laboratories of Biomedicine-Pharmaceutics of China), Harbin Medical University, China;* [2]*College of Bioinformatics Science and Technology, Harbin Medical University, Harbin, China;* [3]*Department of Microbiology, Immunology and Infectious Diseases, University of Calgary, Calgary, Canada*

Received November 15, 2014; Accepted January 20, 2015; Epub January 15, 2015; Published February 1, 2015

Abstract: Factors within the tissue of breast cancer (BC) may shift the polarization of CD4+ T cells towards Th2 direction. This tendency can promote tumor development and be enhanced by the use of tamoxifen during the treatment. Thus, the patients with low levels of tumor-induced Th2 polarization prior to tamoxifen treatment may better endure the immune-polarizing side effects (IPSE) of tamoxifen and have better prognoses. Estimation of Th2 polarization status should help predict the IPSE among tamoxifen-treated patients and guide the use of tamoxifen among all BC patients before the tamoxifen therapy. Here, we report profiling of differentially expressed (DE) intratumoral cytokines as a signature to evaluate the IPSE of tamoxifen. The DE genes of intratumoral CD4+ T cells (CD4 DEGs) were identified by gene expression profiles of purified CD4+ T cells from BC patients and validated by profiling of cultured intratumoral CD4+ T cells. Functional enrichment analyses showed a directed Th2 polarization of intratumoral CD4+ T cells. To find the factors inducing the Th2 polarization of CD4+ T cells, we identified 995 common DE genes of bulk BC tissues (BC DEGs) by integrating five independent datasets. Five DE cytokines observed in bulk BC tissues with dysregulated receptors in the intratumoral CD4+ T cells were selected as the predictor of the IPSE of tamoxifen. The patients predicted to suffer low IPSE (low Th2 polarization) had a significantly lower distant relapse risk than the patients predicted to suffer high IPSE in independent datasets ($n = 608$; $HR = 4.326$, $P = 0.000897$; $HR = 2.014$, $P = 0.0173$; $HR = 2.72$, $P = 0.04077$). Patients predicted to suffer low IPSE would benefit from tamoxifen treatment ($HR = 2.908$, $P = 0.03905$). The DE intratumoral cytokines identified in this study may help predict the IPSE of tamoxifen and justify the use of tamoxifen in BC treatment.

Keywords: Breast cancer, tamoxifen, immune-polarizing side effects, the CD4+ T cell, gene expression profiles, cytokine

Introduction

It is increasingly recognized that human cancers *in vivo* are not homogeneous collections of neoplastic cells but rather consist of complex multicellular systems [1]. The interplay between tumor cells and stroma has been demonstrated to be a vital factor in cancer biologies [2] and responses to different therapeutics [1]. Infiltrating immune cells, which exert diverse biological functions [3], are frequently observed in all types of breast cancer (BC) [4, 5]. For example, CD4+ T cells are an integral part or 'regulator' in the activation and regulation processes of the host responses to many pathogens and cancers. Of particular interest, subtype polarization of CD4+ T cells (Th1 *vs.* Th2 polarization) has been reported to play a decisive role in tumor immunity [6, 7]. Without the Th1 helper function of CD4+ T cells, it would be impossible for CD8+ or cytotoxic T cells (CTLs) to be competent to kill tumor cells [8]. Numerous lines of evidence have accumulated, showing that the Th2 polarization of CD4+ T cells promotes tumor development and metastasis [9-12]. Additionally, a considerable body of literature illustrates that the CD4+ T cells within the human BC microenvironment may be shifted towards a Th2 phenotype to foster cancer development [10-12]. For instance, in compari-

www.nature.com/scientificreports

SCIENTIFIC REPORTS

OPEN

SOX7 co-regulates Wnt/β-catenin signaling with Axin-2: both expressed at low levels in breast cancer

Received: 09 October 2015
Accepted: 27 April 2016
Published: 18 May 2016

Huidi Liu[1,2,3,4], Emilio Mastriani[1], Zi-Qiao Yan[1], Si-Yuan Yin[1], Zheng Zeng[1], Hong Wang[5], Qing-Hai Li[1], Hong-Yu Liu[6], Xiaoyu Wang[1], Hong-Xia Bao[1], Yu-Jie Zhou[1], Jun-Jie Kou[1,2], Dongsheng Li[1,2], Ting Li[1,2], Jianrui Liu[1,†], Yongfang Liu[1,2], Lin Yin[1,2], Li Qiu[1,2], Liling Gong[1,2] & Shu-Lin Liu[1,3,7]

SOX7 as a tumor suppressor belongs to the SOX F gene subfamily and is associated with a variety of human cancers, including breast cancer, but the mechanisms involved are largely unclear. In the current study, we investigated the interactions between SOX7 and AXIN2 in their co-regulation on the Wnt/β-catenin signal pathway, using clinical specimens and microarray gene expression data from the GEO database, for their roles in breast cancer. We compared the expression levels of SOX7 and other co-expressed genes in the Wnt/β-catenin pathway and found that the expression of SOX7, SOX17 and SOX18 was all reduced significantly in the breast cancer tissues compared to normal controls. AXIN2 had the highest co-relativity with SOX7 in the Wnt/β-catenin signaling pathway. Clinicopathological analysis demonstrated that the down-regulated SOX7 was significantly correlated with advanced stages and poorly differentiated breast cancers. Consistent with bioinformatics predictions, SOX7 was correlated positively with AXIN2 and negatively with β-catenin, suggesting that SOX7 and AXIN2 might play important roles as co-regulators through the Wnt-β-catenin pathway in the breast tissue to affect the carcinogenesis process. Our results also showed Smad7 as the target of SOX7 and AXIN2 in controlling breast cancer progression through the Wnt/β-catenin signaling pathway.

Breast cancer is the most common malignant tumor in female and among the leading cancer deaths worldwide, with the incidence rapidly increasing in both American and Asian countries[1,2]. Breast cancer classification and stage evaluation have traditionally been based on clinicopathological features (patient age, lymph node invasion, tumor size, histological type, and pathology grade)[3], but recent technological advances have made it possible to differentiate breast cancers by molecular markers such as ER (Estrogen Receptor), PR (Progesterone Receptor) and HER2 (Human epidermalgrowth factor receptor-2)[4,5]. Among the high risk genetic factors hitherto known to contribute to the pathogenesis of breast cancer are BRCA1 (Breast Cancer Type 1 Susceptibility Protein), BRCA2 (Breast Cancer Type 2 Susceptibility Protein) and TP53 (Tumor protein p53), which have high penetrance for the disease[6]. Over the past decade, extensive research has been focused on the identification of cellular signaling pathways involved in breast cancer, such as MAPK (Mitogen-activated protein kinases), PI3K/Akt (Phosphatidylinositol-3-kinase/Akt) and Wnt/β-catenin signal pathways[7–10]. However, it still seems far away from a full picture of the molecular mechanisms underlying the breast carcinogenesis, which may involve a much greater variety of pathways and factors to be identified.

[1]Genomics Research Centre, Harbin Medical University, Harbin, 150081, China. [2]Collage of Pharmacy, Harbin Medical University, Harbin, 150081, China. [3]HMU-UCFM Centre for Infection and Genomics, Harbin, 150081, China. [4]Department of Biochemistry and Molecular Biology, University of Calgary, Calgary, T2N 4N1, Canada. [5]College of Bioinformatics Science and Technology, Harbin Medical University, Harbin, 150086, China. [6]Pathology Department, The First Hospital of Qiqihaer City, Qiqihaer, 161006, China. [7]Department of Microbiology, Immunology and Infectious Diseases, University of Calgary, Calgary, T2N 4N1, Canada. [†]Present address: Department of Biomedical Sciences, University of Calgary, Calgary, T2N4N1, Canada. Correspondence and requests for materials should be addressed to S.-L.L. (email: slliu@ucalgary.ca)

www.nature.com/scientificreports

SCIENTIFIC REPORTS

OPEN

Received: 30 March 2016
Accepted: 17 June 2016
Published: 14 July 2016

Live attenuated *Salmonella* displaying HIV-1 10E8 epitope on fimbriae: systemic and mucosal immune responses in BALB/c mice by mucosal administration

Qing-Hai Li[1,*], Gang Jin[1,*], Jia-Ye Wang[2], Hai-Ning Li[1], Huidi Liu[1], Xiao-Yun Chang[1], Fu-Xiang Wang[3] & Shu-Lin Liu[1,4,5]

The HIV-1 membrane proximal external region (MPER) that is targeted by several broadly neutralizing antibodies (BNAbs) has been considered a potential immunogen for vaccine development. However, to date the immunogenicity of these BNAb epitopes has not been made sufficiently adequate. In the present work, we used live attenuated *Salmonella* as a platform to present the HIV-1 MPER 10E8 epitope in the fimbriae. The insertion of the 10E8 epitope into the fimbriae had no significant influence on the expression and the absorption capacity of bacterial fimbriae, nor on the virulence and invasiveness of the attenuated *Salmonella*. After oral administration of the vaccine construct to mice followed by 10E8 epitope peptide boost, specific antibody responses in serum and mucosa as well as memory lymphocytes in spleen and plasma cells in bone marrow were induced. We also found that the live attenuated *Salmonella* vector directed the immunity toward Th1 bias, induced Th1 and Th2 cytokine responses and stimulated significant B cell differentiation into GC B, memory B and plasma cells. Therefore, we propose that the live attenuated *Salmonella* constitutively expressing HIV-1 BNAb epitopes on the fimbriae will be an effective approach to improving immune microenvironment and enhancing the immunogenicity of HIV-1 epitope vaccines.

Developing effective vaccines against human immunodeficiency virus type 1 (HIV-1) still faces considerable challenges three decades after the discovery of the virus[1,2]. Enormous and persistent efforts have been made to generate many vaccine candidates, including the vaccine in trial RV144 that showed modest protection[3,4], but so far none has shown the effects useful for human vaccination. Recent studies on HIV-1 pathogenesis and vaccinology have given rise to a general consensus for vaccine design that an ideal HIV-1 vaccine paradigm should simulate the natural route of viral infection[5-7]. Since the primary site of HIV-1 infection is the mucosal surface[8,9], the elicitation of protective antibody (neutralizing or non-neutralizing antibody) responses not only in systemic but also in mucosal compartments should be taken into consideration for HIV-1 vaccine design.

Most naturally infected individuals develop strain-specific antibodies against HIV-1; of interest, approximately 5–25% of HIV-1 infected individuals may develop broadly neutralizing antibodies (BNAbs), which is the primary goal for prophylactic HIV-1 vaccines[10-12]. Since 2009, a growing number of BNAbs have been reported, with most showing wide breadth and strong potency[13,14]. The targets of such antibodies on the HIV-1 envelope glycoprotein (Env) can be grouped into three parts: gp120, gp41 and the interface region of gp120-gp41[13,15]. Thus, epitopes identified in these regions have been chosen as immunogens for HIV-1 vaccine designs. Among

[1]Systemomics Center, College of Pharmacy, and Genomics Research Center (State-Province Key Laboratories of Biomedicine-Pharmaceutics of China), Harbin Medical University, Harbin, China. [2]Department of Microbiology, Harbin Medical University, Harbin, China. [3]Department of Infectious Diseases, The Fourth Affiliated Hospital of Harbin Medical University, Harbin, China. [4]Department of Infectious Diseases, The First Affiliated Hospital, Harbin Medical University, Harbin, China. [5]Department of Microbiology, Immunology and Infectious Diseases, University of Calgary, Calgary, Canada. [*]These authors contributed equally to this work. Correspondence and requests for materials should be addressed to F.-X.W. (email: wangfuxiang999@hotmail.com) or S.-L.L. (email: slliu@ucalgary.ca)

Appl Microbiol Biotechnol
DOI 10.1007/s00253-016-7626-1

BIOTECHNOLOGICALLY RELEVANT ENZYMES AND PROTEINS

Cloning, expression, and characterization of a four-component *O*-demethylase from human intestinal bacterium *Eubacterium limosum* ZL-II

Jia-Xing Chen[1] · Chao-Yin Deng[2] · Ying-Tao Zhang[1] · Zhen-Ming Liu[3] · Ping-Zhang Wang[4] · Shu-Lin Liu[5] · Wei Qian[2] · Dong-Hui Yang[1]

Received: 13 March 2016 / Revised: 26 April 2016 / Accepted: 10 May 2016
© Springer-Verlag Berlin Heidelberg 2016

Abstract *Eubacterium limosum* ZL-II was described to convert secoisolariciresinol (SECO) to its demethylating product 4,4'-dihydroxyenterodiol (DHEND) under anoxic conditions. However, the reaction cascade remains unclear. Here, the *O*-demethylase being responsible for the conversion was identified and characterized. Nine genes encoding two methyltransferase-Is (MT-I), two corrinoid proteins (CP), two methyltransferase-IIs (MT-II), and three activating enzymes (AE) were screened, cloned, and expressed in *Escherichia coli*. Four of the nine predicted enzymes, including ELI_2003 (MT-I), ELI_2004 (CP), ELI_2005 (MT-II), and ELI_0370 (AE), were confirmed to constitute the *O*-demethylase in *E. limosum* ZL-II. The complete *O*-demethylase (combining the four components) reaction system was reconstructed in vitro. As expected, the demethylating products 3-demethyl-SECO and DHEND were both produced. During the reaction process, ELI_2003 (MT-I) initially catalyzed the transfer of methyl group from SECO to the corrinoid of ELI_2004 ($[Co^{I}]$-CP), yielding demethylating products and $[CH_3\text{-}Co^{III}]$-CP; then ELI_2005 (MT-II) mediated the transfer of methyl group from $[CH_3\text{-}Co^{III}]$-CP to tetrahydrofolate, forming methyltetrahydrofolate and $[Co^{I}]$-CP. Due to the low redox potential of $[Co^{II}]/[Co^{I}]$, $[Co^{I}]$-CP was oxidized to $[Co^{II}]$-CP immediately in vitro, and ELI_0370 (AE) was responsible for catalyzing the reduction of $[Co^{II}]$-CP to its active form $[Co^{I}]$-CP. The active-site residues in ELI_2003, ELI_2005, and ELI_0370 were subsequently determined using molecular modeling combined with site-directed mutagenesis. To our knowledge, this is the first study on the identification and characterization of a four-component *O*-demethylase from *E. limosum* ZL-II, which will facilitate the development of method to artificial synthesis of related bioactive chemicals.

Keywords *O*-demethylase · *Eubacterium limosum* ZL-II · Secoisolariciresinol · Site-directed mutagenesis

✉ Wei Qian
qianw@sun.im.ac.cn

✉ Dong-Hui Yang
ydhui@bjmu.edu.cn

[1] Department of Natural Medicines, School of Pharmaceutical Sciences, Peking University, Beijing 100191, China

[2] State Key Laboratory of Plant Genomics, Institute of Microbiology, Chinese Academy of Sciences, Beijing 100101, China

[3] State Key Laboratory of Natural and Biomimetic Drugs, School of Pharmaceutical Sciences, Peking University, Beijing 100191, China

[4] Department of Immunology, School of Basic Medical Sciences, Peking University, Beijing 100191, China

[5] Genomics Research Center, Harbin Medical University, Harbin 150081, China

Introduction

In recent years, phytoestrogens have attracted widespread attention due to their similarities in structures and biological effects to animal hormone estrogens. Phytoestrogens are superior in causing lower side-effects when administered for the treatment of illnesses (Gonzalez-Vallinas et al. 2013; Hard and Edelstein 2015; Potocka et al. 2013; Sharma et al. 2014). Enterodiol (END) and enterolactone (ENL) are two important lignan-type phytoestrogens, which are associated with reduced risk of acute coronary events and many chronic diseases (Corsini et al. 2010; Hu et al. 2007; Sirotkin and Harrath 2014; Wang 2002). According to pharmacokinetics studies, high concentrations of END and ENL can be detected in the blood circulation after oral administration of

Published online: 29 May 2016

International Journal of Infectious Diseases 49 (2016) 134–140

Contents lists available at ScienceDirect

International Journal of Infectious Diseases

journal homepage: www.elsevier.com/locate/ijid

Genotyping of *Salmonella* with lineage-specific genes: correlation with serotyping

Qing-Hua Zou [a], Ren-Qing Li [b], Gui-Rong Liu [c,d], Shu-Lin Liu [c,d,e,*]

[a] Department of Microbiology, School of Basic Medical Sciences, Peking University Health Science Center, Beijing, China
[b] Institute of Immunology, Beijing Center for Disease Control and Prevention, Beijing, China
[c] Genomics Research Center, Harbin Medical University, 157 Baojian Road, Harbin, 150081, China
[d] HMU-UCFM Centre for Infection and Genomics, Harbin Medical University, Harbin, China
[e] Department of Microbiology, Immunology and Infectious Diseases, University of Calgary, Calgary, Alberta, Canada

ARTICLE INFO

Article history:
Received 14 January 2016
Received in revised form 25 May 2016
Accepted 27 May 2016

Corresponding Editor: Eskild Petersen, Aarhus, Denmark.

Keywords:
Salmonella
Serotyping
rpoB
MLST
Serotype-specific gene

SUMMARY

Background: The bacterial genus *Salmonella* encompasses a large number of serotypes that are genetically very similar but biologically quite different, especially in pathogenic properties and host specificity. Serotyping has been used for the classification, identification, and epidemiological investigation due to its excellent discriminating power, but it cannot distinguish the different pathogenic lineages within a polyphyletic serotype. Additionally, very few institutions have the comprehensive set of antisera for typing. Therefore various studies have been performed to explore alternative assays to differentiate *Salmonella* isolates, such as the search for genes that can be used as potential molecular substitutes for serotyping. However, the genes tested so far have often given inconsistent results.
Methods: In this study, the discriminating power of seven genes to differentiate 309 *Salmonella* strains representing 26 serotypes was evaluated and the results were compared with those of other methods.
Results: The seven newly selected genes have a good power to differentiate different serovars. The tree based on the concatenated sequences of these genes revealed phylogenetic relationships of the bacteria consistent with that of the whole genome tree.
Conclusion: Individual *Salmonella* lineages each have specific genes that can be used to differentiate *Salmonella* isolates on a phylogenetic basis.
© 2016 The Author(s). Published by Elsevier Ltd on behalf of International Society for Infectious Diseases. This is an open access article under the CC BY-NC-ND license (http://creativecommons.org/licenses/by-nc-nd/4.0/).

1. Introduction

Since the divergence from a common ancestor with *Escherichia coli* more than 100 million years ago,[1] *Salmonella* have developed into more than 2600 serotypes that cause a variety of illnesses in humans and other animals. All *Salmonella* lineages are closely related, as revealed initially by DNA–DNA re-association assays[2] and then by physical mapping[3] and genomic sequencing.[4–9] Notwithstanding the observed genetic relatedness among the *Salmonella* lineages, they differ profoundly in host range and pathogenic features,[10,11] causing clinical consequences ranging from no obvious disease to mild gastroenteritis to potentially fatal systemic infections such as typhoid fever in humans. Therefore, the timely and accurate identification of *Salmonella* isolates is of great clinical significance.

Various typing methods, such as multilocus sequence typing (MLST), pulsed-field gel electrophoresis (PFGE), and phage typing, have been developed to discriminate these closely related bacteria,[12–16] of which serotyping has been the most widely used assay owing to its excellent discriminating power. However, serotyping has multiple disadvantages, such as low throughput, high expense, the need for expertise, and the requirement of a comprehensive set of antisera, which is not available to many institutions. Most importantly, however, is the fact that many *Salmonella* serotypes are polyphyletic, containing more than one phylogenetic (and pathogenic) lineage. As a result, alternative methods have been attempted for discriminating *Salmonella*, such as PFGE, ribotyping,[17] sequencing of H antigen genes (*fliC* and *fljB*),[18] and 16S–23S rRNA spacer restriction fragment length polymorphism (RFLP).[19] These methods may yield important information for epidemic analysis, but their discriminating ability is usually insufficient for accurate identification. MLST is an excellent method to discriminate strains based on their sequence

* Corresponding author. Tel.: +86 45186669150; fax: +86 45187502720.
E-mail address: sliu@ucalgary.ca (S.-L. Liu).

http://dx.doi.org/10.1016/j.ijid.2016.05.029
1201-9712/© 2016 The Author(s). Published by Elsevier Ltd on behalf of International Society for Infectious Diseases. This is an open access article under the CC BY-NC-ND license (http://creativecommons.org/licenses/by-nc-nd/4.0/).

1

NRC Research Press ARTICLE

Characterization of *Klebsiella* sp. strain S1: a bacterial producer of secoisolariciresinol through biotransformation

Yu-Jie Zhou, Songling Zhu, Dong-Hui Yang, Dan-Dan Zhao, Jia-Jing Li, and Shu-Lin Liu

Can. J. Microbiol. Downloaded from www.nrcresearchpress.com by UNIV CALGARY on 02/01/17
For personal use only.

Abstract: Secoisolariciresinol (SECO) is a lignan of potential therapeutic value for diseases such as cancer, but its use has been limited by the lack of ideal production methods, even though its precursors are abundant in plants, such as flaxseeds. Here, we report the characterization of a bacterial strain, S1, isolated from the human intestinal flora, which could produce secoisolariciresinol by biotransformation of precursors in defatted flaxseeds. This bacterium was a Gram-negative and facultatively anaerobic straight rod without capsules. Biochemical assays showed that it was negative for production of oxidase, lysine decarboxylase, ornithine decarboxylase, arginine dihydrolase, and β-glucolase. The G + C content of genomic DNA was 57.37 mol%. Phylogenetic analysis by 16S rRNA and *rpoB* gene sequences demonstrated S1's close relatedness to *Klebsiella*. No homologues were found for *wzb* or *wzc* (capsular genes), which may explain why *Klebsiella* sp. strain S1 does not have the capsule and was isolated from a healthy human individual. Based on the percentages of homologous genes with identical nucleotide sequences between the bacteria in comparison, we found that clear-cut genetic boundaries had been formed between S1 and any other *Klebsiella* strains compared, dividing them into distinct phylogenetic lineages. This work demonstrates that the intestinal *Klebsiella*, well known as important opportunistic pathogens prevalent in potentially fatal nosocomial infections, may contain lineages that are particularly beneficial to the human health.

Key words: *Klebsiella*, secoisolariciresinol, biotransformation, flaxseed, lignan.

Résumé : Le sécoisolaricirésinol (SECO) est un lignane doté d'une valeur thérapeutique potentielle dans le traitement de pathologies comme le cancer, mais son usage a été limité par un manque de méthodes de production optimales, malgré l'abondance de ses précurseurs chez les plantes comme le lin. Dans la présente, nous relatons la caractérisation d'une souche bactérienne, S1, isolée de la microflore intestinale humaine, capable de produire du sécoïsolaricirésinol par la biotransformation de précurseurs présents dans des graines de lin déshuilées. Cette bactérie était de coloration Gram négative, en forme de bâtonnet rectiligne, anaérobie facultative et non capsulée. Des analyses biochimiques ont relevé l'absence d'oxydase, de lysine décarboxylase, d'ornithine décarboxylase, d'arginine dihydrolase et de β-glucolase. La teneur en G + C de l'ADN génomique était de 57,37 mol%. Une analyse phylogénétique des séquences de l'ARNr 16S et du gène *rpoB* a mis en évidence une proche parenté avec *Klebsiella*. On n'a repéré aucun homologue des gènes capsulaires *wzb* et *wzc*, ce qui expliquerait l'absence de capsule chez *Klebsiella* S1 et l'isolation de cette dernière chez des sujets humains sains. D'après la proportion de gènes homologues à la séquence nucléotidique identique entre les bactéries comparées, nous avons constaté la formation d'une nette démarcation génétique entre S1 et toutes les autres souches de *Klebsiella* comparées, ce qui les a divisées en lignées phylogénétiques distinctes. Ce travail démontre que les klebsiellas intestinales, réputés pathogènes opportunistes de premier plan et prévalents lors d'infections nosocomiales potentiellement mortelles, peuvent renfermer des lignées particulièrement bénéfiques à la santé humaine. [Traduit par la Rédaction]

Mots-clés : *Klebsiella*, sécoïsolaricirésinol, biotransformation, graines de lin, lignane.

Received 22 April 2016. Revision received 25 June 2016. Accepted 27 June 2016.

Y.-J. Zhou, S. Zhu, D.-D. Zhao, and J.-J. Li. Systemomics Center, College of Pharmacy, and Genomics Research Center (State–Province Key Laboratories of Biomedicine–Pharmaceutics of China), Harbin Medical University, Harbin, People's Republic of China; HMU–UCFM Centre for Infection and Genomics, Harbin Medical University, Harbin, People's Republic of China.
D.-H. Yang. Department of Natural Medicines, School of Pharmaceutical Sciences, Peking University Health Science Center, Beijing, People's Republic of China.
S.-L. Liu. Systemomics Center, College of Pharmacy, and Genomics Research Center (State–Province Key Laboratories of Biomedicine–Pharmaceutics of China), Harbin Medical University, Harbin, People's Republic of China; HMU–UCFM Centre for Infection and Genomics, Harbin Medical University, Harbin, People's Republic of China; Department of Microbiology, Immunology and Infectious Diseases, University of Calgary, Calgary, Canada.
Corresponding author: Shu-Lin Liu (email: slliu@hrbmu.edu.cn).
Copyright remains with the author(s) or their institution(s). Permission for reuse (free in most cases) can be obtained from RightsLink.

www.nature.com/scientificreports

SCIENTIFIC REPORTS

OPEN

Received: 12 October 2016
Accepted: 23 January 2017
Published: 06 March 2017

Conserved intergenic sequences revealed by CTAG-profiling in *Salmonella*: thermodynamic modeling for function prediction

Le Tang[1,2,3,*], Songling Zhu[1,2,*], Emilio Mastriani[1,2,*], Xin Fang[1,2], Yu-Jie Zhou[1,2], Yong-Guo Li[4], Randal N. Johnston[5], Zheng Guo[6], Gui-Rong Liu[1,2] & Shu-Lin Liu[1,2,4,7]

Highly conserved short sequences help identify functional genomic regions and facilitate genomic annotation. We used *Salmonella* as the model to search the genome for evolutionarily conserved regions and focused on the tetranucleotide sequence CTAG for its potentially important functions. In *Salmonella*, CTAG is highly conserved across the lineages and large numbers of CTAG-containing short sequences fall in intergenic regions, strongly indicating their biological importance. Computer modeling demonstrated stable stem-loop structures in some of the CTAG-containing intergenic regions, and substitution of a nucleotide of the CTAG sequence would radically rearrange the free energy and disrupt the structure. The postulated degeneration of CTAG takes distinct patterns among *Salmonella* lineages and provides novel information about genomic divergence and evolution of these bacterial pathogens. Comparison of the vertically and horizontally transmitted genomic segments showed different CTAG distribution landscapes, with the genome amelioration process to remove CTAG taking place inward from both terminals of the horizontally acquired segment.

Bacterial genomes may contain highly conserved short sequences that are lineage-specific, such as the tetranucleotide sequence CTAG in *Escherichia coli* and *Salmonella*[1,2]. Genomic regions containing such conserved short sequences carry information about the evolution and phylogenetic divergence of the bacteria, but so far such information, especially that embedded in the intergenic regions, has not been efficiently extracted, due largely to the lack of theoretical or methodological strategies to reveal such conserved sequences. As a result, intergenic regions of the bacterial genomes have been poorly annotated in contrast to genes, which researchers often compare with those of *E. coli*[3] for annotation, taking the advantage that functions of many of the *E. coli* genes have been validated by molecular biology experiments. Such a situation calls for novel approaches to facilitate genomic annotation, and characterization of conserved short sequences may prove instrumental in the identification of functional intergenic sequences.

For this purpose, we have focused on the identification and characterization of short sequences in the bacterial genome, using representative *Salmonella* lineages as the models. Previously, we reported that the CTAG-containing endonuclease cleavage sites such as that of XbaI (TCTAGA) are highly conserved[4,5]. In a recent study, we found that many of such cleavage sites are located in common intergenic regions across *Salmonella* and *E. coli*[1]. This finding strongly suggests the potential importance of such sequences and brings up the hopes that the identification and functional analyses of such genomic regions may facilitate bacterial genome annotation and functional studies. We anticipate that the highly conserved intergenic regions may be involved in gene expression

[1]Systemomics Center, College of Pharmacy, and Genomics Research Center (State-Province Key Laboratories of Biomedicine-Pharmaceutics of China), Harbin Medical University, Harbin, China. [2]HMU-UCFM Centre for Infection and Genomics, Harbin Medical University, Harbin, China. [3]Department of Ecosystems and Public Health, University of Calgary, Calgary, Canada. [4]Department of Infectious Diseases of First Affiliated Hospital, Harbin Medical University, Harbin, China. [5]Department of Biochemistry and Molecular Biology, University of Calgary, Calgary, Canada. [6]College of Bioinformatics Science and Technology, Harbin Medical University, Harbin, China. [7]Department of Microbiology, Immunology and Infectious Diseases, University of Calgary, Calgary, Canada. [*]These authors contributed equally to this work. Correspondence and requests for materials should be addressed to G.-R.L. (email: grliu.natsumi@gmail.com) or S.-L.L. (email: slliu@hrbmu.edu.cn)

www.impactjournals.com/oncotarget/ Oncotarget, Advance Publications 2017

Cancer killers in the human gut microbiota: diverse phylogeny and broad spectra

Yu-Jie Zhou[1,2], Dan-Dan Zhao[1,2], Huidi Liu[1,2], Hao-Ting Chen[1,2], Jia-Jing Li[1,2], Xiao-Qin Mu[1,2], Zheng Liu[3], Xia Li[1,2], Le Tang[1,2,6], Zhan-Yi Zhao[1,2], Ji-Heng Wu[1,2], Yu-Xuan Cai[1,2], Ya-Zhuo Huang[1,2], Peng-Ge Wang[1,2], Yi-Yue Jia[1,2], Pei-Qiang Liang[1,2], Xue Peng[1,2], Si-Yu Chen[1,2], Zhi-Lin Yue[1,2], Xin-Yuan Yuan[1,2,7], Tammy Lu[1,2,8], Bing-Qing Yao[1,2], Yong-Guo Li[4], Gui-Rong Liu[1,2], Shu-Lin Liu[1,2,4,5]

[1]Systemomics Center, College of Pharmacy, and Genomics Research Center (State-Province Key Laboratories of Biomedicine-Pharmaceutics of China), Harbin Medical University, Harbin, China

[2]HMU-UCFM Centre for Infection and Genomics, Harbin Medical University, Harbin, China

[3]Colorectal Surgery Department, Cancer Hospital, Chinese Academy of Medical Sciences & Peking Union Medical College, Beijing, China

[4]Department of Infectious Diseases, The First Affiliated Hospital, Harbin Medical University, Harbin, China

[5]Department of Microbiology, Immunology and Infectious Diseases, University of Calgary, Calgary, Canada

[6]Current affiliation: Department of Ecosystems and Public Health, University of Calgary, Calgary, Canada

[7]Current affiliation: Bachelor of Science (Honour), Life Sciences, Queen's University, Kingston, Canada

[8]Current affiliation: Bachelor of Health Sciences, Biomedical Science, University of Calgary, Calgary, Canada

Correspondence to: *Shu-Lin Liu,* **email:** *slliu@hrbmu.edu.cn*

Keywords: *cancer, malignancy killer, Actinobacteria, gut microbiota, leukemia*

Received: December 12, 2016 **Accepted:** April 02, 2017 **Published:** April 21, 2017

ABSTRACT

Cancer as a large group of complex diseases is believed to result from the interactions of numerous genetic and environmental factors but may develop in people without any known genetic or environmental risks, suggesting the existence of other powerful factors to influence the carcinogenesis process. Much attention has been focused recently on particular members of the intestinal microbiota for their potential roles in promoting carcinogenesis. Here we report the identification and characterization of intestinal bacteria that exhibited potent anti-malignancy activities on a broad range of solid cancers and leukemia. We collected fecal specimens from healthy individuals of different age groups (preschool children and university students), inspected their effects on cancer cells, and obtained bacteria with potent anti-malignancy activities. The bacteria mostly belonged to Actinobacteria but also included lineages of other phyla such as Proteobacteria and Firmicutes. In animal cancer models, sterile culture supernatant from the bacteria highly effectively inhibited tumor growth. Remarkably, intra-tumor administration of the bacterial products prevented metastasis and even cleared cancer cells at remote locations from the tumor site. This work demonstrates the prevalent existence of potent malignancy-killers in the human intestinal microbiota, which may routinely clear malignant cells from the body before they form cancers.

INTRODUCTION

Cancer includes a large group of malignancies that are believed to occur as a combined consequence of genetic and environmental factors, since many genetic traits have been demonstrated to suppress or promote carcinogenesis as cancer suppressors or oncogenes, and environmental factors may help prevent or promote cancers [1–3]. But individuals born to a family that has high genetic risks to cancers do not necessarily develop cancers in their lifetime. Conversely,

Liu et al. Journal of Ovarian Research (2017) 10:49
DOI 10.1186/s13048-017-0346-z

Journal of Ovarian Research

RESEARCH Open Access

Enterolactone has stronger effects than enterodiol on ovarian cancer

Huidi Liu[1,2,3], Jianrui Liu[1,5], Siwen Wang[1,2], Zheng Zeng[1,2], Ting Li[1,2], Yongfang Liu[1,2], Emilio Mastriani[1,2], Qing-Hai Li[1,2], Hong-Xia Bao[1,2], Yu-Jie Zhou[1,2], Xiaoyu Wang[1,2], Sijing Hu[1,2], Shan Gao[1,2], Yingying Qi[1,2], Zhihang Shen[1,2], Hongyue Wang[1,2], Miao Yu[1,2], Tingting Gao[1,2], Randal N. Johnston[3] and Shu-Lin Liu[1,2,4*]

Abstract

Background: Ovarian cancer is one of the three leading gynecological malignancies, characterized by insidious growth, highly frequent metastasis, and quick development of drug resistance. As a result, this disease has low 5-year survival rates. Estrogen receptor inhibitors were commonly used for the treatment, but only 7% to 18% of patients respond to anti-estrogen therapies. Therefore, more effective therapies to inhibit estrogen-related tumors are urgently needed. Recently, phytoestrogens, such as lignans with estrogen-like biological activities, have attracted attention for their potential effects in the prevention or treatment of estrogen-related diseases. Enterodiol (END) and enterolactone (ENL) are mammalian lignans, which can reduce the risk of various cancers. However, the effects of END and ENL on ovarian cancer are not adequately documented.

Methods: We used in vitro assays on the ES-2 cell line to evaluate the inhibiting effects of END and ENL on ovarian cancer cell proliferation, invasion and migration ability and in vivo xenograft experiments on nude mice to validate the anticancer effects of END and ENL.

Results: The in vitro assays demonstrated that high-dose END and ENL could obviously inhibit ovarian malignant properties, including cancerous proliferation, invasion, and metastasis. Compared to END, ENL behaved in a better time-dose dependent manner on the cancer cells. The in vivo experiments showed that END (1 mg/kg), ENL (1 mg/kg) and ENL (0.1 mg/kg) suppressed tumor markedly, and there were statistically significant differences between the experimental and control groups in tumor weight and volume. Compared to END, which have serious side effects to the animals at high concentration such as 1 mg/kg, ENL had higher anticancer activities and less side effects in the animals than END at the same concentrations, so it would be a better candidate for drug development.

Conclusion: END and ENL both have potent inhibitory effects on ovarian cancer but ENL possesses a more effective anti-cancer capability and less side effects than END. Findings in this work provide novel insights into ovarian cancer therapeutics with phytoestrogens and encourage their clinical applications.

Keywords: Ovarian cancer, Enterodiol, Enterolactone, Anti-cancer

* Correspondence: sliu@hrbmu.edu.cn; slliu@ucalgary.ca
[1]Systemomics Center, College of Pharmacy, and Genomics Research Center (State-Province Key Laboratories of Biomedicine-Pharmaceutics of China), Harbin Medical University, Harbin 150081, China
[2]HMU-UCFM Centre for Infection and Genomics, Harbin, China
Full list of author information is available at the end of the article

BioMed Central

© The Author(s). 2017 **Open Access** This article is distributed under the terms of the Creative Commons Attribution 4.0 International License (http://creativecommons.org/licenses/by/4.0/), which permits unrestricted use, distribution, and reproduction in any medium, provided you give appropriate credit to the original author(s) and the source, provide a link to the Creative Commons license, and indicate if changes were made. The Creative Commons Public Domain Dedication waiver (http://creativecommons.org/publicdomain/zero/1.0/) applies to the data made available in this article, unless otherwise stated.

www.nature.com/scientificreports

SCIENTIFIC REPORTS

OPEN

Received: 11 May 2017
Accepted: 21 August 2017
Published online: 08 September 2017

Differential degeneration of the ACTAGT sequence among *Salmonella*: a reflection of distinct nucleotide amelioration patterns during bacterial divergence

Le Tang[1,2,3], Emilio Mastriani[1,2], Yu-Jie Zhou[1,2,4], Songling Zhu[1,2], Xin Fang[1,2], Yang-Peng Liu[1,2], Wei-Qiao Liu[5,9,10], Yong-Guo Li[6], Randal N. Johnston[7], Zheng Guo[8], Gui-Rong Liu[1,2] & Shu-Lin Liu[1,2,4,5,6]

When bacteria diverge, they need to adapt to the new environments, such as new hosts or different tissues of the same host, by accumulating beneficial genomic variations, but a general scenario is unknown due to the lack of appropriate methods. Here we profiled the ACTAGT sequence and its degenerated forms (i.e., hexa-nucleotide sequences with one of the six nucleotides different from ACTAGT) in *Salmonella* to estimate the nucleotide amelioration processes of bacterial genomes. ACTAGT was mostly located in coding sequences but was also found in several intergenic regions, with its degenerated forms widely scattered throughout the bacterial genomes. We speculated that the distribution of ACTAGT and its degenerated forms might be lineage-specific as a consequence of different selection pressures imposed on ACTAGT at different genomic locations (in genes or intergenic regions) among different *Salmonella* lineages. To validate this speculation, we modelled the secondary structures of the ACTAGT-containing sequences conserved across *Salmonella* and many other enteric bacteria. Compared to ACTAGT at conserved regions, the degenerated forms were distributed throughout the bacterial genomes, with the degeneration patterns being highly similar among bacteria of the same phylogenetic lineage but radically different across different lineages. This finding demonstrates biased amelioration under distinct selection pressures among the bacteria and provides insights into genomic evolution during bacterial divergence.

Bacteria constantly accumulate genomic changes to become increasingly better fit to the changing environment, such as in acquiring new capabilities to exploit nature for available resources, including laterally transferred DNA (LTD, e.g., prophages, genomic islands, etc.) and nucleotide variations (NVs, e.g., base substitutions, short insertion or deletions, etc.). The acquisition of LTD is mostly acute, occasionally bringing in beneficial

[1]Systemomics Center, College of Pharmacy, and Genomics Research Center (State-Province Key Laboratories of Biomedicine-Pharmaceutics of China), Harbin Medical University, Harbin, China. [2]HMU-UCFM Centre for Infection and Genomics, Harbin Medical University, Harbin, China. [3]Department of Ecosystems and Public Health, University of Calgary, Calgary, Canada. [4]Translational Medicine Research and Cooperation Center of Northern China, Heilongjiang Academy of Medical Sciences, Harbin, China. [5]Department of Microbiology, Immunology and Infectious Diseases, University of Calgary, Calgary, Canada. [6]Department of Infectious Diseases of First Affiliated Hospital, Harbin Medical University, Harbin, China. [7]Department of Biochemistry and Molecular Biology, University of Calgary, Calgary, Canada. [8]College of Bioinformatics Science and Technology, Harbin Medical University, Harbin, China. [9]Present address: Division of Neurology, Department of Medicine, University of British Columbia, Vancouver, Canada. [10]Present address: Department of Clinical Neurosciences, University of Calgary, Calgary, Canada. Le Tang, Emilio Mastriani and Yu-Jie Zhou contributed equally to this work. Correspondence and requests for materials should be addressed to Z.G. (email: guoz@ems.hrbmu.edu.cn) or G.-R.L. (email: grliu@hrbmu.edu.cn) or S.-L.L. (email: slliu@hrbmu.edu.cn)

CANCER BIOLOGY & THERAPY
2017, VOL. 18, NO. 12, 990–999
https://doi.org/10.1080/15384047.2017.1394542

Taylor & Francis
Taylor & Francis Group

RESEARCH PAPER

Check for updates

Main components of pomegranate, ellagic acid and luteolin, inhibit metastasis of ovarian cancer by down-regulating MMP2 and MMP9

Huidi Liu[a,b,d,&], Zheng Zeng[a,b,&], Siwen Wang[a,b], Ting Li[a,b], Emilio Mastriani[a,b], Qing-Hai Li[a,b], Hong-Xia Bao[a,b], Yu-Jie Zhou[a,b], Xiaoyu Wang[a,b], Yongfang Liu[a,b], Wei Liu[a,b], Sijing Hu[a,b], Shan Gao[a,b], Miao Yu[a,b], Yingying Qi[a,b], Zhihang Shen[a,b], Hongyue Wang[a,b], Tingting Gao[a,b], Lingqin Dong[a,b], Randal N. Johnston[d], and Shu-Lin Liu[a,b,c]

[a]Systemomics Center, College of Pharmacy, and Genomics Research Center (State-Province Key Laboratories of Biomedicine-Pharmaceutics of China), Harbin Medical University, Harbin, Heilongjiang Province, China; [b]HMU-UCFM Centre for Infection and Genomics, Harbin Medical University, Harbin, Heilongjiang Province, China; [c]Department of Microbiology, Immunology and Infectious Diseases, University of Calgary, Calgary, Alberta, Canada; [d]Department of Biochemistry and Molecular Biology, University of Calgary, Calgary, Alberta, Canada

Downloaded by [Haerbin Medical University] at 14:39 04 December 2017

ABSTRACT
Ovarian cancer is the third most common cancer in the female reproductive organs and epithelial ovarian cancer has the highest lethality of all gynecological cancers. Pomegranate fruit juice (PFJ) has been shown to inhibit the growth of several types of cancer other than ovarian cancer. In this study, we exposed the ovarian cancer cell line A2780 to PFJ and two of its components (ellagic acid and luteolin). MTT and wound healing assays demonstrated that all three treatments suppressed the proliferation and migration of the ovarian cancer cells. In addition, western blotting and ELISA assays showed that the expression levels of MMP2 and MMP9 gradually decreased after treatment with increasing concentrations of ellagic acid and luteolin. To confirm our findings in the *in vitro* experiments, we used another ovarian cancer cell line, ES-2, in nude mice experiments. All three treatments inhibited tumor growth without obvious side-effects. Furthermore, compared with the control group, the expression levels of MMP2 and MMP9 were depressed. Ellagic acid induced a greater effect than luteolin, suggesting that ellagic acid might be a promising candidate for further preclinical testing for treatment of human ovarian cancer.

ARTICLE HISTORY
Received 16 June 2017
Revised 21 September 2017
Accepted 15 October 2017

KEYWORDS
ellagic acid; luteolin; pomegranate fruit juice; ovarian cancer; MMP2; MMP9

Abbreviations: DMSO, dimethyl sulfoxide; ELISA, enzyme-linked immunosorbent assay; EA, ellagic acid; HRP, horse-radish peroxidase; HE staining, hematoxylin-eosin staining; L, luteolin; MMPs, matrix metalloproteinases; MTT3-(4,5-Dimethylthiazol-2-yl)-2,5-diphenyltetrazolium bromide, 3-(4,5-Dimethylthiazol-2-yl)-2,5-diphenyltetrazolium bromide; PFJ, pomegranate fruit juice; PBS, phosphate buffered saline

Introduction

Ovarian cancer, one of the three major malignant tumors in women, has high incidence and mortality. It is hard to diagnose until very late stages and the five-year survival rate is highly unfavorable,[1] due especially to its distant metastasis. The Cancer Statistics 2016 estimated 22,280 new cases of ovarian cancer with 14,240 deaths for year 2016 in the United States.[2] If ovarian cancer is diagnosed early and appropriate surgeries and interventional therapies are provided, 90% of patients will survive for more than five years. However, with advanced and metastasized ovarian cancer, less than 30% of the patients may survive for five years.[3] Although death rate of ovarian cancer was higher in North America and Europe than in Asia and Africa, the difference is narrowing.[4] While the specific etiology of ovarian cancer is still unclear, it might be related to age, fertility, blood type, and mental and environment factors.[5–7] Chemotherapy is currently the most common treatment to inhibit ovarian cancer, but long-term use could result in tumor recurrence and further progression, frequently leading to chemotherapeutic resistance.[8,9] In order to consolidate curative effect, immune therapy and traditional Chinese medicine therapy have been adopted by some authors.[10,11] Paclitaxel, a natural antitumor agent, is in the standard front-line treatment and has significant effects on advanced malignancies including ovarian cancer.[12] Substances like paclitaxel are good examples of how natural compounds may be used to treat cancers, inspiring the discovery of safe and effective approaches in ovarian cancer prevention and therapy.

Matrix metalloproteinases (MMPs) are a family of Ca^{2+}-dependent Zn^{2+}-containing endopetidases, which are capable of degrading extracellular matrix proteins to promote cancer cell migration, invasion and metastasis.[13] Among the more than 20 members of MMPs, MMP2 and MMP9 are correlated with the aggressiveness of cancer.[14] MMPs are regulated by hormones, growth factors, and cytokines, which are all involved in ovarian cancer.[15–17] Thus, MMPs have been considered as significant targets for ovarian cancer therapy.

Pomegranate has been used as medicine in many cultures throughout history but is usually consumed as fresh fruit or commercial fruit juice. It possesses many pharmacological

CONTACT Shu-Lin Liu sliu@hrbmu.edu.cn

© 2017 Taylor & Francis Group, LLC

Future
MICROBIOLOGY

Research Article

For reprint orders, please contact: reprints@futuremedicine.com

Genetic diversity and evolutionary features of type VI secretion systems in *Salmonella*

Hongxia Bao[†,1,2,3], Jian-Hua Zhao[†,1,2,3], Songling Zhu[1,2,3], Shuang Wang[4], Jianjuan Zhang[1,2,3], Xiao-Yu Wang[1,2,3], Bing Hua[1,2,3], Chang Liu[1,2,3], Huidi Liu[1,2,3] & Shu-Lin Liu[*,1,2,3,5]

[1]Systemomics Center, College of Pharmacy & Genomics Research Center, Harbin Medical University, Harbin, PR China
[2]HMU-UCCSM Centre for Infection & Genomics, Harbin Medical University, Harbin, PR China
[3]Translational Medicine Research & Cooperation Center of Northern China, Heilongjiang Academy of Medical Sciences, Harbin, PR China
[4]Department of Biopharmaceutical Sciences, College of Pharmacy, Harbin Medical University, Harbin, PR China
[5]Department of Microbiology, Immunology & Infectious Diseases, University of Calgary, Calgary, T2N 1N4, Canada
*Author for correspondence: slliu@hrbmu.edu.cn
[†]Authors contributed equally

Aim: Type VI secretion systems (T6SS) play key roles in bacterial pathogenesis, but their evolutionary features remain largely unclear. In this study, we conducted systematic comparisons among the documented T6SSs in *Salmonella* and determined their structural diversity, phylogenetic distribution and lineage-specific properties. **Materials & methods:** We screened 295 *Salmonella* genomes for 13 T6SS core components by hidden Markov models and identified 363 T6SS clusters covering types i1, i2, i3 and i4a. **Results:** Type i3 and i4a T6SSs were restricted to *Salmonella enterica* subspecies *enterica* and *Salmonella bongori*, respectively. whereas type i2 T6SSs were conserved between *S. enterica* subspecies, *arizonae* and *diarizonae*. *S. enterica* subspecies *salamae*, *indica* and *houtenae* harbored only type i1 T6SSs, which had wide distribution and high sequence diversity. **Conclusion:** The diverse *Salmonella* T6SSs have undergone purifying selection pressures during the bacterial evolution and may be involved in host adaptation.

First draft submitted: 19 September 2018; Accepted for publication: 30 November 2018; Published online: 18 January 2019

Keywords: genomic evolution • *Salmonella* • type VI secretion system

The secretion of effector proteins into the host cells is a crucial step in bacterial virulence and pathogenesis. Type VI secretion system (T6SS) is one of the most recently recognized cytotoxic organelles to deliver effector proteins, which has been discovered in more than 25% of Gram-negative bacteria known to date [1], including *Vibrio cholerae*, *Pseudomonas aeruginosa*, *Escherichia coli*, *Salmonella* and *Burkholderia mallei* [2–5]. However, the molecular diversity and evolutionary features of the T6SSs among the bacteria have not been fully investigated.

Structurally similar to an inverted bacteriophage tail, the T6SSs deliver effector proteins to prokaryotic or eukaryotic target cells for the adherence, cytotoxicity, host cell invasion and intramacrophage survival of the bacteria [6,7]. Typically, T6SSs consist of 15–25 proteins, which are commonly encoded in clusters and interact extensively with one another [8]. The T6SS core components comprise 13 proteins [1], including structural proteins, such as VgrG and Hcp, forming respective phage tail, spike-like protein and ring-shaped needle structure and secreted effectors. TssE, a T4 phage gp25-like protein, constructs the baseplate [9]. TssL, TssM and TssJ together form a transenvelope complex that connects the T6SS tube and sheath to the membrane [10], Tssk forms a stable complex with TssF and TssG [11,12] and the ClpV complex energizes the system to induce disassembly of VipA/VipB (tssB/tssC) tubules through binding specifically to the N-terminal helix of TssC [13].

Salmonella are a large group of Gram-negative enteropathogenic bacteria and the leading cause of bacterial enteric illnesses in both humans and animals. This genus consists of two species, *Salmonella enterica*, which is further divided into six subspecies: *S. enterica* subsp. *enterica* (I), *S. enterica* subsp. *salamae* (II), *S. enterica* subsp. *arizonae* (IIIa), *S. enterica* subsp. *diarizonae* (IIIb), *S. enterica* subsp. *houtenae* (IV) and *S. enterica* subsp. *indica* (VI) and *Salmonella bongori* [14]. Previously *S. enterica* subspecies VII was described [15] but later was proven

Future Medicine

Molecular Genetics and Genomics
https://doi.org/10.1007/s00438-019-01531-5

ORIGINAL ARTICLE

Distinct evolutionary origins of common multi-drug resistance phenotypes in *Salmonella typhimurium* DT104: a convergent process for adaptation under stress

Le Tang[1,2,6] · Song-Ling Zhu[1,2] · Xin Fang[1,2] · Yong-Guo Li[3] · Cornelis Poppe[4] · Randal N. Johnston[5] · Gui-Rong Liu[1,2] · Shu-Lin Liu[1,2,3,7]

Received: 22 June 2018 / Accepted: 11 January 2019
© Springer-Verlag GmbH Germany, part of Springer Nature 2019

Abstract
Antimicrobial resistance makes pathogenic bacteria hard to control, but little is known about the general processes of resistance gain or loss. Here, we compared distinct *S. typhimurium* DT104 strains resistant to zero, two, five, or more of the tested antimicrobials. We found that common resistance phenotypes could be encoded by distinct genes, on SGI-1 or plasmid. We also demonstrated close clonality among all the tested non-resistant and differently resistant DT104 strains, demonstrating dynamic acquisition or loss (by total deletion or gradual decaying of multi-drug resistance gene clusters) of the genetic traits. These findings reflect convergent processes to make the bacteria resistant to multiple antimicrobials by acquiring the needed traits from stochastically available origins. When the antimicrobial stress is absent, the resistance genes may be dropped off quickly, so the bacteria can save the cost for maintaining unneeded genes. Therefore, this work reiterates the importance of strictly controlled use of antimicrobials.

Keywords *Salmonella typhimurium* · DT104 · Antimicrobial resistance · SGI-1 · P972816 · Convergent process · Pathogenic evolution

Introduction

Pathogenic bacteria may develop resistance to antimicrobials, often devastating the treatment of infectious diseases. Little is known about the dynamic process of resistance gain or loss by the bacteria, especially about the evolutionary origins of the resistance traits: the resistance genes seem to be ubiquitous in the environment and available when bacteria need them. For example, although most *Salmonella typhi* isolates do not have drug resistance plasmids (Liu and Sanderson 1995, 1996; Kothapalli et al. 2005), some strains may acquire them (Parkhill et al. 2001). Different bacteria may have distinct sets of genes to encode resistance to the same antimicrobials, but the same bacteria usually have common genetic basis for the same resistance phenotypes. A well-known case is *Salmonella typhimurium* phage-type DT104, a relatively new pathogenic branch of *S. typhimurium*, isolates of which often exhibit multi-drug resistance to five or more antimicrobials, including ampicillin, chloramphenicol, streptomycin, sulfonamides tetracycline, etc., encoded by SGI-1, a 43 kb genomic island (Threlfall et al. 1994; Boyd et al. 2001;

✉ Gui-Rong Liu
grliu@hrbmu.edu.cn

✉ Shu-Lin Liu
slliu@hrbmu.edu.cn

1 Systemomics Center, College of Pharmacy, and Genomics Research Center, Harbin Medical University, 157 Baojian Road, Harbin 150081, China

2 HMU-UCCSM Centre for Infection and Genomics, Harbin Medical University, Harbin, China

3 Department of Infectious Diseases of First Affiliated Hospital, Harbin Medical University, Harbin, China

4 Laboratory for Foodborne Zoonoses, Public Health Agency of Canada, Guelph, ON, Canada

5 Department of Biochemistry and Molecular Biology, University of Calgary, Calgary, Canada

6 Department of Ecosystems and Public Health, University of Calgary, Calgary, Canada

7 Microbiology, Immunology and Infectious Diseases, University of Calgary, Calgary, Canada

Published online: 01 February 2019

frontiers
in Cellular and Infection Microbiology

ORIGINAL RESEARCH
published: 18 April 2019
doi: 10.3389/fcimb.2019.00112

Dysbiosis of the Gut Microbiome in Lung Cancer

He Zhuang[1,2,3†], Liang Cheng[1,4†], Yao Wang[1,2,3], Yu-Kun Zhang[1,2,3,5], Man-Fei Zhao[1,2,3,6], Gong-Da Liang[1,2,3,6], Meng-Chun Zhang[1,2,3], Yong-Guo Li[7], Jing-Bo Zhao[6], Yi-Na Gao[8*], Yu-Jie Zhou[1,2,3*‡] and Shu-Lin Liu[1,2,3,6,9*]

[1] Systemomics Center, College of Pharmacy, and Genomics Research Center (State-Province Key Laboratories of Biomedicine-Pharmaceutics of China), Harbin Medical University, Harbin, China, [2] HMU-UCCSM Centre for Infection and Genomics, Harbin Medical University, Harbin, China, [3] Translational Medicine Research and Cooperation Center of Northern China, Heilongjiang Academy of Medical Sciences, Harbin, China, [4] College of Bioinformatics Science and Technology, Harbin Medical University, Harbin, China, [5] Department of Colorectal Cancer, The 2nd Affiliated Hospital of Harbin Medical University, Harbin, China, [6] Department of Epidemiology, Public Health School, Harbin Medical University, Harbin, China, [7] Department of Infectious Diseases, The First Affiliated Hospital, Harbin Medical University, Harbin, China, [8] Department of Respiration, The Third Affiliated Hospital of Harbin Medical University, Harbin, China, [9] Department of Microbiology, Immunology and Infectious Diseases, University of Calgary, Calgary, AB, Canada

OPEN ACCESS

Edited by:
Yongqun He,
University of Michigan Health System,
United States

Reviewed by:
Nagendra Singh,
Medical College of Georgia, Augusta
University, United States
César López-Camarillo,
Universidad Autónoma de la Ciudad
de México, Mexico

***Correspondence:**
Shu-Lin Liu
slliu@hrbmu.edu.cn
Yu-Jie Zhou
yjzhou@ccmu.edu.cn
Yi-Na Gao
gaoyina_HMU@163.com

† These authors have contributed equally to this work

‡ Present Address:
Yu-Jie Zhou,
Department of Immunology, Capital
Medical University, Beijing, China

Specialty section:
This article was submitted to
Microbiome in Health and Disease,
a section of the journal
Frontiers in Cellular and Infection
Microbiology

Received: 20 December 2018
Accepted: 01 April 2019
Published: 18 April 2019

Citation:
Zhuang H, Cheng L, Wang Y,
Zhang Y-K, Zhao M-F, Liang G-D,
Zhang M-C, Li Y-G, Zhao J-B,
Gao Y-N, Zhou Y-J and Liu S-L (2019)
Dysbiosis of the Gut Microbiome in
Lung Cancer.
Front. Cell. Infect. Microbiol. 9:112.
doi: 10.3389/fcimb.2019.00112

Lung cancer (LC) is one of the most serious malignant tumors, which has the fastest growing morbidity and mortality worldwide. A role of the lung microbiota in LC pathogenesis has been analyzed, but a comparable role of the gut microbiota has not yet been investigated. In this study, the gut microbiota of 30 LC patients and 30 healthy controls were examined via next-generation sequencing of 16S rRNA and analyzed for diversity and biomarkers. We found that there was no decrease in significant microbial diversity (alpha diversity) in LC patients compared to controls (P observed = 0.1422), while the composition (beta diversity) differed significantly between patients and controls (phylum [stress = 0.153], class [stress = 0.16], order [stress = 0.146], family [stress = 0.153]). Controls had a higher abundance of the bacterial phylum *Actinobacteria* and genus *Bifidobacterium*, while patients with LC showed elevated levels of *Enterococcus*. These bacteria were found as possible biomarkers for LC. A decline of normal function of the gut microbiome in LC patients was also observed. These results provide the basic guidance for a systematic, multilayered assessment of the role of the gut microbiome in LC, which has a promising potential for early prevention and targeted intervention.

Keywords: lung cancer, gut microbiota, next generation sequencing, 16S rRNA, microbial diversity, biomarkers

INTRODUCTION

Lung cancer (LC) is one of the deadliest malignancies, which has growing morbidity and mortality worldwide. It poses an enormous threat to the human health (Torre et al., 2015). Research on LC genetics and biology has opened opportunities for novel therapeutic strategies against the disease (Allison, 2015; Chowdhury et al., 2018; Hendriks and Besse, 2018; Herbst et al., 2018; Lissanu Deribe et al., 2018; Wei et al., 2018), but the knowledge about the etiology remains incomplete, making precision treatment or prevention a moving target. To date, the major etiological causes or risk factors facilitating the pathogenesis of cancers have been mostly focused on genetic

Rakov *et al. BMC Genomics* (2019) 20:429
https://doi.org/10.1186/s12864-019-5809-8

BMC Genomics

RESEARCH ARTICLE Open Access

Association of *Salmonella* virulence factor alleles with intestinal and invasive serovars

Alexey V. Rakov[1,5], Emilio Mastriani[2,3], Shu-Lin Liu[2,3,4] and Dieter M. Schifferli[1*]

Abstract

Background: The role of *Salmonella* virulence factor (VF) allelic variation in modulating pathogenesis or host specificity has only been demonstrated in a few cases, mostly through serendipitous findings. Virulence factor (VF) alleles from *Salmonella enterica* subsp. *enterica* genomes were compared to identify potential associations with the host-adapted invasive serovars Typhi, Dublin, Choleraesuis, and Gallinarum, and with the broad host-range intestinal serovars Typhimurium, Enteritidis, and Newport.

Results: Through a bioinformatics analysis of 500 *Salmonella* genomes, we have identified allelic variants of 70 VFs, many of which are associated with either one of the four host-adapted invasive *Salmonella* serovars or one of the three broad host-range intestinal serovars. In addition, associations between specific VF alleles and intra-serovar clusters, sequence types (STs) and/or host-adapted FimH adhesins were identified. Moreover, new allelic VF associations with non-typhoidal *S.* Enteritidis and *S.* Typhimurium (NTS) or invasive NTS (iNTS) were detected.

Conclusions: By analogy to the previously shown association of specific FimH adhesin alleles with optimal binding by host adapted *Salmonella* serovars, lineages or strains, we predict that some of the identified association of other VF alleles with host-adapted serovars, lineages or strains will reflect specific contributions to host adaptation and/or pathogenesis. The identification of these allelic associations will support investigations of the biological impact of VF alleles and better characterize the role of allelic variation in *Salmonella* pathogenesis. Most relevant functional experiments will test the potential causal contribution of the detected FimH-associated VF variants in host adapted virulence.

Keywords: *Salmonella enterica*, virulence factors, allelic variation, host adaptation, FimH, STs, iNTS

Background

In recent years, it has been shown that adaptation of pathogen to certain niches is accompanied by genome degradation [1]. One of the models used for this observation is *Salmonella enterica*, a versatile Gram-negative *Enterobacteriaceae*, that includes over 2,500 different serovars and accounts for a vast number of human and animal infections [2, 3]. *S. enterica* strains causing human disease are divided into human-restricted typhoidal serovars (Typhi and Paratyphi) and nontyphoidal (NTS) serovars (e.g. Enteritidis, Typhimurium, Newport and most others *S. enterica* serovars). The latter serovars are designated generalists, since they also infect a broad-range of mammals and birds, causing gastroenteritis and/or persistent infections with potential for long-term shedding. Animals have also more invasive serovars capable of extra-intestinal spread responsible for septicemia, such as *S.* Gallinarum, which is restricted to poultry and many wild birds [4], and *S.* Dublin and *S.* Choleraesuis, that are mostly adapted to cattle and pigs, respectively, with rarer human or other mammalian infections. Some *Salmonella* serovars can cause invasive NTS infections (iNTS) by septicemic spread [5], and are often not associated with diarrhea. In the last decade, such strains were isolated mostly from Africa, frequently in malaria or HIV-infected patients. Genomic studies have shown that they are mainly caused by specific lineages of *S.* Typhimurium [6] and *S.* Enteritidis [7].

From an evolutionary point of view, the most parsimonious explanation for the host-restricted serovar is that they emerged from an ancestor with a broad host range [8]. The *Salmonella* adaptation process to a reduced number of hosts and a more efficient escape from the microbial competitive intestinal milieu by invading

* Correspondence: dmschiff@vet.upenn.edu
[1]Department of Pathobiology, School of Veterinary Medicine, University of Pennsylvania, Philadelphia, Pennsylvania, USA
Full list of author information is available at the end of the article

BMC

© The Author(s). 2019 **Open Access** This article is distributed under the terms of the Creative Commons Attribution 4.0 International License (http://creativecommons.org/licenses/by/4.0/), which permits unrestricted use, distribution, and reproduction in any medium, provided you give appropriate credit to the original author(s) and the source, provide a link to the Creative Commons license, and indicate if changes were made. The Creative Commons Public Domain Dedication waiver (http://creativecommons.org/publicdomain/zero/1.0/) applies to the data made available in this article, unless otherwise stated.

Wang *et al. BMC Genomics* (2019) 20:930
https://doi.org/10.1186/s12864-019-6259-z

BMC Genomics

RESEARCH ARTICLE Open Access

Genetic boundaries delineate the potential human pathogen *Salmonella bongori* into discrete lineages: divergence and speciation

Xiaoyu Wang[1,2,3], Songling Zhu[1,2,3], Jian-Hua Zhao[1,2,3], Hong-Xia Bao[1,2,3], Huidi Liu[1,2,3], Tie-Min Ding[4], Gui-Rong Liu[1,2,3], Yong-Guo Li[5], Randal N. Johnston[6], Feng-Lin Cao[1,7*], Le Tang[1,2,3,8*] and Shu-Lin Liu[1,2,3,5,9*]

Abstract

Background: *Salmonella bongori* infect mainly cold-blooded hosts, but infections by *S. bongori* in warm-blooded hosts have been reported. We hypothesized that *S. bongori* might have diverged into distinct phylogenetic lineages, with some being able to infect warm-blooded hosts.

Results: To inspect the divergence status of *S. bongori*, we first completely sequenced the parakeet isolate RKS3044 and compared it with other sequenced *S. bongori* strains. We found that RKS3044 contained a novel T6SS encoded in a pathogenicity island-like structure, in addition to a T6SS encoded in SPI-22, which is common to all *S. bongori* strains so far reported. This novel T6SS resembled the SPI-19 T6SS of the warm-blooded host infecting *Salmonella* Subgroup I lineages. Genomic sequence comparisons revealed different genomic sequence amelioration events among the *S. bongori* strains, including a unique CTAG tetranucleotide degeneration pattern in RKS3044, suggesting non-overlapping gene pools between RKS3044 and other *S. bongori* lineages/strains leading to their independent accumulation of genomic variations. We further proved the existence of a clear-cut genetic boundary between RKS3044 and the other *S. bongori* lineages/strains analyzed in this study.

Conclusions: The warm-blooded host-infecting *S. bongori* strain RKS3044 has diverged with distinct genomic features from other *S. bongori* strains, including a novel T6SS encoded in a previously not reported pathogenicity island-like structure and a unique genomic sequence degeneration pattern. These findings alert cautions about the emergence of new pathogens originating from non-pathogenic ancestors by acquiring specific pathogenic traits.

Keywords: *Salmonella*, Bacterial pathogens, Genomic divergence, Genetic boundary

Background

Salmonella bacteria are ubiquitous pathogens, with over 2600 serotypes documented to date [1]. Based on different levels of relatedness, the *Salmonella* bacteria are categorized into eight subgroups, e.g., Subgroups I, II, IIIa, IIIb, IV, V, VI and VII [2, 3]. Human salmonellosis is primarily caused by *Salmonella* Subgroup I lineages but may occasionally be elicited also by bacteria of the other subgroups, which usually infect cold-blooded hosts [4]. Bacteria of Subgroup V (also known as *Salmonella bongori*; see the dynamic changes of *Salmonella* taxonomy and nomenclature in previous publications [5, 6]) lineages are among the least likely human salmonellosis agents, partly due to their lack of *Salmonella* Pathogenicity Island 2, which is required for the bacteria to survive in phagocytes and invade the deep tissues of the host [7, 8]. However, *S. bongori* infections do occur in humans or other warm-blooded hosts [9–11], opening a question about whether certain *S. bongori* lineages with special genetic traits might have facilitated such infections. A first step toward answering this question is the

* Correspondence: sliu@hrbmu.edu.cn; le.tang@ucalgary.ca; CFL023@163.com
[1]Systemomics Center, College of Pharmacy, and Genomics Research Center (State-Province Key Laboratories of Biomedicine-Pharmaceutics of China), Harbin Medical University, 157 Baojian Road, Harbin 150081, China
Full list of author information is available at the end of the article

BMC

© The Author(s). 2019 **Open Access** This article is distributed under the terms of the Creative Commons Attribution 4.0 International License (http://creativecommons.org/licenses/by/4.0/), which permits unrestricted use, distribution, and reproduction in any medium, provided you give appropriate credit to the original author(s) and the source, provide a link to the Creative Commons license, and indicate if changes were made. The Creative Commons Public Domain Dedication waiver (http://creativecommons.org/publicdomain/zero/1.0/) applies to the data made available in this article, unless otherwise stated.

frontiers
in Oncology

ORIGINAL RESEARCH
published: 30 January 2020
doi: 10.3389/fonc.2019.01570

Overexpression of IGF2BP3 as a Potential Oncogene in Ovarian Clear Cell Carcinoma

Huidi Liu[1,2,3,4,5†], *Zheng Zeng*[1,2,3†], *Mitra Afsharpad*[6], *Caiji Lin*[1,2,3], *Siwen Wang*[1,2,3], *Hao Yang*[7], *Shuhong Liu*[6], *Linda E. Kelemen*[8], *Wenwen Xu*[1,2,3], *Wenqing Ma*[1,2,3], *Qian Xiang*[1,2,3], *Emilio Mastriani*[1,2,3], *Pengfei Wang*[1,2,3], *Jiali Wang*[1,2,3], *Shu-Lin Liu*[1,2,3,9*], *Randal N. Johnston*[4,5*] and *Martin Köbel*[5,6*]

[1] Genomics Research Center (State-Province Key Laboratories of Biomedicine-Pharmaceutics of China), College of Pharmacy, Harbin Medical University, Harbin, China, [2] HMU-UCCSM Centre for Infection and Genomics, Harbin, China, [3] Translational Medicine Research and Cooperation Center of Northern China, Heilongjiang Academy of Medical Sciences, Harbin, China, [4] Department of Biochemistry and Molecular Biology, University of Calgary, Calgary, AB, Canada, [5] Arnie Charbonneau Cancer Institute, University of Calgary, Calgary, AB, Canada, [6] Pathology and Laboratory Medicine, Calgary Laboratory Service, University of Calgary, Calgary, AB, Canada, [7] Department of Pathology, Harbin Chest Hospital, Harbin, China, [8] Hollings Cancer Center and Department of Public Health Sciences, Medical University of South Carolina, Charleston, SC, United States, [9] Department of Microbiology, Immunology and Infectious Diseases, University of Calgary, Calgary, AB, Canada

OPEN ACCESS

Edited by:
San-Gang Wu,
First Affiliated Hospital of Xiamen University, China

Reviewed by:
Jianbo Yang,
University of Minnesota Twin Cities, United States
Luis Schwarz,
Auna Oncosalud, Peru
Sophia H. L. George,
University of Miami, United States

***Correspondence:**
Shu-Lin Liu
sliu@hrbmu.edu.cn
Randal N. Johnston
mjohnst@ucalgary.ca
Martin Köbel
mkoebel@ucalgary.ca

† These authors have contributed equally to this work

Specialty section:
This article was submitted to Women's Cancer, a section of the journal Frontiers in Oncology

Received: *13 July 2019*
Accepted: *27 December 2019*
Published: *30 January 2020*

Citation:
Liu H, Zeng Z, Afsharpad M, Lin C, Wang S, Yang H, Liu S, Kelemen LE, Xu W, Ma W, Xiang Q, Mastriani E, Wang P, Wang J, Liu S-L, Johnston RN and Köbel M (2020) Overexpression of IGF2BP3 as a Potential Oncogene in Ovarian Clear Cell Carcinoma. Front. Oncol. 9:1570. doi: 10.3389/fonc.2019.01570

Ovarian Clear Cell Carcinoma (OCCC) displays distinctive clinical and molecular characteristics and confers the worst prognosis among all ovarian carcinoma histotypes when diagnosed at advanced stage, because of the lack of effective therapy. IGF2BP3 is an RNA binding protein that modulates gene expression by post-transcriptional action. In this study, we investigated the roles of IGF2BP3 in the progression of OCCC. We used 328 OCCCs from the AOVT (the Alberta Ovarian Tumor Type study) and the COEUR (the Canadian Ovarian Experimental Unified Resource) cohorts to elucidate the associations between IGF2BP3 expression and clinicopathological parameters, with positive IGF2BP3 expression defined as diffuse block staining, being more frequently observed at stage III ($P = 0.0056$) and significantly associated with unfavorable overall survival (HR = 1.59, 95% CI 1.09–2.33) in multivariate analysis. *IGF2BP3* mRNA gene expression was markedly increased in OCCC cell lines compared to normal tissues such as ovarian surface epithelium. We chose two IGF2BP3-overexpressing cell lines ES2 and OVMANA for *in vitro* and *in vivo* knockdown experiments. The proliferation and viability of both cell lines were significantly inhibited by two IGF2BP3 siRNAs and similar suppression was observed in cell migration and invasion by Wound Healing and Transwell assays. The percentage of apoptotic cancer cells was enhanced by both IGF2BP3 siRNAs. *In vivo* experiments showed significantly reduced sizes of tumors when treated with IGF2BP3 siRNA compared to controls. Furthermore, cancer metastasis-indicators MMP2 and MMP9 proteins were down-regulated. In conclusion, our study shows that IGF2BP3 expression is a promising biomarker for prognostication of women diagnosed with OCCC with multiple effects on key cell functions, supporting its role as an important cellular regulator with potential oncogenic activity, and as a potential target for future intervention strategies.

Keywords: ovarian cancer, clear cell carcinoma, IGF2BP3, IMP3, prognosis, metastasis, MMPs

Tang *et al. BMC Medical Genomics* (2020) 13:59
https://doi.org/10.1186/s12920-020-0704-3

BMC Medical Genomics

RESEARCH ARTICLE Open Access

E. coli diversity: low in colorectal cancer

Le Tang[1,2,3†], Yu-Jie Zhou[1,2,4†], Songling Zhu[1,2], Gong-Da Liang[1,2,5], He Zhuang[1,2], Man-Fei Zhao[1,2,5], Xiao-Yun Chang[1,2], Hai-Ning Li[1,2], Zheng Liu[6,7], Zhi-Rong Guo[8], Wei-Qiao Liu[9,10], Xiaoyan He[8], Chun-Xiao Wang[1,2], Dan-Dan Zhao[1,2], Jia-Jing Li[1,2], Xiao-Qin Mu[1,2,11], Bing-Qing Yao[1,2], Xia Li[1,2,11], Yong-Guo Li[12], Li-Bo Duo[13], Li Wang[13], Randal N. Johnston[14], Jin Zhou[15], Jing-Bo Zhao[5], Gui-Rong Liu[1,2*] and Shu-Lin Liu[1,2,8,9,11,12*]

Abstract

Background: *Escherichia coli* are mostly commensals but also contain pathogenic lineages. It is largely unclear whether the commensal *E. coli* as the potential origins of pathogenic lineages may consist of monophyletic or polyphyletic populations, elucidation of which is expected to lead to novel insights into the associations of *E. coli* diversity with human health and diseases.

Methods: Using genomic sequencing and pulsed field gel electrophoresis (PFGE) techniques, we analyzed *E. coli* from the intestinal microbiota of three groups of healthy individuals, including preschool children, university students, and seniors of a longevity village, as well as colorectal cancer (CRC) patients, to probe the commensal *E. coli* populations for their diversity.

Results: We delineated the 2280 fresh *E. coli* isolates from 185 subjects into distinct genome types (genotypes) by PFGE. The genomic diversity of the sampled *E. coli* populations was so high that a given subject may have multiple genotypes of *E. coli*, with the general diversity within a host going up from preschool children through university students to seniors. Compared to the healthy subjects, the CRC patients had the lowest diversity level among their *E. coli* isolates. Notably, *E. coli* isolates from CRC patients could suppress the growth of *E. coli* bacteria isolated from healthy controls under nutrient-limited culture conditions.

Conclusions: The coexistence of multiple *E. coli* lineages in a host may help create and maintain a microbial environment that is beneficial to the host. As such, the low diversity of *E. coli* bacteria may be associated with unhealthy microenvironment in the intestine and hence facilitate the pathogenesis of diseases such as CRC.

Keywords: *Escherichia coli*, Genetic diversity, Intestinal microbiota, Colorectal cancer, Longevity

Background

Escherichia coli had been generally known as commensal bacterial components of the normal microbiota in the gastrointestinal tract of humans and animals until the 1940s, when a variety of pathogenic strains began to be reported [1]. Pathogenic *E. coli* have different types, causing intestinal (see a nice review in [2]) or extra-intestinal infections [3–6]. New pathogenic types of *E. coli*, such as *E. coli* strains associated with Crohn disease [7–9] as well as those associated with colorectal cancer (CRC) [10–17], have continually been reported. Bacteria in the *Shigella* genus are closely related to *E. coli* and have been treated as pathogenic branches of *E. coli* [18, 19]; *E. coli* and *Shigella* together are often referred to as *E. coli* complex bacteria. To date, a large number of pathogenic *E. coli* isolates have been extensively studied and categorized into phylogenetic groups or clonal complexes according to their genetic differences due largely to their clinical significance [20–23]. However, whether

* Correspondence: grliu@hrbmu.edu.cn; slliu@hrbmu.edu.cn
†Le Tang and Yu-Jie Zhou contributed equally to this work.
[1]Systemomics Center, College of Pharmacy, and Genomics Research Center (State-Province Key Laboratories of Biomedicine-Pharmaceutics of China), Harbin Medical University, 157 Baojian Road, Harbin 150081, China
Full list of author information is available at the end of the article

BMC

© The Author(s). 2020 **Open Access** This article is licensed under a Creative Commons Attribution 4.0 International License, which permits use, sharing, adaptation, distribution and reproduction in any medium or format, as long as you give appropriate credit to the original author(s) and the source, provide a link to the Creative Commons licence, and indicate if changes were made. The images or other third party material in this article are included in the article's Creative Commons licence, unless indicated otherwise in a credit line to the material. If material is not included in the article's Creative Commons licence and your intended use is not permitted by statutory regulation or exceeds the permitted use, you will need to obtain permission directly from the copyright holder. To view a copy of this licence, visit http://creativecommons.org/licenses/by/4.0/. The Creative Commons Public Domain Dedication waiver (http://creativecommons.org/publicdomain/zero/1.0/) applies to the data made available in this article, unless otherwise stated in a credit line to the data.

Phytomedicine 76 (2020) 153267

Contents lists available at ScienceDirect

Phytomedicine

journal homepage: www.elsevier.com/locate/phymed

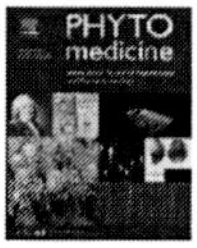

Suppressive activities of mangiferin on human epithelial ovarian cancer

Zheng Zeng[a,b,d], Caiji Lin[a,b,c], Siwen Wang[a,b,c], Pengfei Wang[a,b,c], Wenwen Xu[a,b,c], Wenqing Ma[a,b,c], Jiali Wang[a,b,c], Qian Xiang[a,b,c], Yiting Liu[a,b,c], Jiaming Yang[a,b,c], Fan Ye[a,b,c], Kaihong Xie[a,b,c], Jian Xu[a,b,c], Yao Luo[a,b,c], Shu-Lin Liu[a,b,c,e,*], Huidi Liu[a,b,c,d,*]

[a] Genomics Research Center (State-Province Key Laboratories of Biomedicine-Pharmaceutics of China), College of Pharmacy, Harbin Medical University, No. 157, Baojian Road, Harbin, China
[b] HMU-UCCSM Centre for Infection and Genomics, Harbin, 150081, China
[c] Translational Medicine Research and Cooperation Center of Northern China, Heilongjiang Academy of Medical Sciences, Heilongjiang, China
[d] Department of Biochemistry and Molecular Biology, University of Calgary, Calgary, T2N 4N1, Canada
[e] Department of Microbiology, Immunology and Infectious Diseases, University of Calgary, Calgary, T2N 4N1, Canada

ARTICLE INFO

Keywords:
Epithelial ovarian cancer
Mangiferin
Metastasis
MMP2
MMP9

ABSTRACT

Background: Epithelial carcinoma is a subtype of ovarian cancers, with the highest lethality among all ovarian cancer subtypes. Hitherto surgical excision combined with chemotherapy has been the most extensively employed method in clinical treatment. However, the disease relapses very frequently, calling for more effective therapies. Mangiferin, a natural xanthone glucoside, has displayed promising anti-cancer activities by *in vitro* studies, but its therapeutic value in epithelial ovarian cancer treatment, either by *in vivo* or *in vitro* studies, remained to be known.

Purpose: This study aimed to determine the suppressive activities of mangiferin on human epithelial ovarian cancer and elucidate the underlying molecular mechanisms.

Study design and methods: We employed the 3-(4,5-dimethylthiazol-2-yl)-2,5-diphenyltetrazolium bromide (MTT) assay and the crystal violet assay to determine the half maximal inhibitory concentration (IC_{50}) values of mangiferin with paclitaxel as a positive control and the inhibitory effects of mangiferin on the proliferation of two human epithelial ovarian cancer cell lines. Wound healing and Transwell assays were used to determine anti-metastastic activities of mangiferin. ES-2 xenograft nude mouse model was used for the *in vivo* experiments. Western blotting, enzyme-linked immunosorbent assay (ELISA) and immunohistochemistry (IHC) assays were carried out for evaluating the expression level of matrix metalloproteinase 2 (MMP2) and matrix metalloproteinase 9 (MMP9).

Results: In the present study, we demonstrated by both *in vitro* and *in vivo* assays that mangiferin suppressed the progress of epithelial ovarian cancer in a dose-dependent manner. In the animals treated with mangiferin, the tumor volume and weight were reduced significantly. Analyses of involved molecular events demonstrated that mangiferin down-regulated the expression of metastasis-associated proteins MMP2 and MMP9.

Conclusion: Mangiferin strongly inhibited the progression of human epithelial ovarian cancer by down-regulating MMP2 and MMP9.

Introduction

Ovarian carcinoma is among the three most common gynecological malignancies and is the deadliest (Collins et al., 2014). According to the American Cancer Society, there were 22,530 new cases of ovarian carcinoma and 13,980 disease-related deaths in 2019 (Siegel et al., 2019). Ovarian cancers could originate from epithelial, sex cord stromal or germ cells. Those of the epithelial origin take up 80%-90% of all ovarian cancers and comprise five main histotypes: high- and low-grade serous, mucinous, endometroid and clear cell carcinoma. The 5-year

Abbreviations: ANOVA, analysis of variance; DMSO, dimethyl sulfoxide; ELISA, enzyme-linked immunosorbent assay; FBS, fetal bovine serum; H&E staining, hematoxylin and eosin staining; HRP, horseradish peroxidase; IC_{50}, half maximal inhibitory concentration; IHC, immunohistochemistry; MA, mangiferin; MMPs, matrix metalloproteinases; MTT, 3-(4,5-dimethylthiazol-2-yl)-2,5-diphenyltetrazolium bromide; RIPA, radioimmunoprecipitation assay; PBS, phosphate buffered saline; PFA, paraformaldehyde; PVDF, polyvinylidene fluoride; SDS, sodium dodecyl sulfate

* Corresponding authors.
E-mail addresses: sliu@hrbmu.edu.cn (S.-L. Liu), hdliu@hrbmu.edu.cn (H. Liu).

https://doi.org/10.1016/j.phymed.2020.153267
Received 17 January 2020; Received in revised form 31 May 2020; Accepted 13 June 2020
0944-7113/ © 2020 The Authors. Published by Elsevier GmbH. This is an open access article under the CC BY-NC-ND license (http://creativecommons.org/licenses/BY-NC-ND/4.0/).

Microbiological Research 241 (2020) 126591

Contents lists available at ScienceDirect

Microbiological Research

journal homepage: www.elsevier.com/locate/micres

Salmonella secretion systems: Differential roles in pathogen-host interactions

Hongxia Bao[a,b,c,1,*], Shuang Wang[d,1], Jian-Hua Zhao[a,b,c], Shu-Lin Liu[a,b,c,e,*]

[a] *Genomics Research Center, College of Pharmacy, Harbin Medical University, Harbin, China*
[b] *HMU-UCCSM Centre for Infection and Genomics, Harbin Medical University, Harbin, China*
[c] *Translational Medicine Research and Cooperation Center of Northern China, Heilongjiang Academy of Medical Sciences, Harbin, China*
[d] *Department of Biopharmaceutical Sciences (State Province Key Laboratories of Biomedicine Pharmaceutics of China), College of Pharmacy, Harbin Medical University, Harbin, China*
[e] *Department of Microbiology, Immunology and Infectious Diseases, University of Calgary, Calgary, Canada*

A R T I C L E I N F O

Keywords:
Salmonella
Secretion system
Host-pathogen interaction

A B S T R A C T

The bacterial genus *Salmonella* includes a large group of food-borne pathogens that cause a variety of gastrointestinal or systemic diseases in hosts. *Salmonella* use several secretion devices to inject various effectors targeting eukaryotic hosts, or bacteria. In the past few years, considerable progress has been made towards understanding the structural features and molecular mechanisms of the secretion systems of *Salmonella*, particularly regarding their roles in host-pathogen interactions. In this review, we summarize the current advances about the main characteristics of the *Salmonella* secretion systems. Clarifying the roles of the secretion systems in the process of infecting various hosts will broaden our understanding of the importance of microbial interactions in maintaining human health and will provide information for developing novel therapeutic approaches.

1. Introduction

Salmonella are Gram-negative, facultative intracellular pathogens ordinarily 2–5 microns by 0.5–1.5 microns in average size (Andino and Hanning, 2015). The *Salmonella* genus consists of two species, *S. enterica* and *S. bongori*, the latter of which was formerly known, and is still often referred to, as *Salmonella* subspecies V (Grimont, 2007). *S. enterica* was subdivided into six subspecies (I, II, IIIa, IIIb, IV and VI) based on biochemical and genetic properties (Brenner et al., 2000). *Salmonella* as a genus contains over 2600 known serotypes distributed among the species/subspecies and certain serotypes of *S. enterica* subspecies I frequently cause food-borne diseases ranging from gastroenteritis to life-threatening systemic infections such as typhoid fever (Crump et al., 2004). Non-typhoidal *Salmonella* were estimated to cause 93.8 million cases of gastroenteritis and 155,000 deaths each year, while typhoid fever led to over 21 million illnesses and more than 200,000 deaths globally in only 2000 (Crump et al., 2004; Majowicz et al., 2010).

Innate immune response, involving phagocytic cells such as macrophages and dendritic cells (DCs), is the first line of defense against invading pathogens (Kumar et al., 2009). Host Toll-like receptors (TLRs) are a family of evolutionarily conserved receptors located on the plasma membrane and endosomal membranes of immune and non-immune cells, which could recognize pathogen-associated molecular patterns (PAMPs) including proteins, lipids and nucleic acids (Kumar et al., 2009; Uehara et al., 2005). The activated receptors will further trigger downstream signal transduction cascades and the antimicrobial effector gene transcription to counteract bacterial infections. Host phagocytes utilize acidification of phagosomes, generation of reactive oxygen (ROS) and reactive nitrogen species (RNS), and production of antimicrobial proteins and peptides to kill internalized pathogens (Winterbourn et al., 2006; Jha et al., 2017).

To accomplish the infection to the host, *Salmonella* requires to attach and adhere to the host cell surface first and subsequently release bacterial factors to facilitate their invasion, multiplication in host cells and overcome host antimicrobial defense (Fig. 1) (Wiedemann et al., 2014; Ilyas et al., 2017). Despite the presence of various antimicrobial mechanisms in the host, *Salmonella* have evolved multiple strategies to break these defense mechanisms (Flannagan et al., 2009). For example, the

* Corresponding authors at: Genomics Research Center, College of Pharmacy, Harbin Medical University, Harbin, China.
E-mail addresses: wulantuya2@163.com (H. Bao), slliu@hrbmu.edu.cn (S.-L. Liu).

[1] These authors contributed equally to this work.

https://doi.org/10.1016/j.micres.2020.126591
Received 8 June 2020; Received in revised form 24 August 2020; Accepted 29 August 2020
Available online 5 September 2020
0944-5013/© 2020 Elsevier GmbH. All rights reserved.

frontiers in Oncology

ORIGINAL RESEARCH
published: 21 October 2020
doi: 10.3389/fonc.2020.574552

Check for updates

Isobaric Tags for Relative and Absolute Quantitation in Proteomic Analysis of Potential Biomarkers in Invasive Cancer, Ductal Carcinoma *In Situ*, and Mammary Fibroadenoma

Hao Wu[1,2,3,4,5], *Xian-Yu Zhang*[1,5,6], *Ming Niu*[1,5,6], *Fei-Feng Li*[1,4,5], *Song Gao*[1,5,6], *Wei Wei*[1,5,6], *Si-Wei Li*[1,5,6], *Xing-Da Zhang*[1,5,6], *Shu-Lin Liu*[1,4,5,7]* and *Da Pang*[1,2,3,5,6]*

[1] Genomics Research Center, College of Pharmacy, State-Province Laboratory of Biomedicine and Pharmaceutics of China, Harbin Medical University, Harbin, China, [2] Sino-Russian Medical Research Center, Harbin Medical University Cancer Hospital, Harbin, China, [3] Heilongjiang Academy of Medical Sciences, Harbin Medical University, Harbin, China, [4] HMU-UCCSM Centre for Infection and Genomics, Harbin Medical University, Harbin, China, [5] Translational Medicine Research and Cooperation Center of Northern China, Heilongjiang Academy of Medical Sciences, Harbin, China, [6] Department of Breast Surgery, Harbin Medical University Cancer Hospital, Harbin, China, [7] Department of Microbiology, Immunology and Infectious Diseases, University of Calgary, Calgary, AB, Canada

OPEN ACCESS

Edited by:
Yi-Zhou Jiang,
Fudan University, China

Reviewed by:
Umberto Malapelle,
University of Naples Federico II, Italy
Svetlana Tamkovich,
Novosibirsk State University, Russia

***Correspondence:**
Shu-Lin Liu
sliu@hrbmu.edu.cn
Da Pang
pangda@ems.hrbmu.edu.cn

Specialty section:
This article was submitted to Women's Cancer, a section of the journal Frontiers in Oncology

Received: *20 June 2020*
Accepted: *23 September 2020*
Published: *21 October 2020*

Citation:
Wu H, Zhang X-Y, Niu M, Li F-F, Gao S, Wei W, Li S-W, Zhang X-D, Liu S-L and Pang D (2020) Isobaric Tags for Relative and Absolute Quantitation in Proteomic Analysis of Potential Biomarkers in Invasive Cancer, Ductal Carcinoma In Situ, and Mammary Fibroadenoma. Front. Oncol. 10:574552. doi: 10.3389/fonc.2020.574552

Objectives: Breast malignancy is a serious threat to women's health around the world. Following the rapid progress in the field of cancer diagnostics and identification of pathological markers, breast tumor treatment methods have been greatly improved. However, for invasive, ductal carcinomas and mammary fibroadenoma, there is an urgent demand for better breast tumor-linked biomarkers. The current study was designed to identify diagnostic and/or therapeutic protein biomarkers for breast tumors.

Methods: A total of 140 individuals were included, comprising 35 healthy women, 35 invasive breast cancers (IBC), 35 breast ductal carcinomas *in situ* (DCIS), and 35 breast fibroadenoma patients. *Isobaric tags for relative and absolute quantitation* (iTRAQ) proteomic analysis was employed to characterize differentially expressed proteins for potential biomarkers in IBC, DCIS, and fibroadenomas by comparisons with their matched adjacent tissues and/or normal breast tissues. The public databases Metascape and String were used for bioinformatic analyses.

Results: Using the proteomics approach, we identified differentially expressed proteins in tissues of different breast tumors compared to normal/adjacent breast tissues, including 100 in IBC, 52 in DCIS, and 44 in fibroadenoma. Among the 100 IBC differentially expressed proteins, 37 were found to be specific to this type of cancer only. Additionally, four proteins were specifically expressed in DCIS and four in fibroadenoma. Compared to corresponding adjacent tissues and normal breast tissues, 18 step-changing proteins were differentially expressed in IBC, 14 in DCIS, and 13 in fibroadenoma, respectively. Compared to DCIS and normal breast tissues, 65 proteins were differentially expressed in IBC with growing levels of malignancy.

INTERNATIONAL JOURNAL OF
SURGERY ONCOLOGY

Article

OPEN

Anticancer effects of dietary administration of secoisolariciresinol diglucoside in a patient of gastrointestinal stromal tumor: a case report

Hao Wu, MD, MS[a,b,c,d,e,f], Yao Wang, BS[a,d,e], Jia-Tao Chen, BS[a,d,e], Li-Ping Wang, MD[b,g], Gui-Rong Liu, BS[a,d,e], Shu-Lin Liu, MD, PhD[a,d,e,f,*]

Introduction: Gastrointestinal stromal tumor (GIST) is among the leading malignancies of the digestive system. GIST is not susceptible to chemotherapies and is prone to recurrence or metastasis after surgical operation. Secoisolariciresinol diglucoside (SDG) was suggested to have potential anticancer effects, but no clinical evidence had been available. Here we report successful treatment of a postoperative GIST case with dietary SDG.

Presentation of Case: The patient was a 58-year-old man. He had GIST and received resection of small intestinal lesions 1 year before. He was diagnosed with postoperation of GIST and presented with high level of serum carbohydrate antigen 72-4 (CA72-4). The patient was then treated with dietary administration of SDG with his voluntary acceptance for 5 months, and underwent 2 serum CA72-4 measurements during this period. CA72-4 level of the patient was restored to normal range after treatment with dietary SDG for 1 month. There was no aberrant CA72-4 level, recurrence or metastasis after the treatment with dietary SDG.

Discussion: This is to our knowledge the first report on application of dietary SDG on a postoperative GIST patient with aberrant level of serum CA72-4. SDG can be transformed into active substances with antitumor effects by human gut bacteria. Dietary SDG might inhibit tumorigenicity and malignant behavior of GIST cells.

Conclusion: The excellent effects suggest dietary SDG to be a potential therapy for GIST, especially against recurrence or metastasis.

Keywords: GIST, CA72-4, Dietary SDG, Recurrence, Metastasis, Case report

Key points

(1) Dietary secoisolariciresinol diglucoside (SDG) shows potent anticancer effect reflected by complete patient recovery.

(2) Carbohydrate antigen 72-4 (CA72-4) level becoming normal correlated very well with the recovery of the patient.

(3) SDG is easily edible and may be used widely for cancer prevention and treatment.

[a]Genomics Research Center (State-Province Key Laboratories of Biomedicine-Pharmaceutics of China), College of Pharmacy, Harbin Medical University, [b]Sino-Russian Medical Research Center, Harbin Medical University Cancer Hospital, [c]Heilongjiang Academy of Medical Sciences, [d]HMU-UCCSM Centre for Infection and Genomics, [e]Translational Medicine Research and Cooperation Center of Northern China, Heilongjiang Academy of Medical Sciences, Harbin, China, [f]Department of Microbiology, Immunology and Infectious Diseases, University of Calgary, Calgary, AB, Canada and [g]Kangyuan Hospital, 9 Tongfatoudao Street, Harbin, China

This manuscript has been peer reviewed.

Sponsorships or competing interests that may be relevant to content are disclosed at the end of this article.

*Corresponding author. Address: Genomics Research Center, Harbin Medical University, Harbin 150081, China. Tel: +8645186692236; fax: +8645187086735. E-mail address: sllu@hrbmu.edu.cn (S.-L. Liu).

Copyright © 2021 The Authors. Published by Wolters Kluwer Health, Inc. on behalf of IJS Publishing Group Ltd. This is an open access article distributed under the terms of the Creative Commons Attribution-Non Commercial-No Derivatives License 4.0 (CCBY-NC-ND), where it is permissible to download and share the work provided it is properly cited. The work cannot be changed in any way or used commercially without permission from the journal.

International Journal of Surgery Oncology (2021) 5:e103

Received 3 August 2020; Accepted 16 September 2020

Published online 20 January 2021

Supplemental Digital Content is available for this article. Direct URL citations appear in the printed text and are provided in the HTML and PDF versions of this article on the journal's website, www.IJSOncology.com.

http://dx.doi.org/10.1097/IJ9.0000000000000103

Introduction

Gastrointestinal stromal tumor (GIST) is one of the most common mesenchymal malignancies in the gastrointestinal tract, with no specific clinical manifestations to be used for diagnosis at early stages[1]. The incidence rate of GIST is ~0.001%–0.0015% but a trend of increase is obvious in recent years[2]. GIST is mostly seen in men over 50 years old, occurring in the stomach (60%–70%), the small intestine (25%–36%), colon (5%) or esophagus (5%)[3]. About 10%–30% of the GIST patients develop metastasis[4], most commonly in the liver (65%), followed by the peritoneum (21%), the bone (10%), and lung (10%)[5]. The treatment for GIST is quite challenging, as GIST is not susceptible to radiotherapy or chemotherapy. As a result, surgical resection is almost the only method left to treat the disease. However, over half of the patients would face recurrence or metastasis after the surgical operation[6]. Multiple genetic changes have been identified for their associations with GIST, including C-KIT mutations in 70%–80% and PDGFR-α mutations in 5%–10% of the examined cases. The downstream signaling pathways of C-KIT include PI3K/ART, Src family kinases, RAS-ERK, and JAK-STAT6[7].

Currently, tyrosine kinase inhibitors (TKIs) as routine targeted drugs[8], with Imatinib as a representative, are often used after GIST surgery. Imatinib can inhibit the activities of both C-KIT

Journal of Alzheimer's Disease xx (2021) x–xx
DOI 10.3233/JAD-210259
IOS Press

Altered Gut Microbiota in Adults with Subjective Cognitive Decline: The SILCODE Study

Can Sheng[a,*], Li Lin[a], Hua Lin[a], Xiaoni Wang[a,*], Ying Han[a,b,c,*] and Shu-Lin Liu[d,e,f,g]
[a]*Department of Neurology, Xuanwu Hospital of Capital Medical University, Beijing, China*
[b]*Biomedical Engineering Institute, Hainan University, Haikou, China*
[c]*Center of Alzheimer's Disease, Beijing Institute for Brain Disorders, Beijing, China*
[d]*Genomics Research Center (State-Province Key Laboratories of Biomedicine Pharmaceutics of China), College of Pharmacy, Harbin Medical University, Harbin, China*
[e]*HMU-UCCSM Centre for Infection and Genomics, Harbin, China*
[f]*Translational Medicine Research and Cooperation Center of Northern China, Heilongjiang Academy of Medical Sciences, Harbin, China*
[g]*Department of Microbiology, Immunology and Infectious Diseases, University of Calgary, Calgary, AB, Canada*

Uncorrected Author Proof

Accepted 21 April 2021

Abstract.
Background: Subjective cognitive decline (SCD) is the earliest symptomatic manifestation of preclinical Alzheimer's disease (AD). Gut microbiota may serve as a susceptibility factor for AD. Altered gut microbiota has been reported in patients with mild cognitive impairment (MCI) and AD dementia. However, whether gut microbial compositions changed in SCD remains largely unknown.
Objective: To characterize the gut microbiota in SCD.
Methods: In this study, a total of 105 participants including 38 normal controls (NC), 53 individuals with SCD, and 14 patients with cognitive impairment (CI) were recruited. Gut microbiota of all participants isolated from fecal samples were investigated using 16S ribosomal RNA (rRNA) Illumina Miseq sequencing technique. The gut microbial compositions were compared among the three groups, and the association between altered gut microbiota and cognitive performance was analyzed. To validate the alteration of gut microbiota in SCD, we conducted amyloid positron emission tomography (PET) in selected participants and further compared the gut microbiota among subgroups.
Results: The abundance of phylum *Firmicutes*, class *Clostridia*, order *Clostridiales*, family *Ruminococcaceae*, and genus *Faecalibacterium* showed a trend toward a progressive decline from NC to SCD and CI. Specifically, the abundance of the anti-inflammatory genus *Faecalibacterium* was significantly decreased in SCD compared with NC. In addition, altered bacterial taxa among the three groups were associated with cognitive performance. The findings were validated in SCD participants with positive amyloid evidence.
Conclusion: The composition of gut microbiota is altered in individuals with SCD. This preliminary study will provide novel insights into the pathophysiological mechanism of AD.

Keywords: Alzheimer's disease, gut microbiota, 16S ribosomal RNA, subjective cognitive decline

*Correspondence to: Ying Han, MD, PhD, Department of Neurology, Xuanwu Hospital of Capital Medical University, Beijing 100053, China. Tel.: +86 18515692701; Fax: +86 10 83167306; E-mail: hanying@xwh.ccmu.edu.cn. and Xiaoni Wang, PhD, Department of Neurology, Xuanwu Hospital of Capital Medical University, Beijing 100053, China. Tel.: +86 15010546586; E-mail: wxnanna@163.com. and Can Sheng, PhD, Department of Neurology, Xuanwu Hospital of Capital Medical University, Beijing 100053, China. Tel.: +86 18701257298; E-mail: canyeweiwu2013@163.com.

ISSN 1387-2877/$35.00 © 2020 – IOS Press and the authors. All rights reserved

frontiers in Pharmacology

ORIGINAL RESEARCH
published: 05 November 2021
doi: 10.3389/fphar.2021.706220

OPEN ACCESS

Edited by:
Cecilia Veronica Nunez,
National Institute of Amazonian Research (INPA), Brazil

Reviewed by:
Sahil Sharma,
Sloan Kettering Institute, United States
Patricia Sartorelli,
Federal University of São Paulo, Brazil
Massuo Jorge Kato,
University of São Paulo, Brazil

***Correspondence:**
Chang Li
lichang661@126.com
Yue-Hu Pei
Peiyh@163.vip.com
Shu-Lin Liu
slliu@hrbmu.edu.cn

†Present address:
Yu-Jie Zhou,
Advanced Innovation Center for Human Brain Protection, Beijing Key Laboratory for Cancer Invasion and Metastasis, Department of Immunology, School of Basic Medical Sciences, Department of Oncology, Capital Medical University, Beijing, China

‡These authors have contributed equally to this work

Specialty section:
This article was submitted to Pharmacology of Anti-Cancer Drugs, a section of the journal Frontiers in Pharmacology

Received: *27 May 2021*
Accepted: *29 September 2021*
Published: *05 November 2021*

Citation:
Wang Q, Wang Y, Wang Y-J Ma N, Zhou Y-J Zhuang H, Zhang X-H Li C, Pei Y-H and Liu S-L (2021) Dissection of the Functional Mechanism of Human Gut Bacterial Strain AD16 by Secondary Metabolites' Identification, Network Pharmacology, and Experimental Validation. Front. Pharmacol. 12:706220. doi: 10.3389/fphar.2021.706220

Dissection of the Functional Mechanism of Human Gut Bacterial Strain AD16 by Secondary Metabolites' Identification, Network Pharmacology, and Experimental Validation

***Qin Wang*[1‡], *Yao Wang*[2‡], *Ya-Jing Wang*[1], *Nan Ma*[1], *Yu-Jie Zhou*[2†], *He Zhuang*[2], *Xing-Hua Zhang*[2], *Chang Li*[1*], *Yue-Hu Pei*[1*] and *Shu-Lin Liu*[2,3*]**

[1]*Department of Medicinal Chemistry and Natural Medicine Chemistry, College of Pharmacy, Harbin Medical University, Harbin, China,* [2]*Genomics Research Center (State-Province Key Laboratories of Biomedicine-Pharmaceutics of China), College of Pharmacy, Harbin Medical University, Harbin, China,* [3]*Department of Microbiology, Immunology and Infectious Diseases, University of Calgary, Calgary, AB, Canada*

Gut microbiota plays important roles in several metabolic processes, such as appetite and food intake and absorption of nutrients from the gut. It is also of great importance in the maintenance of the health of the host. However, much remains unknown about the functional mechanisms of human gut microbiota itself. Here, we report the identification of one anticancer gut bacterial strain AD16, which exhibited potent suppressive effects on a broad range of solid and blood malignancies. The secondary metabolites of the strain were isolated and characterized by a bioactivity-guided isolation strategy. Five new compounds, streptonaphthalenes A and B (1-2), pestalolficins F and G (3-4), and eudesmanetetraiol A (5), together with nine previously known compounds, were isolated from the effective fractions of AD16. Structures of the new compounds were established by 1D and 2D NMR and MS analysis, and the absolute configurations were determined by the CD method. The analysis of network pharmacology suggested that 3, 2, and 13 could be the key components for the anti-NSCLC activity of AD16. In addition to the PI3K–Akt signaling pathway, the proteoglycans in cancer pathway could be involved in the anti-NSCLC action of AD16.

Keywords: gut bacterial, secondary metabolites, network pharmacology, anticancer, AD16

INTRODUCTION

The human gut microbiota is composed of an enormous diversity of microorganisms, including bacteria, fungi, and other microbes, which together play important roles in maintaining the dynamic homeostatic and healthy micro-environment of the host (Johnson et al., 2016; Thomas et al., 2017; Liang et al., 2018). In recent years, numerous discoveries have been reported on the human gut bacteria affecting human health and diseases, such as cardiovascular diseases, inflammatory diseases, obesity, and especially cancer (Hasan et al., 2020; Moritz et al., 2020). There has been mounting evidence supporting the roles of the gut bacteria in response to cancer (Johnson et al., 2016; Li et al.,

References

Bao, H.X., Tang, L., Yu, L., Wang, X.Y., Li, Y,, Deng, X., Li, Y.G., Li, A., Zhu, D.L., Johnston, R.N., Liu, G.R., Feng, Y., and Liu, S.L. 2014. Differential efficiency in exogenous DNA acquisition among closely related *Salmonella* strains: implications in bacterial speciation. BMC Microbiol 14: 157.

Beltran, P., Plock, S.A., Smith, N.H., Whittam, T.S., Old, D.C., and Selander, R.K. 1991. Reference collection of strains of the *Salmonella typhimurium* complex from natural populations. J Gen Microbiol 137: 601-606.

Bennett, A.F., Lenski, R.E. 2007. An experimental test of evolutionary trade-offs during temperature adaptation. Proc Natl Acad Sci USA 104 Suppl 1: 8649-8654.

Berlyn, M.K.B., Low, K.B., and Rudd, K.E. 1996. Linkage Map of *Excherichia coli* K-12, edition 9. In: Neidhardt FC, editor. *Escherichia coli* and *Salmonella*. Washington, D.C.: ASM Press. p. 1715-1902.

Bhagwat, A.S., McClelland, M. 1992. DNA mismatch correction by Very Short Patch repair may have altered the abundance of oligonucleotides in the *E. coli* genome. Nucleic Acids Res 20: 1663-1668.

Boyd, E.F., Wang, F.S., Beltran, P., Plock, S.A., Nelson, K., and Selander, R.K. 1993. *Salmonella* reference collection B (SARB): strains of 37 serovars of subspecies I. J Gen Microbiol 139 (Pt 6): 1125-1132.

Brenner, D.J., McWhorter, A.C., Knutson, J.K., and Steigerwalt, A.G. 1982. *Escherichia vulneris*: a new species of *Enterobacteriaceae* associated with human wounds. J Clin Microbiol 15: 1133-1140.

Chen, F., Liu, W.Q., Eisenstark, A., Johnston, R.N., Liu, G.R., and Liu, S.L. 2010a. Multiple genetic switches spontaneously modulating bacterial mutability. BMC Evol Biol 10: 277.

Chen, F., Liu, W.Q., Liu, Z.H., Zou, Q.H., Wang, Y., Li, Y.G., Zhou, J., Eisenstark, A., Johnston, R.N., Liu, G.R., Yang, B.F., and Liu, S.L. 2010b. *mutL* as a genetic switch of bacterial mutability: turned on or off through repeat copy number changes. FEMS Microbiol Lett 312: 126-132.

Chevance, F.F., and Hughes, K.T. 2008. Coordinating assembly of a bacterial macromolecular machine. Nat Rev Microbiol 6: 455-465.

Chiu, C.H., Tang, P., Chu, C., Hu, S., Bao, Q., Yu, J., Chou, Y.Y., Wang, H.S., and Lee, Y.S. 2005. The genome sequence of *Salmonella enterica* serovar Choleraesuis, a highly invasive and resistant zoonotic pathogen. Nucleic Acids Res 33: 1690-1698.

Clegg, S., Hughes, K.T. 2002. FimZ is a molecular link between sticking and swimming in *Salmonella enterica* serovar Typhimurium. J Bacteriol 184: 1209-1213.

Cohan, F.M. 2002. What are bacterial species? Annu Rev Microbiol 56: 457-487.

Cooke, F.J., Brown, D.J., Fookes, M., Pickard, D., Ivens, A., Wain, J., Roberts, M., Kingsley, R.A,, Thomson, N.R., and Dougan, G. 2008. Characterization of the genomes of a diverse collection of *Salmonella enterica* serovar Typhimurium definitive phage type 104. J Bacteriol 190: 8155-8162.

Crosa, J.H., Brenner, D.J., Ewing, W.H., and Falkow, S. 1973. Molecular relationships among the Salmonelleae. J Bacteriol 115: 307-315.

DeLong, E.F., and Pace, N.R. 2001. Environmental diversity of bacteria and archaea. Syst Biol 50: 470-478.

Deng, W., Liou, S.R., Plunkett, G., 3rd, Mayhew, G.F., Rose, D.J., Burland, V., Kodoyianni, V., Schwartz, D.C., and Blattner, F.R. 2003. Comparative genomics of *Salmonella enterica* serovar Typhi strains Ty2 and CT18. J Bacteriol 185: 2330-2337.

Doolittle, R.F., Feng, D.F., Tsang, S., Cho, G., and Little, E. 1996. Determining divergence times of the major kingdoms of living organisms with a protein clock. Science 271: 470-477.

Doolittle, W.F. 1999. Phylogenetic classification and the universal tree. Science 284: 2124-2129.

Evans, L.D., Hughes, C., and Fraser, G.M. 2014. Building a flagellum outside the bacterial cell. Trends Microbiol 22: 566-572.

Feng, D.F., Cho, G., and Doolittle, R.F. 1997. Determining divergence times with a protein clock: update and reevaluation. Proc Natl Acad Sci USA 94: 13028-13033.

Feng, Y., Johnston, R.N., Liu, G.R., and Liu, S.L. 2013. Genomic comparison between *Salmonella* Gallinarum and Pullorum: differential pseudogene formation under common host restriction. PLoS One 8: e59427.

Feng, Y., Liu, W.Q., Sanderson, K.E., and Liu, S.L. 2011. Comparison of *Salmonella* genomes. In: Porwollik S, editor. *Salmonella* from genome to function. Norfolk: Caister Academic Press. p. 49-67.

Fox, G.E., Stackebrandt, E., Hespell, R.B., Gibson, J., Maniloff, J., Dyer, T.A., Wolfe, R.S., Balch, W.E., Tanner, R.S., Magrum, L.J., Zablen, L.B., Blakemore, R., Gupta, R., Bonen, L., Lewis, B.J., Stahl, D.A., Luehrsen, K.R., Chen, K.N., and Woese, C.R. 1980. The phylogeny of prokaryotes. Science 209: 457-463.

Gauthier, A., Turmel, M., and Lemieux, C. 1991. A group I intron in the chloroplast large subunit rRNA gene of *Chlamydomonas eugametos* encodes a double-strand endonuclease that cleaves the homing site of this intron. Curr Genet 19: 43-47.

Gong, J., Liu, W.Q., Liu, G.R,, Chen, F., Li, J.Q., Xu, G.M., Wang, L., Johnston, R.N., Eisenstark, A., and Liu. S.L. 2007. Spontaneous conversion between mutL and 6 bpDelta*mutL* in *Salmonella typhimurium* LT7: association with genome diversification and possible roles in bacterial adaptation. Genomics 90: 542-549.

Harfe, B.D., and Jinks-Robertson, S. 2000. DNA mismatch repair and genetic instability. Annu Rev Genet 34: 359-399.

Holt, J.G. 1984. Bergey's Manual of Systematic Bacteriology. Volume 1 1.

Holt, J.G., Krieg, N.R., Sneath, P.H., Staley, J.T., and Williams, S.T. 1994. Bergey's Manual of Determinative Bacteriology. New York.

Holt, K.E., Parkhill, J., Mazzoni, C.J., Roumagnac, P., Weill, F.X., Goodhead, I., Rance, R., Baker, S., Maskell, D.J., Wain, J., Dolecek, C., Achtman, M., and Dougan, G. 2008. High-throughput sequencing provides insights into genome variation and evolution in *Salmonella* Typhi. Nat Genet 40: 987-993.

Huen, J., Yan, Z., Iwashkiw, J., Dubey, S., Gimenez, M.C., Ortiz, M.E., Patel, S.V., Jones, M.D., Riazi, A., Terebiznik, M., Babaei, S., and Shahinas, D. 2019. A Novel Single Domain Antibody Targeting FliC Flagellin of *Salmonella enterica* for Effective Inhibition of Host Cell Invasion. Front Microbiol 10: 2665.

Kauffmann, F., Edwards, P.R. 1957. A revised, simplified Kauffmann-White schema. Acta Pathol Microbiol Scand 41: 242-246.

Kothapalli, S., Nair, S., Alokam, S., Pang, T., Khakhria, R., Woodward, D., Johnson, W., Stocker, B.A., Sanderson, K.E., and Liu, S.L. 2005. Diversity of Genome Structure in *Salmonella enterica* Serovar Typhi Populations. J Bacteriol 187: 2638-2650.

Kottilil, S., Chun, T.W., Moir, S., Liu, S., McLaughlin, M., Hallahan, C.W., Maldarelli, F., Corey, L., and Fauci, A.S. 2003. Innate immunity in human immunodeficiency virus infection: effect of viremia on natural killer cell function. J Infect Dis 187: 1038-1045.

Kunkel, T.A., and Erie, D.A. 2005. DNA mismatch repair. Annu Rev Biochem 74: 681-710.

Le Minor, L. 1984. Genus III. *Salmonella*. In: Krieg NR, editor. Bergey's Manual of Systematic Bacteriology. Baltimore: Williams & Wilkins. p. 427-458.

Le Minor, L., and Popoff, M.Y. 1987. Designation of *Salmonella enterica* sp. nov., nom. rev., as the type and only species of the genus Salmonella. Int J Syst Bacteriol 37: 465-468.

LeClerc, J.E., Li, B., Payne, W.L., and Cebula, T.A. 1996. High mutation frequencies among *Escherichia coli* and *Salmonella* pathogens. Science 274: 1208-1211.

Li, G.M. 2008. Mechanisms and functions of DNA mismatch repair. Cell Res 18: 85-98.

Lieb, M. 1983. Specific mismatch correction in bacteriophage lambda crosses by very short patch repair. Mol Gen Genet 191: 118-125.

Liu, G.R., Edwards, K., Eisenstark, A., Fu, Y.M., Liu, W.Q., Sanderson, K.E., Johnston, R.N., and Liu, S.L. 2003. Genomic diversification among archival strains of *Salmonella enterica* serovar typhimurium LT7. J Bacteriol 185: 2131-2142.

Liu, G.R., Rahn, A., Liu, W.Q., Sanderson, K.E., Johnston, R.N., and Liu, S.L. 2002a. The evolving genome of *Salmonella enterica* serovar Pullorum. J Bacteriol 184: 2626-2633.

Liu S-L. 2015. A half century pursuing a dream to uncover the origins of human diseases. Beijing: Science Publishing House.

Liu, S.L. 2007. Physical mapping of *Salmonella* genomes. In. Methods Mol Biol. p. 39-58.

Liu, S.L., Ezaki, T., Miura, H., Matsui, K., and Yabuuchi, E. 1988. Intact motility as a *Salmonella typhi* invasion-related factor. Infect Immun 56: 1967-1973.

Liu, S.L., Hessel, A., Cheng, H.Y., and Sanderson, K.E. 1994. The XbaI-BlnI-CeuI genomic cleavage map of *Salmonella paratyphi* B. J Bacteriol 176: 1014-1024.

Liu, S.L., Hessel, A., and Sanderson, K.E. 1993a. Genomic mapping with I-Ceu I, an intron-encoded endonuclease specific for genes for ribosomal RNA, in *Salmonella* spp., *Escherichia coli*, and other bacteria. Proc Natl Acad Sci USA 90: 6874-6878.

Liu, S.L., Hessel, A., and Sanderson, K.E. 1993b. The XbaI-BlnI-CeuI genomic cleavage map of Salmonella enteritidis shows an inversion relative to *Salmonella typhimurium* LT2. Mol Microbiol 10: 655-664.

Liu, S.L., Hessel, A., and Sanderson, K.E. 1993c. The XbaI-BlnI-CeuI genomic cleavage map of *Salmonella typhimurium* LT2 determined by double digestion, end labelling, and pulsed-field gel electrophoresis. J Bacteriol 175: 4104-4120.

Liu, S.L., Liu, G.R., Li, S.X., Liu, W.Q., Zheng, J.F., Zhu, W.F., Gu, H.X., Guo, X.K., Sanderson, K.E., Zhou, Y.G., and Johnston, R.N. 2002b. Bacterial genome structure: a molecular marker to reveal phylogenetic clusters. Journal of Peking University [Med]. 34: 457-463.

Liu, S.L., and Sanderson, K.E. 1995a. The chromosome of *Salmonella paratyphi* A is inverted by recombination between *rrnH* and *rrnG*. J Bacteriol 177: 6585-6592.

Liu, S.L., and Sanderson, K.E. 1995b. Genomic cleavage map of *Salmonella typhi* Ty2. J Bacteriol 177: 5099-5107.

Liu, S.L., and Sanderson, K.E. 1996. Highly plastic chromosomal organization in *Salmonella typhi*. Proc Natl Acad Sci USA 93: 10303-10308.

Liu, S.L., and Sanderson, K.E. 1995c. I-CeuI reveals conservation of the genome of independent strains of *Salmonella typhimurium*. J Bacteriol 177: 3355-3357.

Liu, S.L., and Sanderson, K.E. 1992. A physical map of the *Salmonella typhimurium* LT2 genome made by using XbaI analysis. J Bacteriol 174: 1662-1672.

Liu, S.L., and Sanderson, K.E. 1995d. Rearrangements in the genome of the bacterium *Salmonella typhi*. Proc Natl Acad Sci USA 92: 1018-1022.

Liu, S.L., Schryvers, A.B., Sanderson, K.E., and Johnston, R.N. 1999. Bacterial phylogenetic clusters revealed by genome structure. J Bacteriol 181: 6747-6755.

Liu, W.Q., Feng, Y., Wang, Y., Zou, Q.H., Chen, F., Guo, J.T., Peng, Y.H., Jin, Y., Li, Y.G., Hu, S.N., Johnston, R.N., Liu, G.R., and Liu, S.L. 2009. *Salmonella paratyphi* C: genetic divergence from *Salmonella choleraesuis* and pathogenic convergence with *Salmonella typhi*. PLoS One 4: e4510.

Liu, W.Q., Liu, G.R., Li, J.Q., Xu, G.M., Qi, D., He, X.Y., Deng, J., Zhang, F.M., Johnston, R.N., and Liu, S.L. 2007. Diverse genome structures of *Salmonella paratyphi* C. BMC Genomics 8.

Marshall, P., and Lemieux, C. 1991. Cleavage pattern of the homing endonuclease encoded by the fifth intron in the chloroplast large subunit rRNA-encoding gene of *Chlamydomonas eugametos*. Gene 104: 241-245.

Mayr, E. 1944. Systematics and the Origin of Species from the Viewpoint of a Zoologist. New York.

Mayr, E. 1996. What is a species, and what is not? Philos Trans R Soc Lond B Biol Sci 63: 262-277.

McClelland, M., and Bhagwat, A.S. 1992. Biased DNA repair. Nature 355: 595-596.

McClelland, M., Sanderson, K.E., Clifton, S.W., Latreille, P., Porwollik, S., Sabo, A., Meyer, R., Bieri, T., Ozersky, P., McLellan, M., Harkins, C.R., Wang, C., Nguyen, C., Berghoff, A., Elliott, G., Kohlberg, S., Strong, C., Du, F., Carter, J., Kremizki, C., Layman, D., Leonard, S., Sun, H., Fulton, L., Nash, W., Miner, T., Minx, P., Delehaunty, K., Fronick, C., Magrini, V., Nhan, M., Warren, W., Florea, L., Spieth, J., and Wilson, R.K. 2004. Comparison of genome degradation in Paratyphi A and Typhi, human-restricted serovars of *Salmonella enterica* that cause typhoid. Nat Genet 36: 1268-1274.

McClelland, M., Sanderson, K.E., Spieth, J., Clifton, S.W., Latreille, P., Courtney, L., Porwollik, S., Ali, J., Dante, M., Du, F., Hou, S., Layman, D., Leonard, S., Nguyen, C., Scott, K., Holmes, A., Grewal, N., Mulvaney, E., Ryan, E., Sun, H., Florea, L., Miller, W., Stoneking, T.,

Nhan, M., Waterston, R., and Wilson, R.K. 2001. Complete genome sequence of *Salmonella enterica* serovar Typhimurium LT2. Nature 413: 852-856.

Miller, J.H. 1998. Mutators in *Escherichia coli.* Mutat Res 409: 99-106.

Ochman, H., and Bergthorsson, U. 1995. Genome evolution in enteric bacteria. Curr Opin Genet Dev 5: 734-738.

Ochman, H., and Wilson, A.C. 1987. Evolution in bacteria: evidence for a universal substitution rate in cellular genomes. J Mol Evol 26: 74-86.

Parkhill, J., Dougan, G., James, K.D., Thomson, N.R., Pickard, D., Wain, J., Churcher, C., Mungall, K.L., Bentley, S.D., Holden, M.T., Sebaihia, M., Baker, S., Basham, D., Brooks, K., Chillingworth, T., Connerton, P., Cronin, A., Davis, P., Davies, R.M., Dowd, L., White, N., Farrar, J., Feltwell, T., Hamlin, N., Haque, A., Hien, T.T., Holroyd, S., Jagels, K., Krogh, A., Larsen, T.S., Leather, S., Moule, S., O'Gaora, P., Parry, C., Quail, M., Rutherford, K., Simmonds, M., Skelton, J., Stevens, K., Whitehead, S., and Barrell, B.G. 2001. Complete genome sequence of a multiple drug resistant *Salmonella enterica* serovar Typhi CT18. Nature 413: 848-852.

Parry, C.M., Hien, T.T., Dougan, G., White, N.J., Farrar, J.J. 2002. Typhoid fever. N Engl J Med 347: 1770-1782.

Pillon, M.C., Dubinsky, M., Johnston, R.N., Liu, S.L., Guarne, A. 2013. Characterization of the defects in the ATP lid of *E. coli* MutL that cause transient hypermutability. DNA Repair (Amst) 12: 864-869.

Popoff, M.Y., Bockemuhl, J., and Gheesling, L.L. 2004. Supplement 2002 (no. 46) to the Kauffmann-White scheme. Res Microbiol 155: 568-570.

Popoff, M.Y., and Le Minor, L.E.. 2005. Genus XXXIII. *Salmonella*. In: Brenner DJ, Krieg NR, Stanley JT, editors. Bergey's Mannual of Systematic Bacteriology: Springer. p. 764-799.

Ravin, A.W. 1960. The origin of bacterial species. Genetic recombination and factors limiting it between bacterial populations. Bacteriol Rev 24: 201-220.

Rayssiguier, C., Thaler, D.S., and Radman, M. 1989. The barrier to recombination between *Escherichia coli* and *Salmonella typhimurium* is disrupted in mismatch-repair mutants. Nature 342: 396-401.

Reeves, M.W., Evins, G.M., Heiba, A.A., Plikaytis, B.D., and Farmer, J.J., 3rd 1989. Clonal nature of *Salmonella typhi* and its genetic relatedness to other salmonellae as shown by multilocus enzyme electrophoresis, and proposal of *Salmonella bongori* comb. nov. J Clin Microbiol 27: 313-320.

Roumagnac, P., Weill, F.X., Dolecek, C., Baker, S., Brisse, S., Chinh, N.T., Le, T.A.H., Acosta, C.J., Farrar, J., Dougan, G., and Achtman, M. 2006. Evolutionary History of *Salmonella Typhi*. Science 314: 1301-1304.

Sanderson, K.E., and Demerec, M. 1965. The Linkage Map of *Salmonella Typhimurium*. Genetics 51: 897-913.

Sanderson, K.E., Hessel, A., Liu, S.L., and Rudd, K.E. 1996. The genetic map of Salmonella typhimurium, Edition VIII. In: Neidhardt FC, editor. *Escherichia coli* and *Salmonella*. Washington, D.C.: ASM Press. p. 1903-1999.

Schofield, M.J., and Hsieh, P. 2003. DNA mismatch repair: molecular mechanisms and biological function. Annu Rev Microbiol 57: 579-608.

Selander, R.K., Caugant, D.A., Ochman, H., Musser, J.M., Gilmour, M.N., and Whittam, T.S. 1986. Methods of multilocus enzyme electrophoresis for bacterial population genetics and systematics. Appl Environ Microbiol 51: 873-884.

Smith, C.L., Econome, J.G., Schutt, A., Klco, S., and Cantor, C.R. 1987. A physical map of the *Escherichia coli* K12 genome. Science 236: 1448-1453.

Sniegowski, P.D., Gerrish, P.J., and Lenski, R.E. 1997. Evolution of high mutation rates in experimental populations of *E. coli*. Nature 387: 703-705.

Song, J., Ware, A., and Liu, S.L. 2003. Wavelet to predict bacterial *ori* and *ter*: a tendency towards a physical balance. BMC Genomics 4: 17.

Spanò, S., Galán, J.E. 2012. A Rab32-Dependent Pathway Contributes to *Salmonella* Typhi Host Restriction. Science Vol. 338: 960-963.

Staley, J.T. 2006. The bacterial species dilemma and the genomic-phylogenetic species concept. Philos Trans R Soc Lond B Biol Sci 361: 1899-1909.

Tang, L., Li, Y., Deng, X., Johnston, R.N,, Liu, G.R., and Liu, S.L. 2013a. Defining natural species of bacteria: clear-cut genomic boundaries revealed by a turning point in nucleotide sequence divergence. BMC Genomics 14: 489.

Tang, L., and Liu, S.L. 2012. The 3Cs provide a novel concept of bacterial species: messages from the genome as illustrated by *Salmonella*. Antonie Van Leeuwenhoek 101: 67-72.

Tang, L., Liu, W.Q., Fang, X., Sun, Q., Zhu, S.L., Wang, C.X., Wang, X.Y., Li, Y.G., Zhu, D.L., Sanderson, K.E., Johnston, R.N., Liu, G.R., and Liu, S.L. 2014. CTAG-containing cleavage site profiling to delineate *Salmonella* into natural clusters. PLoS One 9: e103388.

Tang, L., Mastriani, E., Zhou, Y.J., Zhu, S., Fang, X., Liu, Y.P., Liu, W.Q., Li, Y.G., Johnston, R.N., Guo, Z., Liu, G.R., and Liu, S.L. 2017a. Differential degeneration of the ACTAGT sequence among *Salmonella*: a reflection of distinct nucleotide amelioration patterns during bacterial divergence. Sci Rep 7: 10985.

Tang, L., Wang, C.X., Zhu, S.L., Li, Y., Deng, X., Johnston, R.N., Liu, G.R., and Liu, S.L. 2013b. Genetic boundaries to delineate the typhoid agent and other *Salmonella* serotypes into distinct natural lineages. Genomics 102: 331-337.

Tang, L., Zhu, S., Mastriani, E., Fang, X., Zhou, Y.J., Li, Y.G., Johnston, R.N., Guo, Z., Liu, G.R., and Liu, S.L. 2017b. Conserved intergenic sequences revealed by CTAG-profiling in *Salmonella*: thermodynamic modeling for function prediction. Sci Rep 7: 43565.

Tang, L., Zhu, S., Mastriani, E., Fang, X., Zhou, Y.J., Li, Y.G., Johnston, R.N., Guo, Z., Liu, G.R., and Liu, S.L. 2017c. Conserved intergenic sequences revealed by CTAG-profiling in *Salmonella*: thermodynamic modeling for function prediction. Sci Rep 7: 43565

Taylor, A.L., and Thoman, M.S. 1964. The Genetic Map of *Escherichia coli* K-12. Genetics 50: 659-677.

Thomson, N.R., Clayton, D.J., Windhorst, D., Vernikos, G., Davidson, S., Churcher, C., Quail, M.A., Stevens, M., Jones, M.A., Watson, M., Barron, A., Layton, A., Pickard, D., Kingsley, R.A., Bignell, A., Clark, L., Harris, B., Ormond, D., Abdellah, Z., Brooks, K., Cherevach, I., Chillingworth, T., Woodward, J., Norberczak, H., Lord, A., Arrowsmith, C., Jagels, K., Moule, S., Mungall, K., Sanders, M., Whitehead, S., Chabalgoity, J.A., Maskell, D., Humphrey, T., Roberts, M., Barrow, P.A., Dougan, G., and Parkhill, J. 2008. Comparative genome analysis of *Salmonella* Enteritidis PT4 and Salmonella Gallinarum 287/91 provides insights into evolutionary and host adaptation pathways. Genome Res 18: 1624-1637.

Vos, M. 2011. A species concept for bacteria based on adaptive divergence. Trends Microbiol 19: 1-7.

Woese, C.R. 1987. Bacterial evolution. Microbiol Rev 51: 221-271.

Woese, C.R. 2000. Interpreting the universal phylogenetic tree. Proc Natl Acad Sci U S A 97: 8392-8396.

Woese, C.R., Kandler, O., and Wheelis, M.L. 1990. Towards a natural system of organisms: proposal for the domains Archaea, Bacteria, and Eucarya. Proc Natl Acad Sci U S A 87: 4576-4579.

Wu, H., Wang, Y., Chen, J.T., Wang, L.P., Liu, G.R., and Liu, S.L. 2021. Anticancer effects of dietary administration of secoisolariciresinol diglucoside in a patient of gastrointestinal stromal tumor: a case report. International Journal of Surgery Oncology 5.

Wu, K.Y., Liu, G.R., Liu, W.Q., Wang, A.Q., Zhan, S., Sanderson, K.E., Johnston, R.N., and Liu, S.L. 2005. The genome of *Salmonella enterica* serovar Gallinarum: distinct insertions/deletions and rare rearrangements. J Bacteriol 187: 4720-4727.

Zhuang, H., Cheng, L., Wang, Y., Zhang, Y.K., Zhao, M.F., Liang, G.D., Zhang, M.C., Li, Y.G., Zhao, J.B., Gao, Y.N., Zhou, Y.J., and Liu, S.L. 2019. Dysbiosis of the Gut Microbiome in Lung Cancer. Front Cell Infect Microbiol 9: 112.

Zou, Q.H., Li, Q.H., Zhu, H.Y., Feng, Y., Li, Y.G., Johnston, R.N., Liu, G.R., and Liu, S.L. 2010. SPC-P1: a pathogenicity-associated prophage of *Salmonella paratyphi* C. BMC Genomics 11: 729.